RACING TO A CURE

Other Books by Neil Ruzic

For adults
The Shallow Sea
Where the Winds Sleep
(a Literary Guild selection)
Spinoff

For teenagers
There's Adventure in Civil Engineering
There's Adventure in Meteorology

For scientists and engineers
The Case for Going to the Moon
Stimulus (ed.)
Open-Ocean Polyculture System
A Blueprint for an Island for Science
Technologies Emerged (ed.)

Racing to a CURE

A Cancer Victim
Refuses Chemotherapy
and Finds Tomorrow's
Cures in Today's
Scientific Laboratories

Neil Ruzic

UNIVERSITY OF ILLINOIS PRESS
URBANA AND CHICAGO

Library of Congress Cataloging-in-Publication Data
Ruzic, Neil P.
Racing to a cure : a cancer victim refuses chemotherapy and
finds tomorrow's cures in today's scientific laboratories / Neil Ruzic.
p.   cm.
Includes bibliographical references and index.
ISBN 0-252-02867-8 (cloth : alk. paper)
1. Ruzic, Neil P.—Health.
2. Lymphomas—Patients—United States—Biography.
3. Biological response modifiers.
4. Cancer—Research.
5. Cancer—Alternative treatment.
[DNLM: 1. Lymphoma, Mantle-Cell—therapy—Personal Narratives.
2. Biological Therapy—methods—Personal Narratives.
3. Biomedical Research—Personal Narratives. WH 525 R987r 2003] I. Title.
RC280.L9R89   2003
362.1'96994'0092—dc21   2003000558

To Rade and Leslie Pejic, who saved my life;
to Jon Braun and Phil Koeffler, whose research will save others;
to Steve Schuster, one of the new breed of bio-oncologists;
and to Carol, David, and Shahid,
who helped me when I needed it the most.

Contents

Preface

LIGHT PIPES JOIN A SERIES OF MICROSCOPES SO THE SCIENTISTS AND I can look at the same slides. They are red-stained slides of my bone marrow, and we search for cancer. Cancer cells, as I have seen them before in older slides of my tissue, are busy and ugly. A lot of them will be dividing; they seem disorganized, their centers (nuclei) big and lopsided, and the areas surrounding them out to the boundaries of the cells are small.

By contrast, mine are uniform and arranged regularly. There are no cancer cells in my bone marrow—in spite of five years of my having lived with mantle-cell lymphoma, the worst cancer of the lymph system.

The scientists then perform a test in which DNA in my blood is labeled with fluorescent molecules so that the nuclei of these blood cells show up under the microscope, as has the bone marrow. My blood is cancer-free as well. I have never had chemotherapy. I have never had radiation. Only some of the new biotherapies.

After learning I had mantle-cell lymphoma in 1998, I didn't expect to live more than a year or two. Now I am cured. The word *cure* is anathema to cancer doctors and scientists alike, born of decades of failed therapies. But I use it deliberately because it's time we started thinking about real cures.

In the beginning I was advised at four leading cancer centers to endure aggressive chemotherapy. When I refused, the doctors told me that the experimental therapies I'd started to learn about were dangerous because they had not yet gone through years of clinical trials. Their assumption was that chemotherapy—because it was the "standard" treatment for cancer—was somehow *safer.*

The opposite is more often true. Chemotherapy is the practice of giving poisons in the hope that they will kill the tumors before the patient. For the majority of cancers, chemo is experimental to an extreme. If chemotherapy works, why do 12.7 million Americans still have cancer?

After refusing chemotherapy, I did not slide (as do many others who reject chemo) into the mystic world of "alternative medicine." Instead I visited the nation's cancer-research laboratories to find tomorrow's therapies. I knew that, just as treatments in use today were in research twenty years ago, future therapies—benign biological therapies—must be under development today. And they were. Since learning I had cancer, my full-time occupation has been, and continues to be, the investigation of cancer therapies. These are biotherapies. Not chemotherapies.

This book is the story of what I discovered in that search.

Through my journey to scores of research laboratories, I have come to know the scientists who explore genetics, the immune system, and cell behavior and have developed a great admiration for them. My feelings for the majority of cancer doctors, who never write scientific papers and rarely read them, are exactly the opposite. Scientific cures for cancer exist *now,* and they could save millions of lives if there were more informed medical practitioners who would get their patients into clinical trials, fewer barriers to expanding promising research, and less-Byzantine FDA regulations.

Standards of efficacy range from "remission" a few months after a clinical trial all the way to a complete absence of symptoms for the rest of the patient's life. I don't need to wait another five or ten years, or until I die of old age or from something other than cancer; there are ways of determining real cures, such as sophisticated scientific tests that count cancer cells and antibodies in the body long after a given treatment. Augmented by CAT scans, these tests have determined that I am cured of cancer. I am cured of mantle-cell lymphoma, one of the most persistent, insidious, and aggressive forms of blood cancer.

Because lymphoma, like leukemia, pervades the entire system and not just one or more organs, the biological therapies involved in effecting my cure have application to curing all other cancers.

If you have cancer, you don't need to visit research laboratories, as I did. But if you share my passion for life, you do need to learn everything you can about the new biological therapies reaching clinical trials—specifically for your own disease. You can do this through the internet, by reading the latest scientific papers, and through other means. In my own case, I was determined to spend whatever days I had left in a journey of learning. That journey has revealed dozens of molecular-targeted cures that will become standard treatment someday.

If you have cancer, someday is too late. With your life at stake, you don't need to wait.

RACING TO A CURE

1

Into the Pit

A DEEP ORGANIC SMELL, PART SICKNESS, PART HOSPITAL ANTISEPTIC, awakened me to the world of pain. I felt like the loser in a sword fight, gutted where the sword had ripped my belly apart. My mouth was dry, like ash.

I moved my head a centimeter . . . and groaned.

Through the open blinds I could just make out Lake Michigan, which had gloomed into a tint of lead. I was in St. Anthony's Hospital in Michigan City, Indiana, thirty-five miles from Chicago across the lake's southern shore. It was no longer morning, and I realized that Rade, the sword wielder, must have worked on me for a long time.

It was September 1998. I remember those days well, every minute of every day: my wife's tears, my son's grit, and Rade's determination that I would live.

Rade—Dr. Rade Pejic—came in wearing greens, forcing a smile, "How do you feel, Neil?

"I think I'm still alive," I said weakly.

"Well, you've been through a lot. Your spleen was five times normal size. Now it's gone. I took out three lymph nodes the size of golf balls along your aorta and vena cava—golfing around a little before sewing you back up."

His attempt at flippancy didn't work with me. I knew him too well. Over the years he had become a close friend, but I had never been to see him professionally for anything worse than a wart. It was he who suggested the splenectomy because, as he put it then, "What if you have a rough landing on one of those Bahamian airstrips you're always plowing into? Your seatbelt could rupture your spleen, and you'd bleed to death." No mention, then or now, of cancer. Studious avoidance. "Press this for morphine," he added, handing me a button switch connected to a wire.

I pressed and kept pressing throughout the day.

. . .

I awakened now and then to a slow parade. First came my wife, Carol, putting on a brave face. "Well, I guess you won't put African ice in your tea anymore." Her eyes were bloodshot, and tears glistened on her high cheekbones. The ice-in-tea comment referred to an incident in Cairo a few weeks earlier, when we and our grandson Ryan had visited the city to look at pyramids in 115-degree sunshine. Ryan's father—our only son, David—was in the room too. David had driven up from the University of Illinois at Urbana, where he is a professor of nuclear engineering with a good sense of humor. "Hi, Dad! Hope everything came out all right."

Something had come out, but pain filled the spaces where it had been. I tried to increase my resistance with my brain's own analgesic, but the threshold was too high, and I continued to press the button. I felt the exhaustion of an animal that has escaped again and again and was finally in its cave.

During that day I talked to five doctors who appeared in my room—and to a few who only appeared to have appeared, compliments of the morphine. One of the real ones was a tall and attractive oncologist. She aimed from the hip and shot fast. "The lab analyzed your spleen and lymph-node specimens. You've got non-Hodgkin's lymphoma, Neil, cancer of the lymph system."

There it was. The word finally had been spoken. Cancer.

"It's a disease that's close to and almost the same as leukemia," the oncologist explained. "Fortunately the lab says yours is only a low-grade small B-cell lymphoma, not aggressive. We'll give you a few pills now and twice a year or so, a little CHOP, nothing too toxic, and then . . ."

Unknown to me, Carol, with David's help, was hard at work every night on her computer, going on-line and learning to search the Web with a proficiency never before required. Her beginning education into the mysteries of cancer research heralded my own, which started the day I was released from the hospital. Within the mountain of data that began to accumulate for my later digestion was the unsettling fact, revealed by autopsy on a great many bodies, that 40 percent of abnormalities, including cancer, are not diagnosed during the lives of the people who have them.

Rade and I knew as early as last February that my abdominal lymph nodes were enlarged because, not feeling well, I'd had a CAT scan that revealed nodes somewhat bigger than normal. Each of us has about a thousand lymph nodes, kidney-shaped organs located in the armpits, groin, and neck and scattered throughout the abdomen at junctions of lymphatic vessels. Along with the spleen, which may be thought of as a huge lymph node, they act as a sewer system, filtering waste products. Normally they are about the size of large peas. One indication of disease, not necessarily lymphoma, is when the lymph nodes become swollen, sometimes enormously so, as large as grapefruit. At the time we weren't especially worried, because a node that Rade had removed from my groin, though twice the normal size, tested benign and because swollen nodes could mean a simple infection, not cancer.

But now the oncologist was telling me that a test of my quadruple-sized spleen and abdominal lymph nodes showed "small B-cell lymphoma," one of the more-benign forms of non-Hodgkin's lymphoma. I never suspected that the local laboratory's diagnosis was wrong. None of us knew that my cancer was far worse than small B-cell, that there are more than fifty subsets of non-Hodgkin's lymphoma, and that the local oncologist, misled by the lab, was suggesting a therapy that would do nothing to help me. In the weeks to come I learned that medical labs take the easy way first and, as in my case, diagnose only from the cells' appearance under a microscope.

"What's CHOP?" I asked the oncologist in abject ignorance.

"Cyclophosphamide, hydroxorubicin, Oncovin, and prednisone." She rattled it off like a recipe for her favorite dish. "Now how about letting me take a little of your bone marrow?"

Taking "a little bone marrow" isn't as innocuous as it sounds. At her direction I lay on my side while she used a tool something like a corkscrew to bore through the pelvis, where the bone marrow is deeper than elsewhere.

"Sorry," she said, "we can't anesthetize inside the bone."

I felt a snap as she cored through and into the marrow, but it didn't hurt much. She was good at it, and fast, as I learned later by comparison. She pulled on the syringe plunger, extracted a core, and showed me the tube of thick red marrow speckled with white bone fragments.

"It's a good sample," she said, smiling.

· · ·

The next day her smile was superficial. She handed me a lab report that said the cancer cells had invaded my bone marrow. Stage-four lymphoma. The final stage.

"Of course, when you have lymphoma, you expect it to enter the bone marrow. After all, lymphoma *is* a systemic disease. The good news is that your marrow consists of less than 10 percent cancer cells."

After I left the hospital, a second opinion arrived from the Mayo Clinic, whose pathologists, using a method called "flow cytometry," confirmed the diagnosis of malignant B-cell lymphoma but warned that they couldn't interpret the data without fresh tissue. The report said it *could* be a much more aggressive form of non-Hodgkin's lymphoma. Warnings like this, couched in the impersonal wording of pathology, aren't nearly as strong as the also ignored warnings on cigarette packages; not knowing can insulate you from further searching, especially when what you think you have isn't so bad. I didn't think to question the pathology report, but I did later. The path I was traveling not only led to a devastating disease—the absolute worst and most aggressive kind of lymphoma—but twisted into a long road of education rivaling, in the sheer amount of hard work and new experience involved, the degrees I once earned in science and journalism.

I was a student again.

· · ·

My surgeon and family physician, Dr. Rade Pejic, is a native of Serbia and the son of a Belgrade surgeon. Since I am descended on my father's side from Croatians, our ethnic origins might have been expected to produce some artificial enmity. Far from it. Rade (pronounced *Raid*) had become a close ally as both doctor and friend, and the relationship grew even closer as he and his wife, Leslie, a Ph.D. neuroscientist, continued in these roles. At the time of that first operation, Rade was in his late fifties, a big man with jet-black hair. He had volunteered and served two tours of duty aboard a U.S. Navy hospital ship in Vietnam, where he learned how to expunge every organ, to sever every limb, to reassemble victims of grenades, land mines, and machine guns. After that he returned to school to become a vascular surgeon, learning the intricacies of the body's spaghetti of blood vessels, the perfect specialty for performing my splenectomy. He and Leslie have four sons and a daughter. At this time one of them was in medical school and another in pre-med, continuing the tradition.

Rade shot me a hopeful half-smile as I sat in front of his desk, and he connected to Dr. A at a leading medical center in Chicago (see notes). This highly recommended oncologist agreed to see me, rather strangely telling Rade over the phone, *"I just love lymphoma!"*

. . .

A week later Carol and I met Dr. A in his office, his staff having reviewed my tissue blocks that Rade had sent ahead. The middle-aged physician had sandy hair and wore a tailored suit coat, unbuttoned to reveal a tailored shirt and an expensive tie. His deep voice of experience resonated from behind the desk, a direct voice, but pleasant, managing a tone that was upbeat about his cancer patients. His walls were filled with diplomas, self-congratulatory photographs of himself with people who must have been important, and framed letters from grateful patients, presumably cured.

"Do you have any symptoms? Fever, night sweats, pain, swelling, loss of appetite, weight loss, fatigue?

"Night sweats, pain, fatigue. None of the others."

We fell silent as Dr. A stiffened behind his desk like a judge ready to pronounce my sentence, glancing at a report in front of him, his words vibrating from the base of his chest in a sympathetic chord.

"Our pathologist says that your lymphoma is mantle-cell, diffuse, stage-four." He looked me in the eye. "She is always right."

I had used every minute of the weeks since surgery reading the scientific papers that Carol and David retrieved for me—at that time mostly from university libraries and occasionally from the internet—finding background information in books, and talking to those pathologists who would answer my calls. I learned that the main cells in the lymph system are lymphocytes (literally, lymph cells), of which there are two types: B and T cells, which fight pathogens in different ways. Lymphoma arises when these lymphocytes become diseased and suppress the formation and function of normal cells. Mantle-cell lymphoma (MCL) derives its name from tumors that arise from cells in the normal "mantle zone" of the lymph nodes. This zone, a thin area surrounding the center of a lymph node, looks like a mantle or a shroud under the microscope. The mantle zone is made up of immature B cells, which are cells from the bone marrow that haven't yet turned into functional cells. During those weeks I had felt fortunate not to have this deadly subset of lymphoma. But now?

"Now, essentially, you have two options," Dr. A continued. "You can do nothing, in which case your life expectancy is sixteen months, according to a new Nebraska Medical Center study. Or you can get into a protocol we just happen to be starting for highly aggressive chemotherapy. We give you what's in CHOP plus teniposide, leucovorin, cytarabine, and methotrexate. We infuse you with this chemo combination for forty-two days. You rest for two weeks, then take it again for forty-two more days."

He acted as though he had performed his duty by delivering this message and then added, "Afterwards, if you can tolerate it, we give you a bone-marrow transplant. Otherwise, you take interferon."

Most of these chemo agents are deadly poisons that kill fast-growing cancer cells. The trouble is, I'd learned, they attacked all dividing cells indiscriminately, which is why your hair falls out. "What is my life expectancy if I live through all that?" I asked hesitantly.

"It should add another year to your life, maybe more."

"Another year? *One year?*" The horror of it began to distill in my brain, oozing out of that single syllable, *one*. Just one. When it hit with full force, the distillate was a thick and bitter bile made from clotted lymph fluid and rotted hope. He was telling me that, *provided the therapy worked,* I mostly likely would be dead in . . . what? A year or two? And if it did not work, death would be even sooner. We all know we will die someday, but *someday* is never synonymous with *now.* The optimism that causes us to know in our hearts that only other people die of something besides old age allows us to go cheerfully about our lives, ignoring the threats to our own existence, denying our most powerful instinct, survival, ... until we hear the sentence of death. I felt as though the last breath in this room was being inhaled right now by someone else.

"Well, that's average," he said, seeing my distress. "Who knows? Don't forget, this is an incurable cancer you have. I believe in aggressive treatment. Very aggressive."

"I guess you do," I said. "But why not do another CAT scan first to see whether the lymph nodes have grown since the last scan?"

I had undergone two CAT scans before my splenectomy. CAT stands for "computerized axial tomography." Alternatively called CT, leaving out the *axial,* this imaging technique involves constantly sweeping a narrow beam of X rays across your body, typically after you have drunk two liters of barium and received injections of inert iodine. The large nuclei of barium and iodine atoms scatter the X rays to portray different tissue densities. These values are accessed at thousands of points, integrated by computer, and presented on a monitor or printed out on film.

"You can do all the CAT scans you want, but it won't change anything."

He said it as kindly as he could and handed me two scientific papers, one describing the aggressive "multimodality" protocol and the other, the results of this treatment. I scanned them immediately and focused on a single phrase: "MCL is characterized by inevitable relapse regardless of initial therapy." Their words! Anger began to replace horror. What was the purpose of the regimen then, other than to calm the customer by *doing* something or to obscure medicine's illimitable ignorance?

"Tell me," I said, "how does your pathologist know my lymphoma is mantle-cell?"

"What do you mean, 'how does she know?' *She's always right.*"

I was reasonably certain that his always-right pathologist was correct as usual. If so, however, then the first two diagnoses were wrong. The survival statistics on MCL were, if anything, even less encouraging than he stated, and in my mix of revulsion, anger, fear, and other emotions, the idea of a truly definitive test gave me hope. Certain lymphomas, I had learned, can be defined by a strange occurrence in the chromosomes. Our twenty-three paired human chromosomes consist of strands of nucleic acids that can unfold and break during cell division. Scientists number the chromosomes. When a part of chromosome 11 breaks off and jumps to the position formerly held by a part of chromosome 14, and vice versa, there is no doubt that your lymphoma is mantle-cell. Other translocations define other types of blood cancers: for instance, chromosomes 14 and 18 transpose to give you follicular lymphoma; parts of chromosomes 9 and 22 fuse to produce the "Philadelphia chromosome," causing chronic myelogenous leukemia. I had read that whatever their skill, pathologists cannot truly determine the type of lymphoma until a culture is grown from fresh, unfrozen diseased tissue and examined for translocations.

"I'm sure your pathologist is right," I said, "but the labs both in Michigan City and at the Mayo Clinic said I have a low-grade small B-cell lymphoma. My question is, how did your pathologist decide it's mantle cell? Just by looking at the morphology of the cells? Or did she grow a culture and find the translocation of the 11 and 14 chromosomes?" I had been learning the language.

Dr. A regarded me evenly for a long moment over his half-glasses and then thumbed through the report on his desk. "Her diagnosis was based on the architecture of the cells," he said slowly. "Again, though, believe me; she is always right."

I tried to ignore his certainty. Apparently my first two diagnoses were wrong, and it would take a hell of a lot more than an occasional handful of pills, if anything, to have a chance of curing me. When Dr. A asked me to sign the papers agreeing to the protocol, explaining that if I signed I would be assured of being included in the program—and that I could back out at any time—I signed.

"How much time before I absolutely have to get into therapy?"

"Don't wait too long," he said. "Certainly no longer than three months."

"Are there other options besides chemo?" My final hopeful question.

"Well, you could go to Stanford. Levy out there in California has been working with vaccines. But those things are *experimental*." He inflected the word as though it meant "unsafe" or "hazardous." Could anything be less safe than the chemo protocol he recommended?

• • •

Driving home to Beverly Shores, which is just west of Michigan City, I was infused with a strange mix of fear and melancholy. It pulled at me, rising and falling as the moon draws the sea, and I had to fight to suppress panic. Carol cried in silence beside me. She had been my partner in starting a magazine company and developing our island, and now she was my partner in lymphoma, spending long hours on her computer, new to her, searching the Web and retrieving more data than I could digest.

My intuition gave me more hope than warranted by Dr. A. There *had* to be something better than aggressive poison therapy and a bone-marrow transplant. I had long before learned always to heed my hunches, not as guesses, but as faster ways of solving problems that everyone uses as children and that artists and inventors develop into adulthood, a way of thinking that had proved useful in everything from making a lunar cryostat to growing shrimp. I have never believed that intuition is anything mystic or supernatural. Rather, it is a natural mechanism: a neuronal shortcut in processing information from a wide variety of sources, somewhat like the way an analog computer works. Countless scientists, including James Watson, codiscoverer of the shape of the DNA molecule, have remarked on the sudden, intuitive nature of their ideas.

Now I drove slowly, watching the rain stream down the windows, the wipers a metronome to thought. Those few times I had considered my own death, I had supposed my last thought would be of my last breath, followed by an unfelt swarming of bacteria in a recycling of atoms. I realized now that what it really comes down to is leaving behind those you love. I tried telling myself I had no regrets, that I had lived my share of adventures, from reporting a revolution in Costa Rica while still a student to resisting drug smugglers on my tropical Island for Science. I had started a publishing company, written hundreds of articles and some books on science and technology, and lived to see my recent novel *The Shallow Sea* help topple a corrupt regime in the Bahamas. Not exactly Hemingway or Einstein, but good enough for me. More important, Carol and I had raised a well-rounded, accomplished son. And yet . . .

Yet even after living an exciting life into my late sixties, I had to admit I wanted more time, that I would do everything necessary to climb out of the pit of hopeless cancer where so many others who believe that their doctors know all and therefore let their own need for knowledge be annulled are damned to rot in ignorance and cancer. I felt like Poe's protagonist in *The Pit and the Pendulum,* condemned to a slow death by torture, and I knew I would cling to the last shred of life against all odds, to the last second of the last minute, despite the oncologist's most devastating poisons, despite the pendulum's most hideous slice as it swung closer and closer to my cancerous abdomen. Hope, like love, is hard to explain, but when you have it, you dwell within it.

"But wait," I said to Carol with a glint of my former enthusiasm. "There can't be that much of a hurry. Let's put off this chemo stuff until we look at what's going on at Stanford—and a lot of other places."

I had spent most of my life either publishing research magazines or conducting research in one field or another and had learned that just because a new development is experimental does not mean it doesn't work. In these pursuits I had studiously avoided medical science. Not that I held anything against medicine. It was merely a fence I erected around my own portion of the universe, a feeling that I couldn't learn everything, and because my father, brother, and various uncles and cousins were doctors, medicine was something I didn't need to know. Or so I thought. If you get a strep throat, your doctor gives you the right antibiotic, and it goes away; if you break a leg, your orthopedic surgeon fixes it. You don't have to learn to do it yourself. But those are *curable* ailments. The incurable take longer. Like the war you can't leave to the generals, your own cancer is too important to be left to the doctors. Even worse, while the generals know quite a lot about war, oncologists, I discovered to my alarm, know exceedingly little about MCL.

Even oncologists who love lymphoma.

2

Watch and Learn

I DECIDED TO WAIT BUT NOT MERELY TO "WATCH AND WAIT," AS SO
many patients with less-aggressive lymphomas are advised to do. Nor would
I "watch and worry," as most actually do. Instead I dropped everything else
and began a new life investigating cancer science.

First I needed to visit a large cancer center to have fresh tissue removed
and grown in culture to confirm the diagnosis of mantle-cell lymphoma. My
local pathologist, Dr. Tom Roberts, steered me to the M. D. Anderson Cancer Center, in Houston. Established in 1941 at the University of Texas, Anderson receives more grants from the National Cancer Institute (NCI) and the
American Cancer Society than any other center. It contains more than six
hundred laboratories and employs a thousand scientists among a staff of
eleven thousand, making it the nation's largest operation outside the NCI
itself for the diagnosis, treatment, and research of cancer.

Shahid Siddiqi, aeronautical engineer and consultant to NASA, a true humanitarian and close friend, offered to come with me. The previous year the
two of us had flown my single-engine plane on a three-month trip down
the island chain of the Caribbean, through the jungles of Brazil, along the
east coast of Argentina past the Straits of Magellan to the end of the earth
at Ushuaia, a cold five hundred miles from Antarctica, then back up the west
coast through Chile, Peru, Ecuador, Colombia, and Central America. At the
time cancer was the furthest thing from my mind.

Shahid (pronounced *ShaHID*) is a slight man of impish humor, lean and fit, nimble as his two cats. He is not a vegetarian but prefers fruits and vegetables. He is the ideal companion, especially in an airplane. While we both are instrument-rated pilots, Shahid is an expert; he designs these small airplanes, enhances their avionics, and empathizes with the foibles of their onboard computers better than their own microcircuits do. Shahid's clients—the space agency, an aircraft modification company, and a Seattle-based aircraft instrument maker—constantly try to hire him full time. "I need less responsibility, not more, so I have time for my friends," he explains in his clear and patient diction, with more than a trace of accent from his native India.

With Shahid, David, and Carol helping me retrieve information on cancer, I had a staff again—not a hundred people, as in the days of my magazines, but I wasn't going it alone either. From my years in publishing scientific magazines I knew that tomorrow's answers, at least in the fields of industrial research, are under investigation in the laboratories of today. Could medicine be any different? Had not the chemotherapies in use today been developed a half-century ago? Weren't new-generation therapies somewhere in the medical labs right now? Considering the exponential march of science, wouldn't they be almost ready for use?

In the two months after my splenectomy, we first concentrated on the efficacy of chemotherapy protocols for mantle-cell lymphoma, reading papers from professional journals filled with the mostly broken hopes of patients who achieved PRs or CRs, partial or complete remissions. The word *remission,* of course, implies a temporary state. Reputable scientists, clinicians, and practitioners never use the word *cure* when discussing cancer, and—until the last two or three years—with good reason: the hundred-year war on cancer has mostly been lost, one battle at a time. Nietzsche was dead wrong, for me at least, when he said, "Hope is the worst of evils, for it prolongs the torment of man." At this point in my cancer journey, however, I would have settled in a flash for partial remission.

The statistics for chemotherapy are dismal, especially for mantle-cell lymphoma. Only some 5 percent of MCL patients who underwent chemotherapy achieved long-term remission, about the same as those who did nothing. There seemed to be one notable exception, however, and that was hyper-CVAD, a protocol developed at the M. D. Anderson Cancer Center, which claimed to have placed 38 percent of MCL patients in complete remission and another 55.5 percent in partial remission after four cycles of high-dose chemo. Add up those numbers and virtually all achieved remission! What on earth had they discovered? Why had no other lymphoma researchers throughout the world been able to come anywhere close?

Finding out about hyper-CVAD was high on my list, but first I wanted M. D. Anderson to determine whether my chromosomes 11 and 14 had transposed, whether I truly had mantle-cell lymphoma. The pathologist Tom Roberts had sent my slides and CAT scans ahead by express.

• • •

Shahid took a commercial flight from his home in Virginia to Chicago, where I picked him up in my Commander airplane, "Papa Whiskey"—so-called not because my grandchildren call me Papa (and certainly not because I remind anyone of a whiskey bottle) but because my randomly assigned registration number is 114-PW, and in aviation phonetics PW is "Papa Whiskey." Normally I fly Papa Whiskey alone, but when your mind is focused so wonderfully on the hangman's noose of lymphoma, it helps to have a copilot.

We headed south, stopping first at Cape Canaveral for a night and day so I could attend the National Space Society's annual board of governors' meeting, timed to coincide with John Glenn's return from space. I helped start the NSS some twenty-five years ago, and it had grown into an energetic international society promoting various space goals—scientific outposts on the moon, manned landings on Mars, touchdowns on asteroids, and other ultimate adventures.

Seeing friends—Scott Carpenter, Hugh Downs, and others less famous—injected a note of normalcy into a life that had turned into the netherworld, ending for a while the gnawing self-pity threatening to drag me into the abyss. At the meeting I kept quiet about my cancer for fear I could not reconcile myself with death as stoically as had Wernher von Braun, our society's first president, who one day in 1977 announced to us that he would be dead of bladder cancer before the next meeting. I had read that half of cancer patients die a few years after diagnosis. Wernher had died a month later at age sixty-two.

Wernher said then that if he had to get cancer, it couldn't have come at a better time, when he was at the end of his career and had settled his financial affairs. Now I also had arrived at this dubious nirvana. My magazine company had long before become part of Dun and Bradstreet and then of Cahners Publishing, and most of my island now belonged to Royal Caribbean Cruise Lines. Recently I'd sold shares in my remaining five acres and island lodge and completed some intricate estate planning. Carol and I had come a long way, after working our ways through college, from budgeting five dollars a week for food. I had been about to start a sequel to my recent novel, setting up the characters I hadn't killed off in *The Shallow Sea;* my scientist hero was going to undermine cocaine sales by perfecting and legalizing "the perfect drug" (healthy, nonaddictive stuff with an easy antidote), which is so easy to create in fiction.

When cancer struck I dropped the book like a boulder in a pond, watching its circles of silence widening to the death of its shores. How suddenly the music stops, the flowers wilt, the shallow sea churns into a hurricane. How easily your life turns perpendicular to the life you thought you were living. One day back in Indiana, after a day of such thoughts, I stopped feeling sorry for myself and entered my office, a building located on a dune across from my house and accessible by footbridge. An entire wall of white file cabinets beckoned, a dozen of them with four drawers each, filled with a writer's lifetime accumulation. I threw out hundreds of old files, mostly on technology and the Bahamas, including drug-smuggling clippings for my novel, and relabeled the empty drawers LYMPHOMA, half filling one with scientific papers, printouts of downloaded clinical-trial results, and articles from scientific magazines. Before I would finish, well into the next century, every one of the dozen top drawers would be filled with information on subjects ranging from anti-angiogenesis to Zevalin. The drug I sought now was not to move a story forward but to advance my own survival.

Neighbors whom I would see at the post office or town functions regarded me with sympathy and compassion; in their minds, shaped by endless cancer stories from relatives and friends, I must be riding the elevator of misery that traveled in only one direction, downward to the grave. Most of them said they would pray for me. What else could they do?

One friend, a nonsmoker named Paul, developed lung cancer about the same time I was diagnosed. Paul was too devastated to do anything about it except pray. His wife, not a zealot but normally religious, declined my offers to help her look into new experimental therapies. "We'll trust in God," she said, "and so should you." Paul died six months later. Some years ago a close friend, Wayne, had been diagnosed with mesothelioma, cancer of the pleural cavity outside the lungs. He was wealthy but rejected the idea of attempting to fund studies or otherwise enter experimental therapies in favor of sitting in the warm waters of a Bahamian "health clinic" and taking daily vitamin shots around his navel. Guys with braided dreadlocks and nose rings and even some more-conventional people such as Paul, Wayne, and my only brother—an M.D., no less—slide off the slope of reason into "New Age" or "holistic" patent medicines like megavitamins or, humorously, sleeping on magnets or massaging crystals. Even worse, some try to cure their cancers with connective-energy states, karmic traffic, apricot-pit extracts, moxibustion, colloidal silver, inhalation of radon gas, or other quackery, scams that consume billions that could have been spent sifting science.

Vitamins and herbs may prevent and help reverse some illnesses sometimes, but if they were cures for cancer, they would have been knocking on the door of the pharmacological mainstream, as molecular-targeted drugs are doing now. My brother, who seemed to suffer from every illness *except* cancer, never saw a holistic remedy he didn't try. In the end he died of his irrationality in 1997, one year before my diagnosis of cancer, by literally starving himself to death (see chapter 12).

When it came my turn to attempt a cure, it was easy for me to reject answers unknown to science. I knew intuitively that my therapy would be experimental, but like intuition itself, it would be rooted in reality.

• • •

Flying the Florida panhandle that November 1998, Shahid and I kept the Gulf off our left wing, watching the weather deteriorate. Dark clouds scudded in from an area of low pressure at sea, sucking up water and swirling it in front of us like a brick wall. A band of thunderstorms, wider than either of us had ever seen, stretched from far out into the Gulf and extended inland, covering Florida, Mississippi, and Louisiana and pushing as far north as Missouri, according to weather radar that we accessed by radio. We couldn't fly around it, over it, or under it, although we kept watching for holes through it using my 200-mile-range stormscope. This instrument receives electrical signals from thunderstorms, revealing the location and intensity of lightning. Along with flight-service radars, which indicate where the rain is the heaviest, stormscopes help pilots find the safest, if not the most direct, route to their destinations.

Papa Whiskey fell into a hole and then sprang back up the other side. Downdrafts careened the airplane so much I released the autopilot for fear of overstressing the wings. Both Shahid and I had logged some twenty-five hundred hours piloting small planes, and I began the maneuver that would get us out of trouble: "a one-eighty," that is, turning around one hundred and eighty degrees and going back the way we had come. You always can outrun storms, which move across the ground usually at less than twenty knots, because you fly eight times faster.

"Something's wrong," I said.

"Besides the storm?"

"We've lost communications." The comforting voice of the air-traffic controller dissolved into static. Shahid switched to the other radio. More static.

Lightning highlighted Shahid's black hair sprinkled with silver, the color of Papa Whiskey. He dialed the global positioning system to "nearest airport," setting me up for a landing at New Orleans.

Papa Whiskey started pitching, and I eased off on the turn. I have never had thoughts of death when seeing sharks at a hundred feet deep or reporting a war, much less in more easily controlled situations such as this. But then I never had mantle-cell lymphoma before. The combination of the cancer and the storm produced in me a rare morbidity. Strangely, I feared nothing for myself, because I thought I was going to die anyway, but I wanted Shahid to die of old age. Of course, pilots rarely admit they are worried, not because they are macho, but because they're too busy working. I made myself remember the most basic lesions in flying and recognize that it was only a storm of rain, not a storm of lymphoma cells destroying my body. I concentrated on the airplane's position and what I was doing, until I penetrated those fears and sorrows to my former world of light and optimism.

As if rewarding these thoughts, the clouds opened ahead toward the north, forming a clear tunnel, several miles wide, winding through the dark gray mass. If this path through the storm continued, however, its width wouldn't matter much; even the eye of a hurricane provides plenty of room . . . as long as you stay inside it. We snaked through the tunnel one hundred and fifty miles north, our eyes constantly scanning the stormscope, and followed the pathway west, where it narrowed to a mile or so, its dark walls seeming to brush our wings.

An hour later communications returned. We were on the other side of the storm, headed southwest, and we landed easily into a ruby sunset. The rain had washed Houston clean, its skyline glowing in crystal clarity.

• • •

The next morning we beheld the enormity of the M. D. Anderson complex, which, together with research and teaching units of the University of Texas and Baylor University, sprawls over a square mile south of downtown Houston. Green lawns and elms still held their leaves in November and separated a hundred multistory buildings in which about a thousand research projects were ongoing and some eighteen hundred patients were treated every day. It was here that chromosomal "painting" was first used to pinpoint gene abnormalities, where molecular markers were investigated, and where a molecular link between cigarettes and lung cancer had first been documented earlier in the decade.

With the help of campus maps that somehow materialized in Shahid's adroit hands, we crossed over a misty fairway where weeds were not allowed and, as if obedient, none grew. At our target building we rode an elevator upward, descended some stairs, and found our way through a maze to one of many CAT-scan rooms.

Twice before my surgery and three times since, I had endured the smoldering iodine injections used in CAT scans, having to stay absolutely still, staring at the ceiling. The X-ray pictures continued to show scores of enlarged lymph nodes in my abdomen, most measuring three centimeters, or three-quarters the diameter of a golf ball. Arguably, they seemed to have stopped growing, at least temporarily.

This time under the scanner I was lying not on my back but prone, staring at the vinyl floor tile. They were after more than just pictures today. A radiologist slowly inserted a long thin biopsy needle near my spine deep into my lower back. By craning my neck, I could see his associate following the path of the needle on the monitor, giving left-right, up-down directions to help the pathologist guide the needle aspirator toward a particularly big lymph node. To get at it, they had to circumvent the vena cava, the fire hose that returns the blood to the heart. In this way they were trying to retrieve tiny tissue specimens from a malignant lymph tumor without surgery. Had my two-pound spleen been preserved after its removal in Michigan City, it could have been used for such studies. Unfortunately, nonresearch hospitals, such as the one where I had my spleen excised, routinely throw away organs after tissue blocks and slides are prepared.

Three hours and thirty needle aspirations later, the M. D. Anderson pathologists decided they had harvested enough tissue to grow a culture.

• • •

I went to another department for bone-marrow extraction, an experience that made me appreciate the relatively painless technique of the Michigan

City oncologist who had performed it on me the first time. Now I suffered at the substantial hands of a technician who measured five foot, five—in diameter—and gave me little confidence that she knew what she was doing.

"Have you done this before?" I asked.

"Oh, just about every day," she laughed.

She leaned over my prone body at a forty-five-degree angle, like a linebacker eager for scrimmage, concentrating her nearly three hundred pounds onto the corkscrew as she ground into and through my pelvic bone. As before, there was no anesthetic. I felt like I was on a medieval torture rack. My blood pressure shot up so high that she stopped for a moment, alarmed, and checked the cuff on my arm. She backed off and tried again in a different place because she wasn't getting through the bone. In Michigan City it had taken five minutes to dig out a core. It took this technician an hour.

• • •

While I was idling on the corkscrew workbench, Shahid had been trying to find the phone extensions and locations of the head pathologist and some of the other scientists I wanted to see, but the Anderson operator refused to give out such secret information. She was no match for Shahid, though. He found an unused telephone in an aisle, unplugged it to connect his laptop, and proceeded to hack into the Anderson internal computer network.

"I made a loose appointment with Dr. Jeffrey Medeiros, the chief of pathology." Shahid said it like one of his cats having acquired a mouse.

"How loose?" I asked.

"He said we could come anytime."

Taking advantage of the flexibility, we first met some scientists working on vaccines and immunotherapy, but their work seemed a long way from patient therapy. At the pathology department, Jeff Medeiros himself came to greet us and took us into his office/lab, where he introduced us to some of his colleagues.

He turned to me and said, "You know, I've been doing pathology for twenty years, and you're the first patient who's asked to see me."

The room was small, cluttered with books, reports, and trays of slides.

Medeiros, whose last name is Portuguese, was born in Massachusetts and earned his M.D. at the University of Massachusetts. He proved to possess a rare compassion combined with a vigorous intellectual interest. In his late forties, he has a bushy mustache and movie-star looks, somewhat unusual for a chief of lymphoma pathology. More important, he is a research pathologist who takes nothing for granted. Every tissue specimen the slightest bit unusual that enters his laboratory elicits the same rigorous questions: *Why does it look or react like this? What is different about it?*

A few minutes later I was looking through his microscope at bits of one of my own lymph nodes that my Michigan City pathologist had sent ahead in tissue blocks. "See that pattern, kind of an arcing of the cells into the shape of a mantle?" he asked.

"Yes."

"What else do you see?"

"A sea of blue," I said. The tissue had been stained to show up in living color.

"What else?"

"Well, the cells seem kind of different from each other, not a repetitive pattern like wallpaper."

"Exactly!" He said it with the enthusiasm not only of a good teacher but of a scientist undergoing the eureka experience. "Because the cells are somewhat diverse, I'm not at all sure that you *have* mantle-cell lymphoma. Your bone marrow is involved, sure, but less than 5 percent contains cancer cells. Yours just *may* be a less-aggressive lymphoma. After all, it's behaved in an indolent way so far."

Medical scientists use the word *indolent* to describe the behavior of cancer, just as we might use it to describe the teenager next door as lazy, lethargic, or sluggish. Its opposite, though, is not *industrious* but rather *aggressive,* the regrettably typical and ravaging state of mantle-cell lymphoma.

"Have your symptoms stopped?"

"Not yet." I still had pain in my abdomen, still awakened during the night drenched in sweat.

"Let me know if they do." Jeff clearly was cheering for my side against our deadly but so-far lazy enemy, but I knew his empathy wouldn't cloud his judgment.

"When will we know for sure?" I asked.

"In about a week. The culture for cytogenetics has to grow before we can assess your chromosomes. I'll call you."

. . .

Those first weeks of studying cancer found me streaming into space onto some rocky asteroid circling the sun. Clambering into and up from the craters of this tiny world, I could see the blue earth hanging small in the sky but couldn't manage to get back to it. The only light penetrating the valleys of my asteroid arrives when the sun is directly overhead, at local noon—that is, when I read about a new scientist with a new project, offering new hope. But then the sun dims again while the scientist estimates the time required to complete his experiments. I stumble into some new cavern surrounded by jagged rock and claw my way along yet another shaft in this desolate land, until the spikes of the rock smooth out and I can stand and look beyond the precipices, beyond the peaks, beyond even the other asteroids, toward the other side of the sun, where there is light and knowledge illuminated.

3

The Chemo Culture

RAIN THE NIGHT BEFORE SEEMED TO HAVE WASHED THE M. D. ANDER-
son buildings clean. The campus glittered in the November sunlight as
Shahid and I returned, this time to see the renowned Dr. B, a Latin American whom I had called two weeks before. I described my case and ended it
with a little warm Spanish about my having *visitado sudamerica hace un año*.
At that time, with my life at stake, neither cajolery nor anything else was beyond me. He told me when to meet him in his office in Houston, so I had
sent ahead an autographed copy of my last book, a novel. Any asset you have,
I told myself, must be used. In seeking appointments through the usual
channels of assistants and nurses, sometimes I even gave myself the title
"Doctor," finding it helpful in slicing through the bureaucracy of females
who in hospitals everywhere toil in absolute servitude to the mostly male
practitioners of medicine.

The general reception room where we waited for Dr. B was "classic hospital": the customers were treated as children and made to wear uniformed
gowns, eat lukewarm food, and wait indefinite hours before seeing the
godhead. Worse, along with the usual hospital indignities, these patients were
embedded firmly in the Chemo Culture, having suffered the toxins of chemotherapy and the resultant loss of their immune systems and hair. With
their bald pates glistening over gowns, the patients looked like Roman senators mourning the loss of empire, wearing brave dull faces with no concept

of their futures. Even those who managed to keep their own clothing, the outpatients, were murky and somber, as though they might fall over at any minute. In contrast, the doctors and nurses running this CHOP shop smiled cheerfully as they paused to ask a question of a patient.

When it came our turn to see Dr. B, we found him jovial and sanguine, an oncologist who had received worldwide recognition with aggressive hyper-CVAD therapy. I asked Dr. B why other aggressive chemo protocols, such as the one that Dr. A urged me to enter at Northwestern, achieved comparatively poor results.

"I can't speak for them," he said in only slightly accented English, "but we have good success with MCL and other aggressive lymphomas and leukemias. Our regimen consists of four courses of fractionated cyclophosphamide administered with doxorubicin and dexamethasone—alternated with high-dose methotrexate and cytarabine."

The first part of the name *hyper-CVAD* derives from *hyper-fractionated cyclophosphamide* (tradenamed Cytoxin—literally, "cell killer"). *Hyper-fractionated* means the total dose is spread over an extended period. The rest of the acronym refers to the other components: *v*incristine (an extract of the deadly periwinkle plant); a steroid called dex*a*methasone; and a third, synthetic, toxin developed in the 1950s and called *d*oxorubicin (tradenamed Adriamycin).

"And now we're adding Rituxan to the mix," he said.

Rituxan is the tradename for rituximab, called *Mabthera* outside the United States; it was the first monoclonal antibody (all of which end in the suffix -*mab*) approved for lymphoma and was quickly followed by trastuzumab, or Herceptin, for breast cancer. These "Mabs" (also abbreviated as MAbs, mABs, or MoAbs) target and kill cancer cells selectively instead of wiping out all fast-dividing cells—normal and cancerous cells alike—as occurs with both chemotherapy and radiation.

"That's it?" I asked.

"Well, after that you get total-body radiation," Dr. B said. "Then, if we think you can tolerate it, we recommend a transplant."

Hadn't I heard this before? Except now I could add burn to the formula

of slash and poison—surgery, chemo, and radiation—standard cancer therapies for the past sixty years.

"Bone-marrow transplant?" I asked.

"Stem-cell transplant." He looked solemn. "It's easier on the patient."

I had read about the procedure in detail. Stem cells, from which all blood
cells "stem," or arise, are collected by machine from your own blood or from
your sibling's blood if there is a good match. Afterwards you undergo a few
days of intensive chemotherapy, some ten times the standard dose—
sufficiently toxic to kill you if nothing further were done. The chemo destroys your diseased blood, your bone marrow, and your healthy cells alike.
You then are *rescued* (the word used by transplanters) with stem cells
reinfused into your bloodstream.

The idea is to replenish normal cells; unfortunately, plenty of cancer cells
remain floating around your blood, despite laboratory techniques that reduce their number. Utilizing a donor's blood gets you around that hazard
but presents another: about a third of the time you die from graft-versus-
host disease (GVHD). In GVHD mature T cells—the immune system's
strongest soldiers—go to war against your own allies, the donor's cells, which
they regard as "foreign." The graft, strange as it sounds, rejects the recipient. Despite the hazards, the technique is widely used at major cancer centers to treat aggressive lymphomas and leukemias.

"Doctor, have you written a paper on the results of hyper-CVAD for
mantle-cell lymphoma?" I asked.

"Our department has one right now. It's out for comment before sub-
mission to the *Journal of Clinical Oncology*."

"May I have a copy?"

He said nothing for a moment, so I filled in the silence. "Look, as a former
science-magazine publisher, I realize your colleagues may not want other institutions to see it before they make revisions. I promise I won't show it to
anyone before publication."

He was quiet for a moment but quickly broke out into a smile. "Sure,"
he said. A trusting man; most doctors would make you wait. It would be
difficult to resist any treatment prescribed by this charismatic physician.

"Find out for certain whether you have MCL," he said. "If you do, I rec-ommend our protocol."

"When?"

"Don't 'watch and wait' too long. Three months, max. Provided you *re-ally have* MCL."

· · ·

Flying home, I was alone above the clouds, Shahid having returned to Vir-ginia by commercial airliner. Usually at such times I am truly at rest, released from the earth and floating over terrestrial concerns. But these days my mortality hung close, like a nimbus cloud filled with black rain and malig-nant thunder.

Over the previous two months I had talked to a dozen specialists, either in person or by phone. Despite what I had read about new vaccines and com-mercial monoclonal antibodies coming on stream, these cancer doctors still recommended chemotherapy in one combination or another. Why? They obviously knew more than we, didn't they? Shahid, David, and I continued analyzing the scholarly papers that reported the results of these drastic pro-tocols, finding that over the last half-century new combinations of chemo-therapeutic drugs had advanced the art to the point where they usually drove tumors into remission. But these remissions were almost never permanent and certainly not a cure.

We had spent two-thirds of my allocated three months assessing scores of clinical trials for lymphoma. The more aggressive the chemo, the greater the death of the cancer cells, but also the greater damage to the normal cells, including those of the immune system.

Some of these papers puzzled me, especially the advance copy of the Anderson paper that Dr. B had given me, and since it was a quiet flight, I glanced at it from time to time. The paper stated that thirty-four patients received transplantation and that "all achieved remission." Yet in the next sentence the authors added, "Two died of chronic graft-versus-host disease while they were in CR [complete remission] at seven to ten months."

Technically they are correct. You can be in complete remission and still be killed by the "cure." *But how complete is your remission if you are dead?*

It was only November, but through a broken deck of clouds I could see a faint layer of frost beginning to coat the fields like a smoky veil that grew thicker as I headed north. I couldn't wait to take a closer look at Dr. B's paper and thought about it all the way home. After refueling at Little Rock, I kept St. Louis off to my left and finally landed like an anxious bird on the long runway at Valparaiso, Indiana, Papa Whiskey's home.

I barely said hello to Carol (and our two cats) before we both started reading the Anderson paper thoroughly. We read it twice, looking up words we didn't know. There were forty-five patients in the study, but only thirty-four received the planned bone-marrow transplant. What happened to the other eleven? Did they die? Walk away cured? Why didn't the paper say?

Well, I thought, such questions explain why scientists are reluctant to give you their papers ahead of time; the paper would be peer reviewed, and if it passed that hurdle, the editors of the prestigious journal surely would demand revisions by any of the fifteen Anderson clinicians listed as authors. Months later the paper did appear in the *Journal of Clinical Oncology*. There were no changes.

· · ·

It's no wonder that when cancer doctors read (or speed read) such "results" in their primary journal, they continue to push brute-force chemo against all odds. And those odds are stacked against you. Compiling the results from scores of scientific papers and books, Shahid and I calculated average five-year survival rates following diagnosis and chemotherapy. The mean proportion of five-year survivors with mantle-cell lymphoma was about 10 percent; of other non-Hodgkin's lymphomas, 50 percent; and *all cancers,* some 40 percent. At first glance these figures seem to say that chemotherapy gives you a 10, 50, or 40 percent chance of staying alive for five years, depending on your type of cancer.

Nothing could be further from the truth. As dismal as are these percentages, if it were the chemotherapy that kept 40 percent of cancer patients alive even for only five years, administering these poisons might make some sense.

But you have to ask how many of those 40 percent would have lived five years without chemotherapy?

I phoned an expert in immunology mentioned in several books and articles, Dr. Michael Lotze, and was lucky to find him receptive to my call. Lotze, a widely known M.D., is now the director of protein and gene therapies at GlaxoSmithKlein in King of Prussia, Pennsylvania.

"It is a misconception that chemo does much for most cancers," he told me. "We keep testing notions we should have disposed of years ago."

Lotze explained it this way. The toxins for chemotherapy are chosen to fulfill a simple, scientifically unsophisticated premise: kill the fast-growing cells because cancer cells grow fast. The problem is that many normal cells divide and grow fast as well, not just those in your hair, but also cells in the bone marrow, the reproductive system, and the digestive tract. At dosages strong enough to kill tumor cells, your entire system is literally poisoned.

Between the lines, Lotze and many modern oncologists were telling me that the standard treatment for cancer—chemotherapy—is as dangerous in many cases as the cancer itself. Did that mean I should continue to refuse chemo? That my search for better therapies not only might prove better but could save my life?

• • •

I began to learn that the toxins of chemotherapy are among the deadliest on the planet. The history of chemotherapy is the history of testing poisons, first on animals and then on otherwise hopeless patients. The Chemo Culture engulfed the world slowly, starting in Europe at the end of the nineteenth century when the German scientist Paul Ehrlich used arsenic to treat syphilis. Nitrogen mustard gas, which killed hundreds of thousands in World War I, became the favored cancer weapon after World War II, along with Ehrlich's original arsenic compounds and extracts of lethal plants such as mandrake or of the insecticide DDT.

Beginning in 1966 and continuing to the present, the National Cancer Institute has systematically tested thousands of new toxins annually. Today the most widely used chemotherapies are combinations of three or more agents in doses heavy enough to interfere with enzymes, break DNA strands, or otherwise kill cells. They bear belligerent acronyms such as ICE, MOP, and COP, or exotic names such as CVAD and EPOCH. One of the more popular of these chemo combinations is CHOP, which the oncologist in Michigan City had wanted to give me in small doses when I was first erroneously diagnosed with a more-benign form of lymphoma. The first three letters, I remembered, stood for cyclophosphamide (also called Cytoxan), hydroxydoxorubicin (but usually called Adriamycin), and Oncovin (also called vincristine—that deadly periwinkle again). To fight most cancers, including mantle-cell lymphoma, they are administered by injection in extreme quantities—strong enough, after all, to kill cancer cells.

Now I found out—secondhand, fortunately—that they can damage the heart, lungs, liver, and bladder. They can reduce blood-cell production and may lead to abnormal bleeding, increased risk of infection, and reduced fertility in men. The least toxic in the CHOP combination is prednisone, a powerful anti-inflammatory cortisone given orally and used for everything from rheumatoid arthritis to poison ivy. But even prednisone can be dangerous in the quantities usually used against cancer. Besides producing weight gain and facial swelling—the signature "moon face" that develops about the third week—prolonged use weakens the entire immune system; initiates the process of osteoporosis, which damages bones; and suppresses adrenal function, causing anemia, sluggishness, personality changes, mental impairment, and even death.

The NCI also conducts and sponsors numerous molecular-targeted approaches, as I would find later during my journey to the cancer laboratories. At the same time, the NCI remains rooted in our Chemo Culture, introducing more cell-selective toxins and agents to counteract some of the side effects, yes, but still using the old poisons developed in the three decades after World War II.

I am not being facetious in calling the Western world's reliance on chemotherapy the Chemo Culture. *Culture* is defined as a standard of followings, beliefs, and behaviors, such as the Religious Culture, the Sports Culture, the illegal Drug Culture—mores that, once embedded, take a long time to change or disappear. Because chemotherapy pervades society so thoroughly and, like other "cultures," has become accepted, institutionalized, generally unquestioned, and self-protecting, it has earned the designation. How better to describe this cancer universe—the doctors, the government (through its NCI), the pharmaceutical companies, the textbooks, the popular how-to-cope books, the protocols . . . and the stereotypic bald heads in movie after movie?

Chemotherapy is a dangerous culture to embrace. Chemo toxins attack rapidly dividing cells without differentiation, including not only hair follicles but also dividing cells in the gastrointestinal system and bone marrow. Many of these toxins induce mouth sores, anemia, and brutal nausea to the point where you pray you can vomit. The poisons severely interfere with the functions of the heart, lungs, liver, and kidneys. Even worse, they multiply the damage caused by the cancer itself by wiping out the production of lymphocytes, the white blood cells that include B and T cells, the latter being our most effective disease fighters. As a result, it becomes difficult or impossible to ward off infection. The spread of an infection from its initial site to the bloodstream, called "sepsis," is not uncommon after chemotherapy. In severe sepsis the inflammation rages throughout the body like a fire, interfering with blood flow and shutting down the liver, lungs, and other vital organs.

• • •

Another vicious side effect is "chemo brain." I came across data from studies at Dartmouth University indicating that brain impairment, long suspected by cancer patients, was more severe and prevalent than had been previously thought (see notes and chapter 25). The condition has been found to arise not only from aggressive chemotherapies like hyper-CVAD but from "ordinary" cancer treatments like CHOP. Because their effects are scattered and pervasive among the cells of the body, chemos perform these devastations in the brain and elsewhere not just temporarily but often for the remainder of their victims' shortened lives. Given all these terrors, I asked myself again and again why so many intelligent, experienced, and compassionate cancer doctors like Dr. B were stuck in the Chemo Culture.

I started working the phones to hear the other side of the argument, calling prominent chemotherapists around the country. Most of them seemed startled that I would question the efficacy of the chemo standard. Other than saying without enthusiasm that "chemotherapy helps a lot of patients"—apparently interested primarily in the short term—they were reluctant to talk much. I thought it would be easier talking to those I knew, so I started with the lymphoma enthusiast in Chicago.

His nurse-bodyguard asked, "What is it you want with Dr. A?"

"I want him to defend chemotherapy."

She fell silent, apparently feeling no desire to have this strange statement explained. She returned after two minutes to say that Dr. A was out of town.

Dr. B was the most forthcoming, and his views were more important since he represented M. D. Anderson, arguably the most aggressive chemotherapy center in the country. I told him I was having difficulty trying to reconcile the advice to take chemotherapy with its hazards, especially chemo brain.

"How can I answer?" Dr. B. began. "The dangers you point out are certainly present. But do not forget that every person with cancer reacts . . . differently. Instead of a hundred cancers, you could say maybe that there are millions of cancers, all a little different."

Setting aside the human wreckage I'd been reading about, he started telling me how chemotherapy combinations have effected long-term, if not permanent, remissions in certain cancers. "The chemo success rate against childhood leukemia is 80 percent," he said. "Arsenic trioxide plus steroids and vitamin A produce some benefits for certain leukemias."

"How about lymphoma?" I asked.

"Well, various chemos are effective against Hodgkin's lymphoma, large B-cell lymphoma, and acute lymphocytic leukemia," he said.

"But those are fairly rare, aren't they? I mean compared to other non-Hodgkin's lymphomas, especially MCL?"

As he paused to prepare his answer, I could picture him walking around his office like Papa Whiskey in a holding pattern.

"Yes," he said candidly. "But again, different patients react differently.

Chemotherapy extends life an additional eighteen months for stage-three ovarian cancer and some six months for small-cell lung cancer. Certain chemotherapeutic drugs are effective against embryonic testicular cancer, cutaneous T-cell lymphoma, and Hodgkin's disease."

Chemotherapists, I knew, follow the FDA definition of an effective drug as one that achieves a 50 percent reduction in tumor size for one month. Like the eighteen months awarded to ovarian cancer patients, reduction in tumor size didn't sound much like a cure to me.

"Dr. B, instead of the relentless pounding of all malignancies with chemo, wouldn't it be better to ask *why* these toxins work well against a few cancers?"

"Yes, it would," he said.

"And why chemos don't work against most other cancers?" I felt like a courtroom prosecutor badgering the witness.

"Yes."

"Could it be that the metabolic pathways from the mutated genes that produce these tumors are more easily interrupted?"

"Sure."

"Then why not try less-devastating therapies even on cancers known to be amenable to chemo? Maybe to disrupt the intricate chain of events that must be triggered to achieve uncontrollable cell division?"

"That kind of research is going on in a hundred labs right here, and in thousands of others all over the world," Dr. B reminded me. "Meanwhile, how are we supposed to treat patients? How are we going to treat *you*?"

• • •

An honest man, I thought once again. I thanked him and returned to my studies, looking up each of the cancers he said were put into remission by chemo. I soon found that those malignancies are relatively rare, collectively representing something less than 5 percent of all cancers. And even in these comparatively easy to cure cancers, secondary tumors can be started by radiation and chemo; in fact, there is a strong possibility that children with Hodgkin's disease will develop a second cancer from their treatment. The big killers—breast, colon, lung, and prostate cancer and many non-Hodgkin's lymphomas—are not stopped and are possibly made worse by chemotherapy. I found something else even more devastating, something that nailed down my decision to reject chemotherapy. Whether I was nailing my own coffin would be a chance I was ready to take.

What I learned was this: *there is absolutely no correlation between shrinking tumors and extending life.*

. . .

This stage of my journey was mired in negativity. Not only do temporary shrinkages of tumors fail to result in increased survival, but reducing tumor size may do more harm than good. According to one of the most methodical critics of chemotherapy, Dr. Samuel Epstein, a professor of environmental medicine at the University of Illinois at Chicago: "Sometimes, a high response rate actually correlates with a *lower* period of survival."

I pondered, discussed the anomalies with the Pejics and David, and read everything I could about chemotherapy, holding constantly in my mind the warning that I was coming to the end of my three months to "get into therapy." But what therapy?

I would take my chances with Mabs or other treatments I was determined to find. It wasn't a happy decision because I knew that what was true at the dawn of the twentieth century remained true at the dawn of the twenty-first. For the vast majority of cancers that have not yet metastasized—and for mantle-cell lymphoma as well—surgery is the most effective option. Radiation (which can produce secondary cancers) extends life in about 10 percent of cases. And chemo at best offers you a few more years. At worst, it kills you even faster.

Its practitioners tell you that even though chemotherapy may not cure your cancer, it may prolong your life, and anyway, there is no other choice. Finding other choices, of course, had become the focus of my journey to the nation's cancer-research laboratories. I couldn't believe this field of inquiry could be so sterile.

I had to go to these labs, meet the scientists, and see for myself.

Every scientific paper I read and every professional I talked to admitted that it is impossible to determine whether chemotherapy can prolong life, except in those malignancies Dr. B had pointed out and a few other rare cancers, for it would be ethically difficult and logistically impossible to conduct blind clinical trials for each kind of cancer, giving chemo to one group and placebos to another. Chemotherapy is given annually to more than a million cancer patients, according to estimates by Ralph W. Moss. Chemo has become "part of the national mythology," he says, and has been awarded "a special place in the commercially organized fantasies of the nation."

Our Chemo Culture.

. . .

When you enter this fantasy as a cancer victim, you undergo chemo and your cancer goes into remission. So far, so good. But in a few months or years, in a typical scenario, the cancer returns. More chemo, more remission. This time, though, the remission lasts only half as long. The next round gives you relief for only a few months, or not at all, because your tumors have mutated to withstand the poisons. In their drive toward immortality, cancer cells mutate, or transform their genetic structure, to avoid the toxins used to try to kill them. Desperate, you submit to a bone-marrow or stem-cell transplant. If you make it, you achieve remission again. If not, you die of fungal, bacterial, or viral infections that run rampant while your immune system is shut down. Fortunately, two-thirds of patients survive their transplants, and it is that statistic that keeps the practice going. Are you are buying time? Or are you only widening the process of dying?

After my visit to M. D. Anderson, talks to dozens of chemotherapists around the country, and nightly reading, I knew about the complex molecular mechanisms of radioactive antibodies and about personalized cancer vaccines but barely understood them. I knew they benefited cancer patients in clinical trials far in excess of poison therapy, but what I didn't realize yet was the full extent of the stranglehold the FDA held on doctors who were willing to try nontoxic, end-of-the-century biotheraputic drugs.

I kept asking myself and the scientists I talked to whether I was being too hard on those who so freely give chemotherapy. Or are most of them simply like bureaucrats in corporations or government, bent on preserving the status quo? After a lifetime of running businesses, I have come to believe that most salesmen are not good at selling, most stock analysts don't analyze, most teachers don't inspire, and most people do their jobs without verve or imagination or creativity or guts. Why should it be different with cancer doctors? Most cancer physicians are not Albert Schweitzers. And most cancer physicians don't read scientific papers, much less visit research laboratories.

Soon I began dividing cancer doctors into two broad categories. The most visible to patients—unfortunately the vastly larger group—consists primarily of "chemotherapists." These physicians are too busy to keep up with advances in genomics, molecular biology, immunology, hematology, biochemistry, or any other science. They rarely communicate with cancer scientists or attend scientific meetings in these fields. Since they administer toxins to their patients, you would think they at least would be expert in toxicology!

The smaller group has earned the name they call themselves: "oncologists," those who study tumors. These doctors are uniquely aware of advances in cancer science and move their patients into appropriate nonchemo clinical trials. Of course, the distinctions between the two groups are mine alone, and there is a discernible shift to science among practitioners as better therapies begin to trickle down from the research laboratories. It is an agonizingly unhurried evolution, though. And the Chemo Culture that has solidified into our society does nothing to accelerate it. Like other physicians, cancer doctors are chosen by most "patients" (an unfortunately appropriate word) on the quality of their bedside manners, not for their scientific prowess, of which the average person knows nothing.

What these health-care customers don't realize, in their pain and confusion, is that their doctors are the plumbers of the cancer business. Just as a plumber can't be expected to start using noncorroding plastic pipe until the chemical engineers develop it and the pipe companies market it, a chemotherapist continues his old methods until new and better remedies are exhaustively tested and approved. Of course, doctors are far more educated, so you expect more from the modern medical community than from plumbers—especially when you are desperate.

When you are desperate, as was I, you see one doctor after another, cling-
ing to every word. You scour each face, watching for a hidden smile, for the
slightest hint that one of them *knows* how to cure you, against all odds,
against what you so reluctantly but relentlessly have learned both in this
possibly final stage of your life and in everything that went before.

Well, this is what occurs in our modern age. It did not happen that way
in past centuries because few people lived beyond fifty years. Is it really so
strange that, even with all its marvels, modern medicine can't do everything
and in its vexation clings to the old? We think of bloodletting as an ancient
and useless remedy once recommended for fevers and most everything else
(including hemorrhages!), and yet it persisted into the twentieth century. It
was recommended as late as 1923 in a widely used edition of a medical text
by Sir William Osler, who was Walt Whitman's physician. At least bloodletting makes its victims feel better for a short time, provided they have high
blood pressure.

The fact is that chemo is safe—for the chemotherapists. They never will
be sued for injecting FDA-approved poisons into their patients' bloodstreams, regardless of the harm they may be doing. The chemotherapists are
misled not only by an occasional research paper whose time limitation
counts dead people in "remission" but also by the extreme proliferation of
chemotherapy trial-and-error protocols themselves. You can't search the
cancer web without reading about still another trial using different combinations of toxins. The reasoning behind the plethora of protocols goes something like this: if a patient has "failed" the poisons of yesterday or becomes
resistant to them, we'll have to try even stronger poisons tomorrow, and
damn the pain and suffering we impose. Einstein could have been talking
about the devastation and pain of chemotherapy when he offered his
definition of insanity: "endlessly repeating the same process, hoping for
different results."

• • •

Rejecting advice to take chemotherapy was not easy when it came from every cancer physician I saw in that desolate winter of 1998–99. When you are

miserable as I was, it is tough to swim against the current, even when you read in one scientific paper after another that chemo does not help mantle-cell lymphoma. It is most difficult when lying awake at night, your guts still sore from surgery and the unrelenting pressure of enlarged lymph nodes on nerves, wrenching with every turn in the bed, with every halting step to the bathroom, drenched in sweat, imagining the nodes growing within, picturing them pus colored, smelling fear as distinct as rotting fish, feeling the tumors pulling at your pain, when you are worried that you will not survive the year, when you feel rage over having become accustomed to health. When you have sunk into such desperation, you advance first through alarm, releasing adrenaline for the fight. Then, when your adrenal cortex is depleted, you experience not denial but a form of resistance: *if only you can fight hard enough, then you have a chance.*

After exposure to such intense levels of stress, these feelings soon segue into exhaustion. Men die every day, you tell yourself; it is a natural cycle. You find yourself wishing not for the end of life but for a different life, an afterlife where you no longer will be tortured. Finally you tell yourself to stop wishing and start working to control your pain. You learned how to do that when you were a kid.

Now you do it again.

4

Life before Cancer

MY FIRST INDOCTRINATION IN PAIN CONTROL—WHICH PROVED USE-
ful in cancer—came from my father, an oral surgeon. I was a student at the
St. Rita High School, on Chicago's South Side, next to my dad's office. He
had a rather interesting way of extracting teeth. The idea was to get them
out in a hurry before the laughing gas (nitrous oxide) wore off. He'd yank a
mouthful of rotted teeth in less than a minute, letting them fly all over the
room. It was my job to pick up the felled teeth, scattered like dead soldiers,
and place them on the dental tray before the patient awakened and wondered
whether the doctor had started. Of course, if you have cancer, you can't laugh
your way out of suffering, with gas or otherwise. But you can learn to abandon the scene of the pain.

On the day when Dad gave me my first pain-control lesson, I was sitting
in the dental chair before going to my evening job in the photolab of the *Chicago Tribune.* His gray eyes twinkled as he said, "Neil, you've tolerated my
drilling to make inlays for your teeth without painkillers. Now you have an
impacted third molar. It's sideways, and I have to split it in half to get it out.
You can have Novocain at any time if you want it. But you don't need it."

I postponed the decision by asking, "Why?"

"Well, what if you're a spy and have to endure torture to save the world?"
He grew serious again. "If you learn to manage pain without narcotics, you'll
have an easier time through life."

That made sense to me. I was already planning a life of adventure. "Okay, how do I do it?"

"Concentrate on your breathing. Space each breath slowly, regularly. Don't try to fight the pain. Ignore it. Go somewhere else in your mind."

I did. I journeyed to Costa Rica on a cloud. I was only fourteen but already in love with what was said to be the most picturesque and democratic country in Central America, and I had floated there before in my imagination. A minute into drilling Dad noticed me struggling not to raise my hand, so he stopped and squirted a stream of water, his arm held high in an acrobatic arch, spraying not only my molars but my face as well. "Are you in Costa Rica yet?" He was always asking questions when it was impossible for me to use my mouth to answer.

As the drill bore deeper into my tooth, the Latin girls smiled at me from behind their long hair. One plucked a mango from a tree and bit into it with her white teeth, which you could tell had never been drilled. Palm fronds rustled on the grassy carpet sloping down the outside of one of the country's seven volcanoes, and jaguars rolled over so I could stroke the fur on their vibrating bellies. I didn't know whether real jaguars purr, but these did. Suddenly I was back in the dental chair. Dad was smiling. "That wasn't so bad, was it?"

It was easy, I thought. And useful in later life, especially when you have cancer. No Zen. No spiritualism. No nether experiences. Just schoolboy cloud travel.

• • •

In high school I designed and built six-foot airplanes, painting the wings with aniline dyes, letting them soar for hours on a half-minute motor run, and then hitching rides with teenage Piper Cub pilots to search for an orange splotch on the green ground. My other hobby was photography, and my first business in high school was developing and arranging X rays for the dentists up and down Sixty-third Street.

Photography won me a scholarship to Northwestern University, which I entered after a year at Loyola, where I started at age sixteen. I became the director of Northwestern's photo lab, which served all the student publications, and that job enabled me to start a bigger business, photographing dances and other events. It was how I met Carol, who also was working her way through college.

After my junior year I took my first summer off, boarding a banana boat to Panama and hitching a ride to Costa Rica in an airplane not much bigger, it seemed to me, than the ones I used to make. I was there to report the tail end of the Costa Rican revolution for the Overseas News Agency, which had issued press passes to journalism graduates and a few students. One highlight of the three-month trip was meeting the revolutionary leader José Figueres, who later became president of the country. A diminutive man, full of energy like Napoléon or Bolívar, he told me, "I too attended Loyola University for my first year! To study English. And then to MIT for the same reason you went to Northwestern—*science!* Journalism and Science!" You could hear his capital letters. "You are a Truth-Seeker in two great professions that—regrettably—rarely meet! *Pura Vida!*" he added, the passionate Costa Rican expression incorporating the idea of living to the fullest—literally, "Pure Life!"

While I was tasting the salt of foreign correspondence, my brother, Jay, my only sibling, two years older, entered the University of Chicago Medical School, from which he graduated at age twenty-one. During a subsequent residency he began to be plagued by an excruciating pain in his head ("like an axe buried in my skull") that gradually descended into a ten-year depression and a lifelong delusion regarding the "research" he conducted to end his pain, dragging our naive mother into the morass behind him.

I look back on his efforts with regret, not for myself but for Jay. They developed in me a lifelong aversion to superstition, to "paranormal" phenomena (outside of science fiction), and to extreme forms of alternative medicine, especially in trying to cure debilitating diseases such as cancer.

• • •

Carol and I were married just before we both graduated from Northwestern with five B.S. degrees between us: mine in the physical sciences, journalism, and psychology; hers in journalism and education. Carol taught first and second grade (in one classroom) as we built our first home in the Indiana sand dunes of Beverly Shores. After working as a crime reporter on the Michigan City daily newspaper, I attended the magnificent Leadership School, first as a student and then as an instructor in the attached armored reconnaissance company, for I had been invited to enlist (or otherwise be drafted) in the U.S. Army during the Korean War. The lessons I learned helped me immeasurably in business (don't make a threat you're not prepared to carry out; never succumb to an enemy's intimidation; never ask a subordinate to do what you yourself haven't done or aren't willing to do; when you fail, try it differently the next time; and above all, be decisive). In fact, the school actually taught "controlled failure" as a subject, since the very idea of armored recon is in a sense to *seek* failure: deliberately draw fire to locate the enemy—and then get the hell away.

• • •

I began my science education in earnest after the army, at the Illinois Institute of Technology (IIT), not as a student, but as the editor of a magazine published by the affiliated IIT Research Institute (IITRI). This technology center, which sprawls across Chicago's near South Side, stands where a slum was cleared to build some fifty modern Mies van der Rohe–designed buildings. My five-year apprenticeship there was like earning degrees in fields as diverse as flame-sprayed ceramics, fiber optics, magnetic levitation, and cryogenics. No medicine, though. No cancer research. IITRI led directly to my starting my own national magazine of science and technology. In fact, the director agreed to loan me the institute's mailing list, as did Battelle, Stanford Research Institute, A. D. Little, and a half-dozen others. We used these lists to promote subscriptions.

Industrial Research was no staid scientific journal. It was a magazine full of news and articles designed to inform readers in technical fields other than their own, with the idea of cross-fertilizing their research. I believed then— and believe now—that nothing in science is so complex that it cannot be explained to nonspecialists. We translated the expositions of researchers so that investigators in other fields not only could understand them but could utilize information or methods applicable to their own work. The first issue in January 1959 forecast $12 billion to be spent that year for industrial research, half from industry and half from government. (The figure for 2003 was $300 billion, still split fifty-fifty.)

After six months of traveling with space salesmen—representatives who sold advertising in a dozen or more magazines—my advertising manager turned in ads totaling ten pages. Not close to breaking even, but not bad for a first issue. Working in the basement of our unfinished house, which I had been building myself over the previous five years, we and our neighbors sorted and placed in mailbags twenty-five thousand copies of that first issue, weighing one pound each. Unlike manufacturing companies, publishers must produce an entirely new product every issue. Now I planned our second product to be more elaborate, more creative, more exciting . . . and more expensive.

Exciting the advertisers was another story. Even those ad managers who had encouraged us after seeing the magazine claimed they had to wait a year or sometimes two before advertising in it, "to make sure the magazine will continue," a prerequisite for failure if there ever was one. Our second issue was to contain more than a hundred editorial pages and be bound with an expensive aluminum-foil cover, but when the closing date arrived, we had only four pages of advertising. My partner, in charge of selling ad space, was sickened by his own failure. "There's no point in continuing," he said with true regret, for he owned an equal share of the company.

Everything I have ever undertaken involved failure first. Today, from the vantage point of having had and cured my own cancer, I have come to believe that you must use whatever assets you have accumulated during your life to learn about, and then find your way into, a modern therapy that gives you a fighting chance. What assets? *Whatever attributes you possess!* Technical knowledge that might be adapted, the ability to use a computer, understanding books and papers you might have thought beyond your scope . . . and—especially—the arts of diplomacy and salesmanship.

Why sales? Because doctors, being human like the rest of us, give preference to those who seek intelligent treatment; because physicians need to be told of new results emanating from cancer research laboratories; because—unaided or unsold—physicians take the time, trouble, or opportunity to get only 3 percent of their adult cancer patients into clinical trials!

The magazine was my first real business, and there was no way I could just abandon it. Carol and I were heavily in debt, having sold our car and borrowed as much as we could on a second mortgage. Even at that time, you didn't normally start a national magazine without a million dollars or so from some rich uncle. Lacking that, I had sold shares to virtually everyone I knew, including the printer, the typesetter, my employees, and friends. How could I let them down? Carol had quit teaching to have our son, David, whose first birthday we had just celebrated. When I came home at night, I would awaken David and play with him, but afterward I couldn't sleep, plagued by new or modified plans. Despite working eighteen-hour days, commuting to the office in Chicago, and writing promotional brochures and letters on Sundays, I couldn't sleep because my heart beat so hard it rocked the bed. I knew nothing of selling advertising space, but I had to try.

As I look back on those times, I see the magazine as preparation for survival. I know what it's like to give everything you have—and everything you didn't know you had. Those who have started companies on a shoestring, or have fought in wars, or have risen out of poverty, or have fulfilled some other difficult dream know what I'm talking about: the heart-thumping risks, the passing of the point of no return. It is not adversity alone; most of us know suffering. It is not only hard work; countless people do that every day. It is achieving a goal despite the odds, tripping and getting up again. It is never considering failure.

Pure life, sure. And pure tenacity to make it happen.

• • •

One morning I asked our paper merchant, one of our shareholders who helped us out on Saturdays as an unpaid bookkeeper, "Milt, who makes the foil we're using on the cover?"

"The Aluminum Company of America," he said.

Long-distance charges were not to be taken lightly. I turned over a three-minute timer filled with sand and picked up the phone, calling Pittsburgh, asking for "the advertising manager of Alcoa," glancing nervously out the thirteenth-floor window of our office in the Borg-Warner Building. Snowflakes fell like grains of sand, melting in the dark canyon of Monroe Street.

"Which one?" replied a female voice from Pittsburgh.

"Oh . . . how many ad managers do you have?"

"There are twenty-three divisions here. Each has its own advertising department."

"How about the division that advertises on aluminum foil?"

I turned over the timer twice before a disembodied voice identified himself as the ad manager of the electromagnetic-equipment division.

"Hi!" I said, giving him my name. "I'm the publisher of *Industrial Research,* the most beautiful technical magazine ever published," adding, "calling from Chicago."

He laughed, surprising me.

"Why are you laughing?"

"Because technical magazines aren't supposed to be beautiful."

"Why not?"

"Well, they're just not."

"How about your ads on foil? Aren't they beautiful, well-designed to grab a buyer?"

"Of course."

"Wouldn't you like to see one of them on the back cover of my magazine, which has as its cover Alcoa foil?"

"Who did you say you were again?"

I told him, and he asked me to wait a minute while he went to his library to find our first issue. I knew it would be there, for we had sent out five thousand copies to potential advertisers in every technical company and every technical advertising agency in the country.

When he returned, he said, "That's quite a remarkable first issue. Exciting."

We talked for what seemed an eternity that dark winter day, his tone growing more and more serious as I turned over the timer ten more times. I made my first sale: two pages—covers 3 and 4, because the text for his foil promotion appeared on the nonfoil side of the page. I told our reps, none of whom wanted to hear that an editor had sold a two-page ad to one of the biggest companies in America on a phone call—much less two pages in seven colors on aluminum foil. These reps had never even heard of a seven-color ad! I extended the advertising deadline two weeks and closed that issue with thirty pages of advertising. We were back in business.

• • •

In 1961 *Newsweek* made an offer for *Industrial Research,* and turning it down was difficult. Although we were losing less with each issue, we were still in the red and desperate for money. Instead I tried, failed, and tried again, eventually building a magazine whose readers looked forward to provocative articles, the two sides of a debate running side by side for a dozen pages. I hung signs around the editors' offices saying, "WE THRIVE ON CONTROVERSY." At that time Soviet-U.S. competition in technology was fierce, and information about their projects was in great demand. This situation spawned an ambitious idea in me. Having written science-fiction stories for *Galaxy* magazine, I had become friends with some of the writers, especially Arthur Clarke and Isaac Asimov. Isaac had been born in Russia, arriving in the United States at age three, so one day I asked him if he spoke Russian, suggesting that we tour the USSR together to do a special edition on Soviet science and technology. Even then Isaac was widely known through his fifty books. (By his death in 1992 he had written more than five hundred.)

"Sure, I know enough Russian to get by, Neil, but how do you plan to get us there?"

"There are ways to pay for—"

"No, I mean *how* will we get there?"

"Why, I fly from Chicago to New York, you fly from Boston to New York, we meet and fly to Moscow, and then—"

"No, I don't fly anywhere!" said Isaac, the prolific inventor of characters who zoom the galaxies. "I am *afraid* to fly."

. . .

Five desperate and dogged years ensued—indelible years of financial hardship and day-and-night work, forcing monthly publication without adequate financing and paying staff members in stock certificates. Like the tides, we fell with each failure and rose with each success. But these were also years of editorial prizes, increased readership, and escalating inquiries to the ads. After five years something strange happened. We actually broke even for an entire year! And afterwards we began making profits in a mirror image of the former losses. We started another magazine, *Oceanology,* and bought *Electro-Technology,* giving us a combined circulation of 300,000. We built an office building in the Beverly Shores sand dunes and became the town's largest employer. It is easy to attract professionals—science writers, commercial artists, bookkeepers, typesetters, space salesmen—when you have money to pay them. They were delighted to move from Chicago or New York to live astride the southern shore of Lake Michigan, where you could walk to work and your kids could grow up in good schools and clean air.

One idea I had to establish *Industrial Research* as a leading magazine was the IR-100, an awards program for the most significant new technical products of the year. Launched in 1966, the annual competition (now the R&D-100) has become the "applied researchers' Nobel Prize," as *The New Yorker* described it after the first event was held at the New York Hilton. Hugh Downs invited me on the *Today* show, and together we demonstrated some of the winning products: a low-light camera for astronauts, a brighter laser, a new oil-prospecting tool, super-soft steel-like copper, metal glue, a three-dimensional holographic camera, and others understandable to a nontechnically oriented audience. As a result of that show, we were asked to hold the annual event at the Museum of Science and Industry in Chicago, where it was held until 2002, when it moved to larger space at Chicago's Navy Pier. One hundred winners, their spouses, their bosses, and well-wishers such as the Illinois governor assemble on an evening in September for the black-tie awards dinner. The one hundred winning products are on display for a month. Wherever you find a high-tech company such as IBM or Hewlett-Packard, chances are you'll see mounted on the lobby walls the signature steel-on-walnut IR-100 plaques. To date, forty years later, some four thousand awards have been made.

. . .

Little by little I turned into a lunar scientist. The space race with the Soviets was on, and I began by explaining the scientific reasons for going to the moon—unlike the press, which fixated on landing Americans there first. I devised ways of using the moon's alien attributes to support a scientific research base. For instance, utilizing the slow-moving line of demarcation between the extremely hot daytime and the ultracold nighttime, I developed a lunar water mill to extract water from hydrous meteorites. Another invention was my "lunar cryostat," further reducing the minus-250-degree temperatures (F) that occur during the fifteen-day lunar night to approach within a few degrees of absolute zero, or minus 459.67 degrees F. You can reach such low temperatures on earth with enormous cooling and pumping efforts, but on the moon, with proper shielding, you could have "free cold." Strange and wonderful things happen at these supercold temperatures: electrons flow forever in a circuit, and frictionless trains could traverse the lunar surface by levitation above superconducting tracks. My efforts won me the first U.S. patent for a device to be used exclusively on the moon.

The magazine attracted an illustrious editorial advisory board, which helped in judging the IR-100 as well as in suggesting articles. Members included Nobel laureates; university presidents; the inventors of radar, the first digital computer, the transistor, stroboscopic photography, the laser, the bathythermograph, and the first commercial electron microscope; and men such as the rocket pioneer Wernher von Braun, the archaeological explorer Thor Heyerdahl, the writer Arthur Clarke, and Bill Lear of corporate jet fame. My son and the magazine, born in the same year, grew up together. David's acquaintance with these famous researchers may have contributed to his becoming a physicist.

. . .

My life's dream had been to set foot on another world, but devising uses for the moon wouldn't land me there, so I did the next best thing. Fourteen years after starting the publishing company, which by now had well over a hundred staff members, I sold all three magazines to Dun and Bradstreet, bought Little Stirrup Cay in the Bahamas, and launched the Island for Science. By writing a monthly column in the magazines I used to publish, I attracted scientists who developed projects in solar desalination of seawater, wave and wind energy, insect biocontrol, and other products of intensive utility to the region.

NASA had offered me a standing invitation to work as a consultant, reporting directly to the administrator. Now, while attracting scientists and developing concepts for the Island for Science, I took them up on it and, along the way, helped several others start the National Space Society. Of course we got Wernher von Braun (who in 1958 had directed the launch of the first U.S. satellite) to become our first president. Started in 1975, the society thrives, with thirty-five thousand members and fifty regional chapters throughout the world. Buzz Aldrin, one of the first two men to walk the moon, is chairman, and Hugh Downs is an active former president. Its mission is to stimulate America to join the adventure and utilize the payback from the exploration of space.

. . .

After six years I left NASA and worked full time developing the island, leading a construction crew and shipping building materials from Florida in our own Korean War landing craft. The one commercial (rather than research) project was a seaweed-shrimp farm off the island's south side, where the water, even at high tide, is no higher than a man's shoulder. We grew seaweed for its valuable gel extracts of carrageenan and agar, used not only in laboratory culture dishes but to thicken, emulsify, or stabilize some ten thousand foods and drugs. I discovered that the red seaweeds grew in a true symbiosis with shrimp. The seaweed photosynthesizes, supplying oxygen to the shrimp, which in turn contribute carbon dioxide and solid wastes as nutrients to the plants.

Of a dozen research projects, one relating to cancer was the mass "bioscreening" of ocean organisms to isolate those worthy of further testing in laboratory mammals. For instance, an organism may have potential as an anticancer drug if, when ground up and placed in an aquarium with a living sea urchin, it literally knocks over the urchin. The urchin was one of several "biofilters." Another was brine shrimp, whose disruption by marine flora or fauna usually indicated that the disrupter would be useful as an insecticide. Some 80 percent of earth's animals—a half-million species or more—live in the water, yet hundreds of thousands of them are unknown. The 1 percent that have been examined for pharmacologic activity contain biotoxins, enzymes, steroids, amino acids, anti-angiogenics, and other useful stuff. Another project was the collection of the Bahamian sea rod, from which hormonelike substances called "prostaglandins" were produced initially. Little did I know then that prostaglandins would play a key role in my cure of lymphoma.

The Island for Science continued on its path toward developing a wide variety of new methods in seafarming and energy that could improve life for Bahamians—until the Bahamian government stopped us. One more failure first. It turned out, according to the U.S. Department of State, that the prime minister himself had been taking commissions on the shipment of illegal drugs in return for free passage through his waters to the Florida coast. The government shut us down, finding our presence disruptive to its clandestine activities. By the time the U.S. Coast Guard built its case, it was too late for the Island for Science.

But changing course is not the same as defeat. It took years, but I found a highly profitable business for the island that the Bahamian government (which derives almost all its taxes from tourism) could not refuse. I contracted with a cruise-ship company, Royal Caribbean Cruise Lines, to add the island to the itinerary of several of its ships that already cruised the Bahamas, and I rebuilt the buildings into facilities for passengers. Now called CocoCay (still Little Stirrup Cay on navigation charts), it is a popular daytime port of call.

The Island for Science, like *Industrial Research* before it, made some important innovations, not the least of which was fostering interdisciplinary research. In project after project on the island we succeeded unexpectedly when scientists from the highly diverse fields of marine biology, wind energy, electronics, aerodynamics, and other disciplines brought their distinctive viewpoints to bear on the other guy's puzzle—a method largely missing in cancer research.

5

Our War Within

RESEARCH IN THE WAR AGAINST CANCER IS ANYTHING BUT INTER-disciplinary. The closest you come to such cross-fertilization is in laboratories where molecular biologists and immunologists work side by side with pathologists and hematologists, and less often with oncologists who see patients. You might think that, in a pursuit so important, clinicians dealing with cancer patients every day would be more involved in discovery. I would go way beyond that. Particle physicists, astronomers, cosmologists, and mathematicians, who regularly construct unusual hypotheses and many of whom would be willing to study cancer biology, could offer insights from vastly different perspectives. Certainly software designers. Physiologists. Chemists. Maybe even a few science writers steeped in scores of disciplines who know how to ask provocative questions. (If nothing else, writers could help get out proposals for the principal investigators, leaving them more time for research.)

Instead, because of the complexity of the human animal, the disciplines of cancer science grow narrower, more specialized, *less* interdisciplinary. Molecular biologists—despite the fact that physicists originally created their field—are bogged down with others of their own kind, buried under immense amounts of data. Biology is mostly a descriptive science, separating out the smallest details. Theoretical physics is theory-driven, synthesizing facts. Physical scientists are accustomed to reducing complex systems to basics. That's what they do. Their presence on interdisciplinary cancer teams might help to make sense of it all.

When I began my quest, curing cancer as such was the furthest thing from my mind. I needed to cure my cancer. Finding experimental therapies was not simply a matter of finding the right doctor, as when you might need to have your gall bladder removed. "Surgeons like you who excise gall bladders know *exactly* what they are doing," I said one day to Rade Pejic, who had seen so many gall bladders in his life that he could detach them blindfolded. "But cancer doctors, for the most part, do not know, and they don't tell you that they don't know!"

Rade looked at me sagely, shaking his head horizontally, which emphasized the contrast between his jet-black hair and pale face; his job left him no time to spend outdoors. "I find it strange, too," he said. "You would think that practitioners of cancer medicine would be at the forefront of research, discussing with you—and me—the new therapies that they have looked into personally."

"The arrogance of so many chemotherapists is exceeded only by their inability to cure cancer," I said. We let it lie there between us like a boulder on the long road ahead.

Before I understood the difference between an oncologist acquainted with science and a chemotherapist mired in toxins, I followed up in Chicago on referrals to several cancer doctors who regarded me and their other patients as though we possessed the intelligence and follower instincts of sheep. You don't just pick up the phone and make an appointment with these guys. You go through questioning by their nurses about the urgency of your case and send ahead the usual stuff—slides, tissue blocks, CAT scans, pathology reports, and opinions. Then you wait to be fitted into their schedule. One especially hard-to-get appointment was with a prominent lymphoma specialist, Dr. C, whom I had heard on a teleconference describing newly approved monoclonal antibodies.

. . .

The day of my appointment in late November of that first year of my lymphoma, 1998, was sweet with promise, the evergreens not yet blanketed in snow, the lake not yet churned into the full froth and ice of a Chicago winter. Carol and I arrived at the appointed time to see Dr. C at a prominent university hospital. We didn't mind the two-hour wait in his reception room because our son, who had driven up from Urbana, met us there.

David has the same football-player physique as I have, although his 180-pound frame positions him more as a quarterback, while my 200 pounds would make me a halfback. With light once-blond hair and Carol's blue eyes and high cheekbones, he is handsome in a rugged sort of way. David is both a physicist studying the plasmas used in semiconductors and fusion reactors and a professor of nuclear engineering. He had been voted the best teacher in his college several years running. We spent our waiting time talking, not about his children or about the absorption of nuclei in a thermonuclear reactor, as once we did, but about the new mission that had intruded into our lives. We now knew what therapy I did *not* want, and we talked about alternatives to chemo, comparing notes on what each of us had learned about monoclonal antibodies, or Mabs.

To understand Mabs requires some understanding of the human immune system. "There are some ten thousand trillion immune cells within our bodies, primarily B and T cells—which make up 20 to 50 percent of the total leukocytes at any one time," I said, reviewing what I had learned, making sure we were all on the same page.

"Leukocytes. Those are the white blood cells, right?" Carol asked.

"Yes, they're derived from stem cells, which are born in the marrow and encased there, inside our bones, for protection."

"I always think of B cells," David said, "as deriving their education, or maturing from stem cells, in the bone, even though they were named after first being discovered in the bursas of chickens—the padlike sacs in the vicinity of bone joints—the place where you get bursitis. Chickens have them too.

"The T cells," David continued, "those are the ones that have gone to college in the thymus, migrating from the bone marrow to that little gland located just above the heart."

"The significant part for my lymphoma," I said, "is to find a way to help the antigens on the surfaces of my cancer cells stimulate B-cell antibodies to attack and kill them." The reason it was so important was that we were seeking a manmade antibody, billions of clones of the right one, to wipe out the cancer cells selectively instead of the carpet bombing of chemotherapy. *Antigens* is a collective term for the molecular signatures of various pathogens that constantly invade us. Our immune system has evolved to become highly decentralized such that each specific antibody actually fits into a specific antigen, like a key fits a lock. Because the antibody fits the antigen, the part of the antigen cell's surface that receives it is called the *receptor*. Further, because certain cell-surface indicators flag the antibodies, this portion of the antigen is referred to as a *marker*. Antigens, receptors, markers— parts of the same cell.

Though we don't normally think about it, there is high drama inside us. The human body vigorously wages an endless war within, and battles are fought every second of our lives. Natural antibodies are the foot soldiers, our first-line of defense against infection. Incredible as it sounds, instead of detonating a general-purpose bomb against cells plagued by viruses, bacteria, fungi, worms, or protozoa, the immune system actually makes special soldier-antibodies to fight every single invader! Constant recruitment by our internal defense department produces ten million new lymphocytes in the white cells every day.

The war analogy is even more striking when comparing cancer to terrorism. Beyond the obvious parallels of mobilization and surgical strikes, there is a misdirected, sluggish defense at first, until something really big comes along, like cancer—or the World Trade Center attack. Terrorists change their form, mutating into something harder to kill, in both warfare and cancer-fare, metastasizing to remote areas to strike again in different places. Both terrorism and cancer can be fought by saturation bombing, the first with aircraft, the second by chemotherapy, but innocent civilians and normal cells die as collateral damage. ("Smart bombs," too, have their cancer-warfare counterparts in manmade antibodies carrying radiation at the cellular level.)

Combination warfare works better against both, such as precision targeting while at the same time cutting off the supply of funds to terrorists.

Or using Mabs while simultaneously cutting off the tumors' blood supply. Good intelligence continues the analogy. Just as governmental agencies track which terrorists have gone where, our sophisticated B and T cells possess memories. Their molecules remember the bad guys that enter our system, so that when an internal terrorist invades a second time, specific antibodies clone themselves into additional millions, which then spread out to search for and destroy the enemy in all the cells it inhabits.

Sometimes antibodies becomes confused and attack normal cells, causing autoimmune diseases such as rheumatoid or even osteoarthritis. I wondered, somewhat casually, whether there could be a link between arthritis and lymphoma. It was a random idea born of nothing except the fact that I seemed to have contracted them both at about the same time. But as I read more and more of the literature of science, I began to see that there are indeed links between the two. I read about a Swedish study indicating that high inflammatory activity increases the risk for lymphoma.

The process goes like this: as the immune system constantly reinvents itself, producing at least a billion new white blood cells every day, it responds to inflammations just as it responds to any invader, such as viruses or bacteria. When these white cells are made, random genetic shuffling causes the antibodies to be put together in subtly different ways. The result is a diverse collection of cells, each of which is specific to a certain antigen. If a receptor binds to the body's own antigens, the triggering of an autoimmune attack is forestalled. But when that fails to happen, you feel it in your joints. Arthritis.

The white cells unused in attacking an antigen die after a few days. The others, those that do the fighting, are still alive and produce antibodies. Don't forget, these cells remember! Having learned to recognize a particular antigen, they retain this knowledge and become "memory cells," surviving for a long time to attack identical "terrorist" cells, or pathogens, that invade even years later. Immunological memory. It is how vaccines work.

The whole progression of inflammation—including arthritis—also subjects the cells to greater random genetic shuffling simply because they are alive so much longer.

So, I thought, since there is some arthritis-lymphoma connection, wouldn't it make sense to lower the inflammations causing the arthritis? The Cox-2 blocker is benign. Why not take it? I had arthritis anyway! So I asked Rade for a prescription and began taking the standard dose of Celebrex for osteoarthritis—200 milligrams.

Over time it altered more than mere arthritis. Its effect was far greater than I could have hoped for as those dark days as 1998 drew to a close.

· · ·

Theory is fine, but what the oncologists—and I—believed necessary at that time was therapy. My gradual divergence from these doctors was not over whether therapy was required; rather, it was over, first, when to stop watching and waiting and, second, what *kind* of therapy. The chemotherapists favored saturation bombing, "the more aggressive, the better," according to Drs. A and B, totally ignoring my patient's preference for the precision strikes of manmade antibodies designed to attack my B-cell lymphoma.

Just as B cells produce antibodies, laboratories can make them by replicating, or cloning, a specific single antibody that appears in the human bloodstream about three days after the first encounter with a specific antigen. These clones of a single antibody—the "monoclonal" antibodies, or Mabs, we were trying to understand—were made originally in 1975 by British scientists in a series of experiments remarkable for the time. First they injected a mouse with human tumor antigens, which produced an immune response consisting of many different types of B-cell antibodies. Second, they selected from those "poly" antibodies found in the mouse's spleen a single, or "mono," B cell that would latch onto and attack a specific antigen they had chosen to target—by attaching, say, to the primary marker for MCL. Third, after irradiating an identical twin of the first mouse to shut down its own immune system, they transferred the B cell into this second mouse. In the absence of immune fighter cells, the injected B cells grew like a tumor and were not rejected. The B cells growing in the second mouse were all of one kind, hence "monoclonal." Voila! Human monoclonal antibodies had been produced in mice.

Researchers throughout the world, especially in the United States, joined the chase and have been making and testing various humanized Mabs since then, resulting in scores of monoclonal antibodies that can be designed to fight *any* antigen, including those presented by *any* cancer. It has been a remarkable quarter-century of antibody experimentation. Yet during those years millions of cancer patients suffered patiently and died, perhaps not so patiently, without benefit of the new biotechnologies. You could argue that the technology was not ready yet, and of course it wasn't proved beyond doubt. Still, couldn't patients at least have been offered a choice between chemo/radiation and the promising experimental therapies?

I thought about what I'd learned and felt that pursuing this latest avenue of knowledge would be fascinating, if only I didn't have to write it in the first person. I passed the days less nervously by focusing my mind intensively on cancer vaccines and how some genes mutate and replicate cells that can't die. Antibodies belong to a protein group called gamma globulins, and "GG," as the doctors refer to it, has been used for years to boost the immune system. Rade Pejic tried to get some GG for me but was told that the supply was limited because of the tremendous demand by AIDS patients. Mabs were coming into use to supplement those made in the body, but at this time the only one oncologists were using was Rituxan, and then only for certain patients with low-grade lymphomas—emphatically not for those with mantle-cell lymphoma.

Earlier in the year the FDA had approved Rituxan for lymphoma and trastuzumab (Herceptin) for breast cancer. These and other Mabs are defined by which antigens, or cell-surface markers, they search for and destroy, the designations termed "CD3," "CD25," or other CDs. The letters stand for "cluster of differentiation," and each numbered CD designates a specific marker on the surface of a diseased—or normal—cell. It is as though such cell markers stick up a white flag and announce to the Mab, or soldier antibody, "I surrender; here I am!" There are many CD markers, and new Mabs to attach to and kill them are devised at least annually. The CD20 marker, for instance, is a terrific target for a manmade Mab because it's "expressed," or turned on, more frequently on cancerous B cells and thus is prevalent in

B-cell lymphomas such as mine, as well as in many kinds of leukemia. Rituxan is an anti-CD20 antibody.

At the standard doses given at the time, Rituxan was widely regarded as being useless for MCL. The chemotherapy combination CHOP was the preferred treatment, with Rituxan added simply to enhance it.

Radioactive Mabs, such as Zevalin and Bexxar, also home in on the CD20 surface marker, much like heat-seeking missiles carrying deadly armaments. After they hunt out the cells expressing CD20, the same way "naked" (non-radioactive active) Mabs do, they also deliver lethal radiation both to the cells so marked and to the surrounding cells. Yet Bexxar, which has been in trials for a decade, was not FDA approved until 2003. At the time of my initial inquiry—and until 2001, when Zevalin finally was approved—you could get a radioactive active Mab only in clinical trials and only under specified conditions, such as having "twice failed" chemo. That dubious standard is still applied for new Mabs coming on stream.

• • •

"I certainly am over-expressing CD20," I said to Carol and David, looking at my path report. "The trouble is, you can't seem to get anyone to give you a Mab alone, even just Rituxan, without taking chemo at the same time."

"They want their chemo 'gold standard' in there," David said. "Don't they realize that just because something is standard practice doesn't mean it's the best option?"

I thought about standard practice for a few seconds, realizing that David's comment was rooted in physical science. Square-rigged sailing ships, hydrogen-filled dirigibles, and direct-current power transmission came to mind. They were considered standards in their time, slow to change. But with so many lives at stake, shouldn't modern health science be different?

"It's more than just standard practice," I said. "It's a standard of beliefs. The Chemo Culture."

Carol shuffled some papers on her lap, half-glasses perched on her small elegant nose. "But when they *have* used Rituxan alone, it's worked in a lot of cases, although I haven't seen any trials specifically for MCL."

Rituxan had been shown to produce response rates of about 50 percent in patients who are refractory. "Refractory patients"—unlike refractory furnace bricks, which resist damage from heat—are not those who have resisted chemo unscathed. Rather, they are the overwhelming majority of patients whose chemotherapies have not prevented their tumors from recurring. Yet in a few isolated clinical trials that used Rituxan alone as a first-line agent against indolent lymphomas, its efficacy rose to 70 percent. Unfortunately for me, these encouraging percentages were shown in trials not to extend to MCL—the numbers weren't even in the same ballpark. What they failed to test at that time, however, were dramatically increased dosages of Rituxan.

"But why not at least *try* Rituxan alone?" Carol asked hopefully. "If it can't do damage and *might* work on you because your MCL is indolent, what's the harm in trying? Maybe Dr. C will give it to you without chemo, at least to see if it can shrink the tumors."

Carol thinks in practical terms, with no pretension. Once I bought for her use our first (and last) luxury car, which she found not useful in her extensive gardening chores, so we gave it to David and bought a pickup truck.

"The problem seems to be more regulatory than scientific," I said. "Taking Rituxan probably would preclude my getting into a trial for something possibly more effective, like Bexxar or Zevalin." Those were important considerations in 1998. Even today myriad FDA rules make patients and oncologists wary of otherwise excellent biotargeted first treatments for fear they will preclude scientifically sound second steps.

The radioactive Mabs sounded to us like a more-intelligent second choice—after first-choice Rituxan—than chemotherapy. For both therapies the target is the same, a specific antigen, but the firepower is greater with radioactivity. While nowhere close to the indiscriminate saturation bombing of chemotherapy, the radiation carried by radio-Mabs kills cancerous and precancerous cells. Some normal cells surrounding the main tumors are irradiated and destroyed to a diameter of some thirty cells. While that might sound like a lot, a cell measures less than a micron, or a thousandth of a millimeter, far too small to be seen without a microscope. Unfortunately, stray gamma rays, such as those conjugated into some radioactive Mabs, can destroy distant normal cells too. Still, using a Mab to wipe out cells that may or may not be diseased is still fairly conservative therapy—not as bad as zapping billions of both diseased and normal cells with chemo that destroys every dividing cell in your body.

For information on Mabs (or any drug) we found we could bypass a lot of misinformation by going directly to a scientific institution's or company's Web site. The anti-CD20 monoclonal antibody Rituxan was developed jointly by IDEC Pharmaceuticals and Genentech. Their radioactive active version, Zevalin, is essentially Rituxan attached to the radioactive isotope yttrium-90. "Hot Rituxan."

Bexxar is another radioactive anti-CD20 antibody, but it is conjugated (or "labeled") with a different radioactive isotope: iodine-131, which seemed to me to be unnecessarily powerful, since it emits powerful gamma rays as well as the more-harmless electrons, or beta rays. Developed by a company now merged into Corixa, it went through clinical trials in more than a thousand lymphoma patients at eighty centers seeking FDA approval. A third radioactive Mab for lymphoma, called Oncolym by its developer, Peregrine Pharmaceutical, uses iodine-131, as does Bexxar, but attaches to a completely different cell-surface marker. I thought Oncolym would constitute a good choice if Rituxan didn't do the job, because it would be attacking vastly different portions of the cancer cells. Zapping the same CD20 cells with Bexxar or Zevalin seemed like unnecessary and possibly dangerous overkill.

"David," I asked, suffering from random thoughts, "what are the half-lives of I-131 and Y-90?" This was the kind of family conversation we were having these days, nothing about Ryan and Brandon. Grandchildren can be enjoyed only by the living.

"Thought you'd get around to that, Dad, so I looked them up last night. Yttrium-90 is only about two and a half days. Iodine-131, eight days. But I don't think their half-lives are as important as the fact that, while they're both beta emitters, I-131 also emits gamma rays."

I had been talking routinely to investigators working on these drugs, learning from them the names and references of scientific papers or trials that indicated efficacy. For instance, a clinical trial in 1998 at Sloan-Kettering

showed that, whereas only 28 percent of lymphoma patients had responded
to their most recent chemo, 65 percent responded to Bexxar, and their response was substantially longer.

"I've been exchanging e-mail with a lot of MCL patients who were in
some of these trials," Carol said. "Of course, they've all had chemo. They
say that Zevalin and Bexxar are a breeze to take compared to the poisons of
chemotherapy . . ."

The conversation trailed off as we looked up to the arrival of a stone-faced
woman in white. She ushered us into the doctor's presence.

Dr. C's office wasn't oval but stretched presidentially into the horizon at
the far end of the room. Thick carpet. Big desk. Wall papered with diplomas. Tall, spectacled, hurried, Dr. C seemed to speak not to any one of us
but *through* us, perhaps to some unseen nemesis hiding in back. His features
were sharp, his manner a parody of a caring doctor resolutely leading his
patients into a hopeful future while maintaining professional detachment.

"So you have mantle-cell lymphoma," he said. Not a question. A question has too many possible answers.

"Apparently. But the tests at M. D. Anderson haven't—"

"Chromosomal translocation tests?"

"Yes. The pathologist there says I may not be expressing cyclin D1 because—"

"Doesn't matter. You've got to get into therapy. Don't wait too long."

"What kind of therapy?

"Chemo. CHOP is as good as the rest of them."

"How about monoclonal antibodies?"

"We'll give you that, too."

"Why not Mabs first *instead of* chemo?" I was thinking of the radioactive Mabs.

"No, they don't do enough alone."

He was so refractory to argument, so relentless in his pessimism, I found
it hard to believe he was the same guy I'd heard on a telephone conference
pontificating about the benefits of radioactive monoclonal antibodies. I
didn't know how to avoid antagonizing him and manage to get any of these

antibodies without chemo, even Rituxan. I was reminded of once having quarreled with the prime minister of the Bahamas with disastrous results. So I asked the usual, "How much time before I need to start therapy?"

"For MCL? *Not more than three months.*"

Is this some stock reply learned in chemotherapy school? At least I was gaining time, I thought wryly, for a full month had passed since Dr. A first gave me "three months." But in truth he had shattered my fragile hope. I expected more from someone as prominent and erudite as Dr. C.

• • •

After saying goodbye to David, who returned to Urbana, we drove to our next appointment in cocooned silence, the windshield wiper beating time like a metronome. Suddenly I asked Carol, "I wonder if he meant *just* Rituxan when he agreed to give me a Mab?"

Abruptly I swerved the car through sclerotic traffic, did a U-turn, and drove back to the university building. I encountered the busy doctor striding down the hallway toward me. He stopped short, bridling at my unexpected reappearance.

"Dr. C, please, one quick question. When you said you would give me a monoclonal antibody, did you mean only Rituxan—or one of the radioactive antibodies?"

"Rituxan, of course. I can't give you unapproved drugs!"

"How about clinical trials?"

His eyes were gray and as hard as ball bearings, and he tightened them into a squint, taking me apart like a specimen, section by section. "Look, Mr. . . ."

"Ruzic. Rhymes with 'music.'"

"Look, you've got your program. *Now stick to it!*" With that he marched brusquely away as though suffering from something. You didn't have to be a physician to diagnose his disease. It was CGS: Chronic God Syndrome.

A Half-Billion for Proof

AFTER SEEING DR. C, WE DROVE FROM THE NEAR NORTH SIDE TO THE near South Side and arrived at the Chicago campus of the University of Illinois as snow began falling softly, like rice. We had come here to meet Michael Blend, whom I had called for an appointment after hearing him talk about radioactive monoclonal antibodies on Chicago television. He had answered the phone himself. The contrast between these two men of medicine could not have been stronger.

In his office, perched on the edge of a desk overflowing with reports and books, Dr. Blend leaned forward and told us he was conducting trials on two radioactive monoclonal antibodies. Both a physician and a Ph.D. radiation biologist, Mike Blend is the director of nuclear medicine at the university. An unassuming man in his fifties. Six foot, with big shoulders, flat gut. Graying hair. Studious, glasses, yet vigorous, muscular. The opposite of pretentious, working in shirtsleeves. I liked him instantly.

I told him we had come here from seeing Dr. C.

"Dr. C. likes to give CHOP."

"I had hoped for more. He has such a good reputation." I started thinking of him as Dr. CHOP.

"He does. You can't blame Dr. C entirely for not wanting to stick his neck out. The main problem is the Food and Drug Administration. When Kessler was commissioner, he did a lot to bring the FDA out of the dark ages. He cut the time in half that it takes for new drugs to be approved, but it's still too long."

He was referring to David Kessler, the doctor, lawyer, and chief of the FDA (now dean of the Yale School of Medicine). For eight years he had fought the tobacco industry before resigning in disgust—not over lack of progress against tobacco but over the political forces that made his own bureaucracy so cumbersome. I had followed the tobacco fight from a position of virtue, having quit smoking when the health warnings first came out in force.

"The first surgeon general warning was in 1964," Mike Blend said, pushing thin glasses back up his nose. "Since then, twelve million Americans have died from smoking." He winced as though he'd known them personally. This was clearly a subject of interest to a cancer researcher.

"Why is the FDA so stuck on chemo?" I asked.

"The short answer is that they inherited it as the standard," he said.

"Sure, but now that we have targeted biological therapies, why does it take so long to approve them? I know they're worried about safety, but compared to chemo . . ."

"People think the FDA is here to protect them from ruthless pharmaceutical companies that otherwise would sell them unsafe drugs. Sure, you hear about drugs being pulled off the market every so often, but those cases are one in a thousand, if that. Proving safety is relatively easy, in quick phase-one studies. Phase-two trials are performed to prove the drug is efficacious, that it really works. They cost more than phase one, but universities can still do them because we use small numbers of patient volunteers who have no other hope. I'd like to see a lot more cancer patients enroll in clinical trials."

He stood up from his desk and glanced out the window. The snow had grown deeper, grayer.

"I suppose more people don't enter trials," Carol said, "because they're afraid of getting a placebo."

"You're right that some of them believe that. The main reason, though, is that patients are unaware of the clinical trials going on for their specific cancers. Getting a placebo in a cancer trial these days is an unfounded fear."

Placebo, I remembered, comes from Latin meaning "I will please," but it hardly is pleasing to patients worried that, while they might not get a placebo, they might land in a control group receiving something other than the drug being tested. Sometimes, as Mike said, the worry is unfounded. You have to know you want the therapy you request. In an extreme example, gunshot wounds in the sixteenth century routinely were treated with boiling oil until an army surgeon ran out of oil and used an ointment of egg yokes, oil of roses, and turpentine, which kept far more patients alive. Curtis Meinert, a professor at the Johns Hopkins center for clinical trials, who told that story, asks: "Who were the guinea pigs in the experiment? Those who got boiling oil or those who got the ointment?"

"And it's not ethical to administer a placebo to someone dying of cancer," Mike was saying, "although I admit that in phase-three trials they sometimes give *standard of care* therapies to control groups. That's not as bad as it sounds because sometimes the control-group therapy turns out to be better than the new therapy being tried."

"Then how do you control the experiment?" I asked.

"We compare results of new drugs with past records of patients who received other therapy or had none at all."

I was happy to hear that we have advanced since the sixteenth century.

"It's phase-three trials that take the real money," Mike said. "These are big, randomized studies representative of thousands of patients with a given disease, and they're held at dozens of cancer centers at the same time. The pharmaceutical companies spend enormous effort and money proving their drug isn't merely safe and efficacious, but that it is *better than the standard.*"

"In other words, better than chemo."

"Right, that's the accepted standard for cancer."

I fell silent.

"What's wrong?" Mike asked.

Every time I hear about having to take chemo in order to get this or that new therapy, I suppose my body language turns combative. Carol looked at me knowingly. She knew exactly what was wrong. "Maybe I'm just looking for something to hate," I said. For the thousandth time I wondered how so many cancer doctors could be wrong, using chemo to the exclusion of new-generation therapies, rarely enrolling their customers in free trials.

"You have good reason to fear chemotherapy," he said simply. "Especially for MCL."

"This business of comparing a radiolabeled Mab or a vaccine with the standard," I said. (*Radiolabeled* means coupled to the antibody, a term slightly more precise than *radioactive*.) "It seems to me that it's a question of time. I mean, chemo always works to shrink tumors, right? But then you become refractory, and it's less and less effective. Some lymphoma patients, even some with MCL, do well on chemo for a long time, maybe five years or more. Do you have to wait five years to make the comparison?"

"I'm afraid so."

The dying horse of chemo was dead, at least for me, and there was no point in kicking it any more. I asked Mike about the last in the series of clinical trials, phase four.

"Those trials are even bigger—extending a new drug sometimes to hundreds of thousands of people—but they're completely different from the first three. They come *after* a drug is marketed. The companies pay fees to oncologists to track whether their patients on the drug are reacting better or worse than noted in the first phases. Patients don't exactly *enter* a phase-four trial; they don't even know they're included. Phase-four trials blend into the selling effort because when a pharmaceutical company invites a doctor or pays him to report on a drug, that usually induces him to try it on his patients for the first time."

New drugs usually go through at least the first three phases prior to approval. It wasn't until May 2001 that the FDA showed it can respond fast when presented with overwhelming evidence of a cure, such as happened with Gleevec after a clinical trial actually cured almost everybody in enrolled in it—an unusual occurrence for a phase-one trial. The press heralded Gleevec as the first of a new generation of "smart drugs"—those that target and change an intracellular signaling molecule and in the process wipe out the cancer cells. What the media failed to state was that Gleevec's phase-one trial was to be the beginning of a second round of larger trials. Gleevec had been in human trials for three years.

"Mike, you hear people say it's the drug companies that resist change because they're getting rich on selling the chemo chemicals. I've been an investor in pharmaceuticals and other industries for years. The profits of Merck or Lilly aren't out of line with, say, those of GE or Intel. With all the money they spend on research for better drugs, why on earth would pharmaceutical companies want to sell relatively inexpensive chemo toxins?"

"They don't," he said. "Think of the money a company could make if it developed a drug that would *cure* any kind of cancer!"

He's right. Companies don't work for the overall good of their competitors. They're all trying for the blockbuster, spending billions, racing to all kinds of cures.

"The blame for continuing chemo belongs to the chemotherapists who are slow to change. The way it is now, the drug business is a hell of a financial risk. Only one in every five thousand drugs tested is eventually approved by the FDA. And only three out of ten that are approved ever make a profit."

"I've read that it costs as much as $500 million and takes ten years to bring out a major new drug," I said.

Mike nodded. Right ballpark.

In effect, I thought, it means that the FDA says to the drug companies: Pay out a half-billion dollars developing and testing a new drug for ten years, and we'll think about approving it. No wonder consumers find drugs so expensive. Such statistics had reached my consciousness before, but barely, like the background noise of a distant waterfall suddenly noticed, and it was strange now to be personally involved.

"It's not confirmed yet, but if I find my lymphoma is truly mantle-cell, which would be likely to work better, Zevalin or Bexxar?"

"We're getting good results with both for many subsets of lymphoma . . ." He paused, standing up, flexing his leg muscles, clearly reluctant to continue. "But not with MCL," he said, and hurried to answer my question so that the disappointing news would not linger. "The higher energy and shorter half-life of the yttrium isotope in Zevalin would seem to be superior, but not necessarily. It depends on your tumors—maybe you want less energy over a longer period of time, as with Bexxar. On the other hand, if yours turns out to be a typical mantle-cell lymphoma, that is, if it starts getting really aggressive, we may *want* the higher energy of Zevalin. In most protocols—not MCL, I'm sorry to say—we see an 80 percent complete response rate compared to about 50 percent for Rituxan." He stopped for a moment to rub his eyes behind his glasses and run a hand through his thinning hair. Mike Blend didn't look tired, but I could tell he worked long hours.

"Complete response? For how long?" I said.

"After three years more than half the patients are still in remission."

That beat the hell out of chemo's eighteen or thirty-six months to sudden death. In 2001 Thomas Witzig of the Mayo Clinic completed a clinical trial comparing Zevalin plus Rituxan to Rituxan alone in patients with low-grade but refractory lymphomas. The randomized, controlled study showed an 80 percent response rate, nearly twice the 44 percent for Rituxan alone— almost exactly matching Mike Blend's results of three years earlier. But, I reminded myself, those studies were for low-grade lymphomas, not for mantle-cell lymphoma.

"How about Oncolym?" I asked about the radioactive Mab that uniquely targets a vastly different series of cell-surface markers—the HLA-DRs.

"We don't have much data on it yet. I'm trying to get a clinical trial going here."

"Do you think Neil ought to try it?" Carol asked, emphasizing what *should* be done, not whether I could bypass the labyrinth of FDA regulations to get the drug.

"Not yet. Watch and wait."

"If I start developing symptoms again, can I get into any protocol for radioactive Mabs?" I said.

"Maybe by the time you need one, the FDA rules will change. Unfortunately, right now for any of these radio-Mabs, you must have twice failed chemo."

A patient must have twice failed chemo. This wasn't Mike's phraseology; it pervaded the scientific literature, the FDA's quaint way of putting it. A lesser love affair with chemo and the FDA at least would have reversed its decree as *chemotherapy must have twice-failed the patient.* Both Bexxar and Zevalin had been available through clinical trials for years. Yet only a tiny percentage of lymphoma patients had been enrolled in the protocols that their oncologists *could have told them about.* It would take another three years before Zevalin beat Bexxar as the first FDA-approved radioactive antibody against cancer. I began to see the FDA as a bureaucracy first and an agency protecting people against bad food and bad drugs second. Bureaucracies concentrate on self-perpetuation and self-protection, their officials overly concerned with covering their asses.

"It takes the FDA a long time to approve these drugs in particular," Mike said, seeming to read my thoughts, "not only because of inherent bureaucratic make-work but because the public is worried about anything radioactive." He was right. Fear of radiation, so pervasive in this country, had stopped safe nuclear-power reactors from being built over the past twenty years, camouflaging the real hazards, the coal-fired plants that assist genes in mutating to cause lymphoma, lung cancer, and emphysema.

Mike Blend described a typical scenario: an FDA statistician asks Corixa to run more analyses on the clinical data on Bexxar already reviewed. The company scientists then drop everything and spend a month doing the analyses. Then the FDA takes three more months to examine the results. At that point some official invariably requests a review of other data, sometimes for no reason other than an "academic interest" unconnected to the hypothesis being tested . . . , and so it goes. Finally, following years of this interplay after the clinical trials are completed, the drugs are approved. It would be great if you could just go to an oncologist and he or she would determine which of the several existing radioactive antibodies would benefit your particular subset of lymphoma. The way it works now, you don't *know* which of these drugs are suitable, and you have to fight your way into clinical trials to find out.

• • •

Mike Blend led us past RADIATION DANGER signs to his radiological and animal labs. A technician was feeding caged guinea pigs and white rats, and they began leaving their exercise treadmills for dinner.

"People think they're going to be guinea pigs, that clinical trials are risky,"

Mike said as he watched the animals. "But human trials start only after vigorous testing in animals. Only one out of a thousand compounds tested in animals is ever approved for phase-one testing. If there's any toxicity, it will show up before human trials."

Any fatigue I had been feeling stopped at my muscles. My mind was spinning with possibilities for my entry into clinical trials. "I think of it as a way to jump into the future," I said, "like having your own time machine."

Mike smiled. "It is. Clinical trials are just about your only chance to get a therapy years before it hits the market. Keep in mind, even after the trial is over, the patient can still get the drug. And you can always quit midstream if there's something you don't like."

"How about already approved drugs for something that might work on all or most cancers, something I could try for MCL?" I said, looking for a shortcut.

"They are starting to give *high-dose* Rituxan experimentally," Mike said encouragingly. He was full of information. "Higher doses of Rituxan have been infused in patients up to six times the usual quantity with far greater results. High doses of Rituxan are being clinically tested at M. D. Anderson and elsewhere and found to be safe. They produced no cumulative toxicity and were effective against more than just low-grade lymphomas."

I followed Carol's glance out the window. It had stopped snowing. A single beam of light from a hidden setting sun fell across the white-clad campus like a blessing. Life seemed more hopeful now that I had met Michael Blend.

We talked for hours, Mike doing his best to answer my barrage of questions, taking the time necessary to explore the cancer scene in detail and referring us to new scientific papers. By the time we finished, it was dark. We thanked him and left, trudging through the snow toward our car. I could picture Mike working all night.

• • •

Clinical trials weren't always as receptive and patient-oriented as they are today. In the old days it was accepted practice to keep patients in the dark. In

1789 Edward Jenner injected children with pus from a milkmaid's cowpox pustule, hoping they wouldn't get the much worse disease of smallpox. It worked to prevent smallpox. Jenner had developed the first vaccine! Louis Pasteur was the first to consider ethics in his experiments. In 1884 he came up with an antidote for rabies, testing various combinations on animals for years to make it safer. Only when a woman begged him to try it on her infected, dying son did he agree to treat the boy—doing so successfully. For forty years starting in 1930, researchers in a now infamous clinical trial in Tuskegee, Alabama, withheld treatment from a control group of syphilitic black men, without their knowledge, to see how the disease would progress. As late as the 1960s doctors fed live hepatitis viruses to mentally retarded patients.

The turning point came in 1973 when Congress passed a law charging the FDA to protect human subjects. Ever since, the government has taken from researchers the role of policing new therapies, demanding a host of good practices, such as informed consent of patients, assessment of risks, and fair selection of those who agree to clinical trials. Like many other social forces in American life, the pendulum swings—from no regulation, to welcomed regulation, to overregulation.

Looking into clinical trials and the reasoning behind them consumed our days, and I read doggedly into each night. Carol would find the Blend references and other scientific papers I'd asked for, often by enlisting David to hunt articles at the University of Illinois library or by working the phones like a reporter at deadline. Carol, who would be happier digging in the dirt planting her gardens surrounding our house, had learned to use a computer, but you couldn't get scientific papers that way then, although clinical trials were easily accessible on-line.

Several trials on anti-angiogenesis (literally, "against blood-vessel formation") were getting started. Dr. Judah Folkman, a surgeon-turned-scientist at Children's Hospital at Harvard, had been working since age twenty-eight—in 1961—on his theory of starving cancerous tumors by cutting off their blood supply. In the beginning his ideas were thought to be preposterous, not only because he was a "mere" surgeon doing scientific research, but because at the time little was known about how cancer spreads. For most of the following forty-some years Folkman and colleagues have been experimenting relentlessly to isolate naturally occurring substances in the body that he called "angiostatin" and "endostatin." The word ending -*statin* (from the Latin "to stand still," as in *status*) generally is applied to chemical structures that stop specific enzymes or protein activities (such as lovastatin or pravastatin, used to inhibit cholesterol enzymes). Similarly, Folkman's anti-angiogenic statins disrupt the enzymatic activity associated with vascular growth. Remove the statins, and the microvessels feeding the tumors start growing again. While Folkman's research proved that other agents—such as chemotherapeutic drugs taken in small but frequent doses—could achieve the same goal, he concentrated on the naturally occurring angio- and endostatins because he felt they were less likely to harm the immune system when used over many years.

Folkman also called attention to epidemiological studies demonstrating that ordinary NSAIDs—the nonsteroidal anti-inflammatory drugs, such as aspirin or ibuprofen—reduce the risk of a wide range of cancers. NSAIDs mainly inhibit cyclooxygenase-1 (the Cox-1 enzyme) but also somewhat block formation of Cox-2. In the process, Cox-2 inhibitors reduce inflammation with less risk of creating peptic or other ulcers in the stomach. The Cox-2 enzyme is found in all white blood cells—neutrophils, macrophages, and others.

Sudden flash!

Here was the arthritis-cancer connection I had been looking for, at least partially explained. The mechanism was the Cox-2 conversion of a fatty acid (arachidonic acid) to prostaglandins—local modulators of biochemical activity first isolated (coincidentally, from the Bahamian sea whip that we had been growing off my Island for Science). Celebrex had been developed as a Cox-2 blocker at the G. D. Searle Division, now a division of Pfizer/Pharmacia. When there was time, I would go to its research lab in St. Louis to learn more about it.

Checking the literature carefully, I looked for links between Cox-2 inhibition and Folkman's concept of killing of the tiny blood vessels feeding tumors. My idea was somewhat intuitive, but inchoate, and no more than one of at least a dozen unrelated concepts I wanted to explore in this field so new to me—localized radiation on the larger lymph nodes, monoclonal antibodies in higher doses or in conjunction with other Mabs targeting different cell markers, ways of turning up the immune system, and treatments against other cancers that might be adapted to lymphoma. I was not a cancer scientist, but in a practical sense I had an advantage over them, for I was not stuck at a bench or directing a laboratory devoted to a single concept. I could and did scour all strategies and results, becoming en route a researcher of research, akin to the life I'd led before in extending the prowess of *Industrial Research* magazine. The idea that an arthritis drug could help against blood tumors did not appear in any of the scientific papers we found at that time. But it meshed with the rationale of my journey into this strange new land of cancer research: if I could find anything rooted in science, anything beyond the hopeful but inane nonsense of the mystics, I need not wait years for proof or disproof. And there was every reason not to restrict my therapy to any single regimen.

• • •

Ten days after my series of needle biopsies at M. D. Anderson, Jeff Medeiros phoned me from Houston. It was November 18, 1998.

"Sorry to tell you this, Neil, but *you have unequivocal MCL.*"

The pathologist's words clapped like a lightning bolt, dropping my stomach a thousand feet in a heartbeat. The news gave me a fierce headache, and I swallowed a couple of aspirin, thinking at the time that it would take more than aspirin—or Celebrex—to ascend from my plunge. I pushed down hard on emotions that scurried around recklessly, calming myself with thoughts of the past. You have been here before, many times, I told myself. You have only to work harder, to keep searching, asking questions. Asking the right questions. "Then why is my lymphoma indolent?" I said, a final grasp at a final straw.

"Good question. Are you still having symptoms—fatigue, night sweats, and so on?"

"They are subsiding. No more fevers, no chills, no extreme fatigue like before, just some sweating at night, and I'm down to 10 mg of codeine at night for pain. I'll be getting another CAT scan in a couple of weeks."

"Sounds like your MCL is still indolent, especially if the new scan shows more shrinkage. Everybody else who has MCL *overexpresses* cyclin D1." He meant that the presence of this enzyme, or catalyst, is abnormally high in mantle-cell lymphoma. "We did an immuno-histochemical stain on your tissue, and it was *negative*. You don't appear to be expressing cyclin D1 at all! Maybe that accounts for why your disease is indolent. I was in Japan recently talking to a research pathologist who has been studying the cyclins—"

"Yatabe? Yasushi Yatabe?"

"Yes. You know him?"

I told Jeff that I'd read Dr. Yatabe's paper about cyclin D1, a cell-growth regulator. The gene that begets cyclin D1 plays a central role during the cell-division cycle and has been noted in breast and other organ cancers in addition to lymphoma and other blood cancers. The word *cyclin* derives from "cell cycle," and there are many forms, designated A, B, C, D, and so on, followed by numbers indicating various subtypes. When D1 was absent, lymphomas were usually a lot less aggressive. I had written to Yatabe in Nagoya, and he answered in genuine sympathy for my illness.

"Did he have any ideas on how to turn off D1?" Jeff Medeiros said.

"No, but he thinks MCL with and without cyclin D1 overexpression are different diseases."

"Well, if they are, it looks like you've got the better of the two," Jeff said. "No cyclin D1."

It was good news if it continued. Fully 86 percent of cyclin D1–negative MCL patients in a Yatabe study lived more than five years, whereas only 30 percent of cyclin D1 positives lasted that long. If my cyclin D1 was negative, if I could partake of one of the modern therapies, or both, I might live until someone got to the bottom of this puzzle. A race against time. Lymphoma, it has been said "never loses." Like gravity to a skydiver, the best you can hope for is a draw, and at the time I would have settled for one in flash.

"Yatabe is going to leave Japan and come to work on this problem next year at USC," Medeiros said encouragingly.

Here was the brain drain we hear about in action, talent exported from Asia for the benefit of the University of Southern California. Their drain, our gain. A third of our graduate students in science and engineering have come from other countries. If more young Americans fail to enter these admittedly demanding fields, it could mark the beginning of the decline and fall of the United States when the foreigners return to their increasingly affluent homelands (as occurred later with Yatabe when he went back to Japan).

The conversation with Jeff Medeiros drew to a close. When he said goodbye, I heard the unmistakable lengthening of the two syllables as though he meant it in a final, terminal sense. I put down the phone and raised a hand to the back of my neck, kneading it hard, as if rubbing away frustration. All I had heard from every voice was the same mantra: there certainly was hope, there would be a cure, but it would be a future cure, leaving . . . what for the present? I felt exhausted.

But only for a moment.

Researchers such as Jeff Medeiros and Yasushi Yatabe constitute a category of cancer doctors separate from chemotherapists or oncologists, separate even from Mike Blend, an unusually scientifically aware practitioner of radioactive antibodies. Seeking truth through basic science, they belong to the global fraternity of explorers who discover how the universe works, how we are made or how God made us. Asking, always asking. And slowly answering the questions one at a time, questions that always lead to more questions and along the way gradually expand mankind's boundaries of knowledge. Whether we would learn how blood cancers advance, and how to stop them, in time was for me the ultimate question, but I felt intuitively that I could survive without those breakthroughs, that there was knowledge enough out there.

I had only to find it.

7

The Language of Medicine

THE WEEK BEFORE CHRISTMAS I MADE AN APPOINTMENT WITH AN-
other practitioner of radioactive antibodies. He was Mark Kaminski, director of leukemia and lymphoma at the University of Michigan's Cancer Center in Ann Arbor. I had planned to detour to Champaign to pick up David,
but the weather was so bad, I couldn't dream of flying. "Christmas Carol"
was busy in Santa's workshop (our basement), and I didn't want my cancer
to destroy her holiday preparations any more than it already had, so I drove
alone to Ann Arbor at night through a blinding snowstorm. I stayed at a hotel
right on the university campus and saw Dr. Kaminski in the morning.

Like Mike Blend, Mark Kaminski had come to my attention via Chicago
television, and he had granted me an appointment immediately. Also like
Mike, Mark Kaminski is a warm, friendly, outgoing clinician who was achieving excellent results with radioactive monoclonal antibodies. In his late forties, Mark has a round face, high forehead, and wears big glasses through
which he sees his patients as human beings in trouble instead of as an "MCL"
or a "CLL." He is both a professor of medicine and the director of the lymphoma clinic, a small part of a huge health network that includes the medical school, 3 hospitals, and 120 outpatient clinics. Some 2,000 physicians and
an equal number of nurses handle 38,000 hospital admissions and more than
1.2 million outpatient visits a year.

He showed me his clinic on the way to his office. I saw patient beds separated from one another and from hallways with four-foot lead-lined walls to prevent radiation from striking passers-by. An excessive precaution, I thought, for the harmless electrons of Zevalin's beta rays, but perhaps not so for the stronger gamma rays of Bexxar, on which Dr. Kaminsky was conducting trials.

In his office Mark looked at my CAT scans and pathology reports and confirmed Mike Blend's findings that Bexxar had helped only a minority of mantle-cell lymphoma patients so far. Instead of recommending either Bexxar or Zevalin in his ongoing trials, he suggested seeing Ron Levy at Stanford for a custom-made vaccine. Whereas monoclonal antibodies such as Rituxan attack only a single target on the surface of malignant cells, lymphoma vaccines recruit the entire immune system to attack the cancer wherever it appears in the body. Like so many others I would meet in my journey, Mark Kaminski not only knew the lymphoma-vaccine pioneer Ron Levy but was one of his protégés.

When I told Mark I was hoping to get a vaccine without first taking toxins, he was surprised to find that I had not taken chemotherapy in the three months since diagnosis, which made it at least a year since the onset of the disease.

"How did you get away without chemo?" he asked. "Mantle-cell lymphoma is the more aggressive of lymphomas."

"I'm not sure," I said, "but I suspect my splenectomy had something to do with it."

He thought about that for a moment and said, "Unfortunately, one of the prerequisites of a vaccine trial is that you must have twice failed chemo." He said it slowly, knowing it was not what I wanted to hear yet letting me know that he was not a member of the Chemo Culture. Seeing my disappointment, he added, "I agree with you about the dangers of chemo—in case the vaccine doesn't work—especially now when we have Mabs that might lower the tumor burden as effectively."

He paused, the fingers of his mind seeming to tug at something he wondered whether to reveal. At length he said, "I've been in contact over the last few months with a scientist-oncologist at one of the big federally funded cancer centers who has agreed to start a Bexxar-first trial."

I thought of Mark's initiative as a revolt, and I was all for revolution in this field of endeavor. Confronting and changing the entrenched protocols of cancer treatment appeared to entail as much salesmanship, diplomacy, and tenacity as had my former business life.

"You mean so MCL patients could take Bexxar instead of chemotherapy, not in addition to chemo, to shrink their tumors while the vaccine is being made?"

"Sure. Everybody knows chemo doesn't help MCL in the long run. It's about time for a breakthrough in primeval thinking . . ."

Mark suggested I call the scientist myself to see whether input from an "informed patient" might catalyze the project. We parted on that hopeful note.

· · ·

The snow, no longer blinding, fluttered to the ground like wisps of cotton out of a navy blue sky, blanketing the roadway, muffling traffic noise. Silver smoke spiraled upward from chimneys, which soon gave way to rolling farmland along the 230 miles back from Ann Arbor.

At home I told Carol what had transpired and then strode over a footbridge that David and I had built to span the valley between the two sand dunes on which I had built our house and my small office building. I ignored an inquisitive deer I usually stop to admire, ignored the winter-gray lake beyond, and entered my one-room office, were I immediately called the scientist Mark had mentioned. He answered and passed the buck to a clinical oncologist, a Dr. D at the same institution, who had taken on the voluminous paperwork of getting the trial started. I redialed and reached a woman whose job it was to get rid of people like me.

"Dr. D is busy seeing patients . . . if you'd care to leave your number, he will call you back."

I always do, and they usually don't. But after my fourth attempt later in the week I was rewarded when Dr. D called me back. My concern and that of other patients, I told him, was being forced into chemotherapy to get a vaccine. He sounded angry, muttering something about my using the name of his colleague to get him to call. It was only two days before Christmas and he might have been trying to get away from the office, I thought. In any event, he seemed to thaw and took the time to ask me whether I was certain that I had mantle-cell lymphoma.

"Yes, I'm certain," I said. "I had bio-cell studies done at M. D. Anderson. It confirmed the 11-14 chromosomal translocation."

"Look, if you have that translocation, and if you're positive for CD20 and CD5, negative for CD23, and overexpress cyclin D1, then you've got mantle-cell lymphoma!"

I was all those things, except cyclin D1 positive, or so I thought at the time, but I didn't want to sidetrack the conversation, despite his asperity. "I understand you are working on getting a trial started to use Bexxar instead of chemo to lower the tumor burden before vaccine—"

"Look," he commanded. "I don't have much interest in that plan. Besides, you're a patient! You can't influence these things!" He hung up.

His attitude was directly opposite that of Kaminski or Blend. Dr. D suffered from the rampant arrogance of the in-group: you are either a professional or you are nothing.

• • •

Since then I talked several times to Mark Kaminski and increasingly to Mike Blend, who has become a friend and frequently stops at our home with his wife, Lesly, on their way to Michigan, where they have a getaway cabin. As 1998 was about to end, now knowing both Kaminski and Blend, I decided I had seen my last practitioner who was not a scientist. It wasn't their personalities that bothered me: Dr. A had been forthright; Dr. B, cordial; Dr. C, transparent; and Dr. D, intransigent. What repelled me was their great leap backward, their science-by-tradition reminiscent of darker ages when Galileo's sun was condemned to orbit the earth.

A right turn from chemotherapeutics to targeted drugs was in progress everywhere I looked. You could read about biotherapies. You could feel them like fresh snowflakes in the air. But you couldn't *get* them.

The top four drug companies—Pfizer/Pharmacia, GlaxoSmithKline, Johnson and Johnson, and Novartis—spend $22 billion annually for research, averaging 16 percent of sales. Most physicians receive their information on upcoming drugs from such pharmaceutical giants, but these are not the only organizations at the forefront of biotherapies. It is the smaller biotechs and the universities that are leading us out of the Chemo Culture. It was not easy in those bleak days of my urgency to find an oncologist, let alone a chemo-therapist, who knew much about radioactive antibodies or vaccines, who would help me get into a clinical trial, or who would give more than the standard dose, if needed, of the naked and harmless antibody Rituxan.

From now on I would seek out the experimentalists, the test pilots of science like Mike Blend and Mark Kaminski who were proving the biotherapies, determining doses, suggesting combinations with other new targeted agents, and amassing data. In addition, I would call on the basic researchers, the molecular biologists and immunologists who seek to understand exactly how our bodies work. It wouldn't be easy to get past their front doors, for these people are chronically pressed for time. But maybe, just maybe, I could make that jump into the future by finding out what these scientists were in the process of discovering.

• • •

The "three-months" until I was supposed to get into therapy had run out. A hundred days had passed since my splenectomy, and 1999 was approaching fast. If my treatment was to be something other than chemo, there wasn't time to find a cure. I was desperate. In the past whenever I've been stressed, I have sought refuge in work, thereby subjugating worry to overcoming the problem that produced the anxiety in the first place. It had been that way in launching my magazines and in battling the Bahamian government to continue the science island. Striving. Fighting. Turning liabilities into assets. I thought of what I was doing as living a mystery story, seeking clues that would keep me, the reluctant detective, alive.

Every waking moment—and there were plenty of them because normal sleep was impossible—was filled with reading journals or textbooks, talking to scientists, or e-mailing other mantle-cell lymphoma patients. As cancer had changed their lives, so now had it changed Carol's and mine. We were studying *medical* research of all things! Old nonscientific friends were abandoned temporarily. We spent half our evenings with Rade and Leslie Pejic and many others with Mike and Lesly Blend discussing the molecular biology behind new therapies. The data deluge from e-mail attachments, scientific papers, and books was torrential, and it had to be sorted and digested. The top drawers of a dozen white filing cabinets along one wall of my office were rapidly filling with reports and clippings on hundreds of subjects related to lymphoma. I bought a faster computer with more memory. Although fascinated by the numerous avenues of cancer research, and vindicated by my first assumption that better answers to cancer could be found in today's laboratories, I was overwhelmed by work.

Carol took off time from decorations and gifts and discovered "the MCL Group" on the internet. Some six hundred mantle-cell lymphoma victims interact every day by e-mail and sometimes by phone. Forced to it by their therapists' reliance on chemo, members of the group search the scientific literature themselves, ask one another questions, compare notes, and devise their own strategies. Then they try to sell their doctors on helping them join a new clinical trial for an experimental drug. Usually it's a moot point, because most group participants have had round after round of chemo and now are less than ideal candidates for the new therapies being tried.

An exciting prospect under discussion by the MCL Group was the vaccine work pioneered by Ronald Levy, which Mark Kaminski had recommended. I recalled the scornful remarks about Levy's research made by Dr. A, the man who "loved lymphoma" and had warned me that vaccines are experimental (no doubt connoting in his mind unsafe) while at the same time advising me to take unsafe, highly aggressive chemotherapy followed by an even more dangerous bone-marrow transplant.

I faxed Dr. Levy a letter describing my case and asking for an appointment. Replying by e-mail, he agreed to see me and then phoned to warn me that I might not want to make the trip to California because I couldn't get into his protocol without having twice failed chemo. In my publishing days I had learned something of salesmanship, mostly that a sale starts with the first no and that unsuspected new opportunities often arise. I wanted to meet the famous Ronald Levy. I told him I would appreciate seeing him anyway, and afterward I tenaciously devoured the papers he and his team had published over the last few years.

The "literature" of medicine isn't as easy to comprehend, of course, as the literature of Nabokov or Updike, but I can learn new words as well as anyone. With medical dictionaries, learning "Medical" came considerably faster than learning Spanish or French, which I had been studying on and off throughout my life, and these Latin-based languages helped me with etymologies. I already understood metric from my former life in the physical sciences. On this planet water freezes at 0 degrees C and boils at 100 C. Shrimp die at 30 C. A milliliter is about five teaspoonfuls. Metric is the language of most of the world, so we ought to know it anyway.

If foreigners can learn English, deciphering such thorns as "The bandage was wound around the wound, making it hard to polish the Polish furniture," we certainly ought to be able to learn Medical, a mere dialect. It is, after all, still English, with some extra Latin and Greek words added. The language of medicine harks back to the days when doctors, priests, and other mystics didn't want their followers to understand what they were discussing because it was mostly nonsense and because they wanted to establish an insider's cult. Confronted with a language other than the vernacular, their ignorant patients would stay that way, a tradition that too often carries on to this day even in the United States. The outsider, of course, is the health customer, or "patient," a word derived from the French "sufferer," and first used by Chaucer in the late fourteenth century to describe those who "suffered from disease patiently." Doctors can't go around saying "skin tears" or "effectiveness"; they mystify these terms into "lacerations" or "efficacy," which mean exactly the same things, and imprecisely refer to "fluids" when they mean only liquids—*fluids* properly denoting both gases and liquids.

However, these roots in dead languages allow the creation of new words to describe newly discovered phenomena. The phrase *single cell* takes on a more-specific meaning when you name it a *monocyte*. Monocytes roam the lymphatic system relentlessly gobbling up the terrorist invaders, the pathogens ("disease producers"), for breakfast, lunch, dinner, and late-night snacks. Doctors might take the term *big eaters* to refer to their corpulent colleagues, so they translated it into the Greek *macrophages*. Words such as *lymphoma* and *sarcoma* denote kinds of *omas,* or tumors—respectively, of lymph and flesh. *Melanoma,* which refers to the deadly skin cancer, literally means "black tumor," and *carcinoma* means "cancer-tumor"; this last form involves the epithelial tissue, which comprises cells that cover skin and membranes or form the secreting portion of glands. Most of us are familiar with the term *carcinogenic* in reference to substances, such as tobacco smoke, that "produce cancer." Two people who don't reject each other's kidneys or bone marrow are histocompatible, the prefix *histo-* coming from the Latin for tissue.

The word *cancer* originated from the Latin for "crab" because the swollen veins around a surface tumor looked like the legs of a crab (which is also the rough shape of the constellation in the night sky between Gemini and Leo).

The Levy papers started with the concept of custom-made personal, or idiotype, vaccines; the Greek roots of *idiotype* mean "unique," and the term refers to the peculiar determinants of your antibodies that make them different from everyone else's. *Vaccine* entered the language uniquely, jumping into Medical from the Latin *vaca,* or "cow," because the first infectious agent to be inoculated in people was cowpox. Of course *vaccine* and *vaccination* have dropped their bovine origins and apply to immunotherapies against other diseases as well. One day you may call your special antibodies "my idiotype" as routinely as some novelists now use *phenotype,* which is the expression of your total genes, or genetic makeup, such as your blood group, hazel eyes, brown hair, or environmental mutations.

My problem was not in comprehending the words; it was in understanding the extreme complexity of the body. Leslie Pejic, who had just earned a Ph.D. in neural science specializing in Alzheimer's disease, became my tutor. Leslie, an energetic mother of five with a fine sense of humor who at this time was in her late forties, helped me immensely in my drive to comprehend the intricacies of molecular biology and immunology and even talked to some of the researchers on my behalf. At this stage of my new education, as in past endeavors, I was acutely aware of Alexander Pope's warning from the late seventeenth century that

A little learning is a dangerous thing.
Drink deep, or taste not the Pierian spring.

I determined to drink deep, through the layers of therapies that were effective and were not effective, right down to the bottom of that sacred spring in Pieria where the Muses would confer learning on those who drank from it—and now to the depths of biological action seen in the molecules themselves.

• • •

Andy Raymond, who lives in San Diego, came to Chicago for the sheer pleasure of flying back to California with me in Papa Whiskey as I went to visit Ronald Levy in Palo Alto. A bright young man of David's age, Andy had been my mainstay when he was in his late teens and I was constructing the Island for Science. These days Andy is a mature and experienced manager (whose phenotype includes brown eyes, a ready smile, and a weight-lifter's body). He works for the Steris Corporation directing the conversion of hundreds of hospital operating rooms throughout the western states to withstand the rigors of earthquakes.

To fly to California from the Chicago area in a small plane, you skirt the Rocky Mountains and stop for fuel in the Texas Panhandle. We didn't make it that far the first day, however, because my alternator stopped alternating. No sputtering engine. Nothing amiss except a reading on an instrument, as when a person becomes a patient after some instrument reveals an abnormality. A warning.

We landed in a town along the Kansas-Colorado border, not too far from Columbine. The alternator problem sounds more dangerous than it was since at worst it could affect only the instrument panel and not the engine, which operates on an independent and redundant electrical system. Airport repair shops don't stock the diverse alternators used in different aircraft, and it would take a day or two to locate the right one and have it sent by express. We solved the problem as we had done so often on boats in the Bahamas. We bought a charger, two very large twelve-volt batteries, and short cables from K-Mart. We charged the batteries in our motel room while we slept and in the morning wired them in series with the aircraft battery to produce twenty-four volts.

We took off into a clear morning with crisp white clouds against a bright blue sky. From above the patchwork of farms and ranches of the Great Plains was like a relief map flushing a dozen shades from burgundy to brown. The roads between them, too far below to see the potholes and dirt traversed by wingless vehicles, became veins and arteries pulsing with sporadic action. After fuel stops in Amarillo and Phoenix, we arrived at the San Francisco Bay area and made Palo Alto in time to have a late dinner with David, who had taken the red-eye from Illinois.

• • •

Over sushi and rice wine we talked about how difficult it was going to be to see scientists instead of oncologists or clinicians.

"After all, these guys don't work for fees and aren't trying to enroll anybody in their protocols. The only thing they have is their time," David said, relishing a small pile of mustard-colored fish eggs wrapped in seaweed. It reminded me of a diseased lymph node.

David was enmeshed firsthand in the pressures of science. It doesn't matter whether you're in the medical or physical sciences, research is no nine-to-five job. Not only do scientists, especially "pure" or basic-research scientists, spend long hours investigating how something works; they also have to write proposals for grants, read the literature in their fields, and serve on committees. Some of them teach as well. And of course they have families like the rest of us, so it's not hard to understand why they can't take time to see every patient who comes knocking, no matter how many compassion genes reside in their chromosomes.

"Either you have something unique to contribute to their intellectual base, or you help fund one of their projects," David said.

"I'll do both," I said. "Levy seems interested because, although I have MCL, it's indolent—at least so far." My latest CAT scan showed the lymph nodes to be neither waxing nor waning, atypical behavior for lymphoma. Only a few nodes were as large as three centimeters. Most were smaller, although still larger than the normal half-centimeter size of a pea.

"I hope Stanford has a way to shrink those tumors other than chemo," David said. "Now on top of the other problems, a preliminary Dartmouth study has been released proving that many people given chemotherapy suffer brain impairment, compared with a control group treated for the same diseases with surgery or local radiation alone. These are *not* patients who had high-dose chemo or bone-marrow transplants. Just standard chemo. They were tested at least five years after chemo, and they were mentally impaired."

"Do they know why?"

"There is speculation that the chemo drugs breach the blood-brain barrier—after all, toxins travel throughout the whole body—but they don't know that for certain," David said.

"What did they test for?" I asked, thinking back to my psychology courses at school and knowing how misleading some tests can be.

"Straightforward tests: memory, learning, concentration, language, motor skills. They ruled out any patients in either group who had depression, fatigue, or anxiety—which could interfere with mental functions. The chemo patients scored significantly lower in every test."

Any alternative to chemo seemed like a good idea to us. In studying manufactured antibodies and then the vaccines under development at the Levy lab, we were moving closer to science. Vaccines lay at the interface between basic and applied research, as had the work on solid-state diodes and transistors in the 1950s. Vaccines have eradicated smallpox and effectively prevent diphtheria, typhoid, tetanus, tuberculosis, polio, pneumococcal pneumonia, hepatitis, flu, and recently chickenpox, and they soon may be available for malaria and cholera. Although some vaccines, such as the one for smallpox, can be administered up to four days after exposure, vaccines normally are given when you are still healthy, that is, before the onset of the disease. Not so with cancer vaccines. A custom-made vaccine often can rid you of your lymphoma, and there are few side effects because the vaccine ingredients come from your own cells.

As I had with David, I told Andy about Kaminski's desire to start a trial using radioactive antibodies to shrink the tumors before inoculation. "The vaccine protocol, of course, requires zapping you with standard chemo first to 'lower the tumor burden,' which I suppose is a reasonable thing to do after you've already ruined a person's immune system by having him twice fail chemo."

"You can't get a vaccine without chemo," David summarized, "and taking standard chemo for MCL might do more harm than good."

"S.O.P.—standard operating procedure," said Andy, who then reverted to island talk. "It's like being fifty feet deep with an empty tank of air and a school of sharks between you and the surface. You can't stay where you are, and you can't improve your position."

Andy was going home to San Diego in the morning. David would stay to see Levy with me.

"But while they're insisting on chemo first," I said, "Kaminski told me they are producing a 100 percent tumor remissions with Bexxar. Seventy percent of them he calls complete remissions—although I hasten to add that complete remissions are far from a complete cure, since the cancer almost always returns."

"Even so, it buys time. Are those remissions for MCL?" David asked, his blue eyes alight.

"No, for low-grade lymphomas, like follicular lymphoma, that usually remain indolent for years before the tumors start growing and you have to do something. But since my MCL is still indolent . . ."

I let the thought hang there, producing a submerged pause as though the three of us were underwater, breathing from the same scuba tank. Why speculate when tomorrow we could ask Levy himself?

8

Cancer Vaccines

TERRORIST CANCER CELLS EVOLVE AND MUTATE TO HIDE FROM OUR defenses much faster than our immune system can clone its "soldiers," the antibodies that find and fight them. By producing B-cell antibodies and the even more-powerful T cells, our defense forces initiate the process of killing the invading pathogens, targeting each antigen specifically via its surface markers. The problem in cancer is that the diseased cells present surfaces that look normal to the immune system. Even when cancer cells display antigens studded with markers designating them for destruction, they manage to escape, perhaps by rapid changes that confuse the attackers or by shedding the cancer-specific antigens that act like free-floating decoys. Some malignant tumors removed from patients have been found to contain killer T cells that seem to be completely inactive.

When the B and T cells do attack successfully, they often kill with double-edged swords. Sometimes B cells (and more rarely T cells) *themselves* mutate by failing to mature completely; that is, they fail to differentiate into specialized cells after being formed in the bone marrow, and instead they clone greater and greater numbers of themselves that crowd out normal blood cells. No wonder cancer is so hard to cure!

It takes *only one* mutated B cell out of millions to start the cloning process that soon overruns the defending lymphatic system—which comprises not only the lymphatic vessels, lymph nodes, and spleen but also the tonsils (including adenoids), appendix, and bone marrow. (Some classifiers include the thymus and liver as well.) Descendants of this single mutant B cell continue to replicate relentlessly, overwhelming the body's ability to filter out infections through the lymph system. The result is B-cell lymphoma. The white blood cells, especially the major component called "neutrophils," are depleted, and sometimes the red cells, which transport oxygen to the rest of the body, become exhausted.

Fortunately my white-blood-cell counts never tested dramatically low, but many people of all ages in the MCL Group were diagnosed initially by a dramatic drop in neutrophils, some measuring 1,000 per cubic millimeter of blood instead of the normal 3,000 to 7,000. When white-cell counts are superlow, you can't ward off infections; you develop fevers, itch severely, and suffer fatigue so bad that you can barely climb out from under your wet sheets. These are symptoms of your body's inability to fight the invading army. Even when it works against some cancers, chemotherapy lowers the white-blood-cell count even further.

High white-cell counts are dangerous, too. When lymphomas enter the "leukemic phase"—that is, when the white cells rapidly divide, sometimes reaching counts as high as 150,000—you are in danger of harming various organs, including the brain, which is a hotbed of metabolic action. I would visit this blazing meteor of white-cell proliferation before my mantle-cell lymphoma was finished with me.

· · ·

In the 1970s the same discovery that allowed the cloning of mouse antibodies against any antigen—that is, tapping the mouse immune system to search for differences between cancer and normal cells—allowed Ronald Levy to analyze antibodies for their ability to recognize antigens on the surfaces of leukemic cells taken from the same person. When a B cell develops into a lymphoma, that lymphoma is a clone of cells that, being identical, bear the same antigen on their surfaces. The unique portion of the B cell, called the *idiotype*, became Levy's target.

In 1981 the Levy lab took idiotype proteins from a patient's tumor, used them to vaccinate a mouse, and treated the patient with the resultant mono-clonal antibodies. That first patient is alive, well, and free of lymphoma to the present day. Afterwards they tried it on fifty lymphoma volunteers, 75 percent of whom mounted a specific, vigorous, and truly astounding at-tack against their lymphoma tumors. The work led Levy and others to found IDEC Pharmaceuticals, which built on Levy's data to make a one-size-fits-all antibody. That antibody became known as Rituxan, truly a wonder drug.

Rituxan doesn't cure every lymphoma victim, however, and long-term usage can lead to depletion of normal B cells. The problem is that each person's tumor constitutes a unique target, and therefore different antibodies must be customized for each patient. In 1997 Levy and colleagues, especially Richard Miller and David Maloney, again took the idiotype protein from a man's tumor. But this time they vaccinated the patient with the protein made in mice and changed its form in a way that would induce him to make his own antibodies and launch a T-cell response to fight his own cancer.

They also began coupling their vaccines with various "adjuvants" (aids) that dramatically increase the production of antibodies. (Strangely, the first anticancer adjuvants, developed in the 1980s, were brews of oil and dishwa-ter detergent containing alum and phosphates, but the new ones are more complex.)

Thus an idiotype cancer vaccine (more precisely, "personalized immu-notherapy") consists of customizing your antibodies—in other words, clon-ing your own antibodies specific to your own cancer antigens. Generalized, nonspecific immune stimulators have proved disappointing in most cases because tumors arise from your own cells and normally are not recognized by the immune system. In idiotype vaccines, however, because the antibod-ies are contoured exactly to your own cancerous B cells, the cancer can be destroyed.

• • •

The waiting room at the Stanford hospital, like those of the other cancer cen-ters, segregated the usual *misérables,* refugees sitting helplessly and reading newspapers or murmuring among themselves. I wondered whether they appeared faceless to their doctors, whether their oncologists saw these patient patients not as fathers or mothers or young men and women with careers and loves and hopes but as carcinomas, melanomas, or lymphomas. Or reservoirs of blood to be transplanted.

Three of Dr. Levy's young white-coated residents examined me, their faces flat and drained of emotion. In medical school they must have taken a course called "Detachment" in order to deal with death and cancer. One of them prodded my right armpit so hard, almost *willing* a lymph node to appear, that I knew it would hurt for days. I reminded myself that he was only trying to help me by finding a lymph node big enough to make an idiotype vaccine. While they required fresh tissue, major surgery was out of the question, so unless you had a large-enough peripheral lymph node— that is, one in your groin, neck, or armpit instead of, as in my case, deep within my abdomen—you couldn't participate in the trial.

Ron Levy came in carrying my CAT scans. The trim, balding, sixtyish Levy sported a short graying beard like an exclamation point. Wearing a suit and glasses and smiling warmly, he spoke with a low and even voice and moved with the unhurried grace of those who spend most of their time in a laboratory. The originator of lymphoma vaccines, Ron Levy is a star of cancer research. If medals to civilians were widespread in this country, he'd be wearing a chestful. We shook hands, and I introduced him to my son, mentioning David's credentials as a physics professor. I felt like adding that David teaches kids soccer, skis, scuba dives, makes beer, and plays racquetball. But of course I didn't.

"Why do you think your MCL is indolent, Neil?"

"The last two CAT scans showed no lymph-node growth," I said.

Levy shook his head slowly, as if not wanting to disappoint me. "I'm not so sure. We compared your scans, and it looks to us like the lymph nodes may be *growing*. But even if they are not right now, don't forget that this disease is characterized by waxing and waning lymph nodes. I wouldn't get your hopes up too high."

At this point my hopes were fragile, waxing and waning like lymphomas.

"I'd really like to enter your protocol, but I don't like the idea of taking chemo for mantle-cell lymphoma. Your friend Mark Kaminski says you ought to consider a vaccine without chemo, using radiolabeled monoclonal antibodies instead to shrink the tumors." I condensed the story of Dr. Kaminski's efforts to initiate a vaccine trial that first would reduce the tumor burden with a radioactive antibody, maybe in conjunction with Rituxan, instead of doing it with the usual chemo. I left out the part about Dr. D's lack of enthusiasm.

Levy seemed to be pulling my way. He looked me over as if seeing not a sufferer who had come to him for help but an ally in fighting lymphoma.

"Sure," he said at length. "Not only is it possible to use a radiolabeled monoclonal antibody instead of chemotherapy, but it's a very good idea. The problem is the FDA won't allow it."

"Why not?"

"Well, neither the radio-Mabs nor the vaccines have been approved. You guys are scientists," he said, glancing at David and me. "How can you figure out what's going on when you mix *two* experiments?"

"Yes, but this isn't just about science," David shot back. "It's about curing people like my dad!"

"Unfortunately that's not the way the FDA sees it." His expression was inscrutable, giving no inkling of his opinion about that bureaucratic regulation.

"Look, David, Neil. Chemotherapy always works, at least temporarily. The strategy is for the chemo to reduce the size of the tumors and for the vaccine to keep them reduced, maybe permanently."

Over the twenty years until then, the last month of 1998, only about six clinical trials had been conducted, at Stanford, the National Cancer Institute, and Yale. These relatively small studies yielded mixed results depending on the type of lymphoma and the history of a patient's prior chemotherapy. Arguably—considering the number of trials you include and the length of time you track them—some 50 percent of vaccinated patients have achieved long-term disease-free survival, including the disappearance of all cancer cells. (Large vaccine trials were underway in 2003 on about a thousand patients that may lead to answering the questions I posed to Levy in 1998.)

"Ron, I've read your papers. The vaccines work in half the cases. What happens if you're in the other half? What damage would be inflicted by chemotherapy?"

"I don't think you can wait for the approval process of new protocols. Mantle-cell lymphoma is no pussycat; you really ought to get into therapy."

"Within three months?"

Ron laughed, acknowledging the standardization of this recommendation. "Yes," he said. "The immediate problem is that you don't have any big peripheral lymph nodes. You need to have one somewhere near the surface that's at least two centimeters. The FDA won't allow major surgery in this protocol for a number of reasons, chief among them being that the chemo is enough of an assault on the system without aggravating it further."

"Isn't there any way around that?"

He stopped for a moment, his eyes shining. Was he suggesting a stunning leap across regulations imposed by a governmental agency that has been accused of slowing science and killing patients? No. Such accusations were made by others, not by Levy, who more than any other scientist I would meet in this field appreciates the safeguards the FDA imposes. At the same time, it was clear that he wanted to help me.

"There is one possibility," he said. "As long as you're here, go see one of my former graduate students, Dan Denney. Dan is starting a company with a process that requires only a small number of tumor cells to be used for our vaccine—so small they can be removed easily by fine-needle aspiration."

• • •

The value of interviewing someone on his own home ground, as I had learned in my youth as a reporter in Costa Rica, is precisely to elicit such an impromptu suggestion as Levy had made. We managed to see Dan Denney that very night at his company in Redwood City, where he was working late. The one-story building had a mostly glass exterior and seemed to have been constructed in a hurry, like so many in the Bay Area that house biotech start-ups. Denney himself met us at the back door and led us past lived-in laboratories where open books and journals were nestled between microscopes, beakers, and chromatographs. We passed cubicles with blackboards, their unerased scribblings echoing postponed debate. At his office he waved us into chairs, took off his sport coat, and lowered himself behind a paper-strewn desk. Tilting back in his chair, he began to tell us in a quiet voice what he and his colleagues were doing.

Dan Denney is youthful but experienced. He had earned Ph.D.s in immunology and microbiology and spoke in a humble way that I was finding to be typical of scientists in this field. Unlike most, he was both scientist and entrepreneur, and he reminded me of myself at his age, starting a company against all odds, working day and night, driving a wedge between the new and the old of established corporations. I was surprised to find his company, Genitope, was further along than Ron Levy had indicated. Already three years old in 1998, the company employed a dozen scientists who worked closely with the Levy lab.

To customize a cancer vaccine at that time cost upward of fifty thousand dollars per patient. While that's no small sum, it is only a tenth of the five hundred thousand it cost to treat the average lymphoma victim with chemotherapy. Some vaccinated patients require booster treatments, which are inexpensive, whereas virtually all patients on chemo—if they live—undergo recurrent treatment. Assuming that half of lymphoma patients treated by idiotype vaccine would require only minimal or no further therapy, the vaccine approach would save a quarter-million dollars per person.

The reason these vaccines are expensive is because they had to be produced by a complex, time-consuming process called "rescue fusion." The first step, after choosing human tumors whose cells have generated remarkable amounts of a certain molecule, is to inject them into mice, fusing human-mouse cells. These are used to produce a new cell line, a strain of abnormal cells that has become standardized, commercially available, and exchanged among the world's laboratories. "Hybridomas" (hybrids of tumors) then are made in the laboratory by fusing tumor cells from the patient with a commercially available fusion partner—cells that themselves are the result of a previous fusion between a mouse and human cell. Unfortunately, rescue fusion does not always work the first time for a variety of technical reasons—such as fragile tumor cells or weak hybridomas—and the scientists may have to start the whole process over again, boosting the cost.

Genitope was working to mass-produce the customized vaccine using a molecular approach instead of rescue fusion to speed up the process and make it far less expensive. Called "molecular rescue," the process skips the mouse process entirely. Instead, it clones the genes coded for the idiotype from a patient's tumor and transfers them to another cell that produces the protein, which is then modified; the resultant vaccine is then injected back into the patient. Not only would Dan Denney's molecular-rescue method eliminate the need for surgery, but because a sample from a needle biopsy can be frozen with dry ice, bits of cancer tissue from anywhere in the world theoretically could be shipped to the company for processing, after which the custom-made vaccine would be returned to the hospital of origin and inoculated into the patient. That dramatic goal was a dream, but an extremely practical dream.

Dan Denney and his scientists have two patents on their system, one for the production of cell lines used in the immunotherapy manufacturing process and one for the isolation of tumor-specific genetic materials used to produce the cell lines. Genitope was conducting two clinical trials at the time of our visit, both in phase two. One was at the Levy lab; the other, at the University of Nebraska Medical Center, was directed by Dr. Julie Vose, who became yet another Ronald Levy protégé when she took a sabbatical to study under his direction.

However, chemotherapy was required in both trials. No one at the time seemed interested in trying to shrink the tumors with Mabs instead.

Three years later I was heartened to learn that both Levy and Genitope had started small clinical trials using a vaccine without requiring chemo *or* Mabs first. Indeed, Levy found, at least with follicular lymphoma, that "even relatively large tumor burdens can undergo regression following . . . vaccination." That is, vaccination alone.

• • •

With a potential market of a quarter-million patients diagnosed with non-Hodgkin's lymphoma in the United States alone—growing by ninety thousand a year just here and in Europe—any biotech company that devised truly effective cancer therapies would leap into the billion-dollar class overnight.

The average age of onset for non-Hodgkin's lymphoma, formerly thought to be sixty-two, has been decreasing as more of the population is affected each year, and it is already the fourth-costliest cancer. Lymphoma is no longer an old-people's disease. The average age of onset is now fifty-five—the same for mantle-cell lymphoma, according to a recent "roll call" of the MCL Group. Lymphoma thus strikes men and women younger than the average for all cancers taken together, 80 percent of which are diagnosed at age fifty-five or older. New diagnoses of lymphoma have grown by 81 percent over the last two decades, with a 51 percent mortality rate at five years and 44 percent at ten years, the second highest mortality (next to lung cancer) of any malignancy. That does not mean that the mortality rate for lymphoma is growing; it means that the mortality in the population is growing because the incidence of the disease is increasing. Yet it is epidemic by any standard. Lymphoma is more rampant than any other cancer except those you can avoid by not smoking or staying out of the sun.

I was excited about the prospects for biotech companies entering this field, but not as a businessman anticipating his grail or a scientist within reach of a long-sought goal. Having lived through and awakened exultant from both those dreams long ago, I knew intuitively that what lay beneath the surface would prove larger in scope, more complex, more scientifically sophisticated, a breakthrough in the glacial mass of cancer science.

My excitement, if I would permit it to flower, was fueled by something else: the most ancient instinct—survival—for I saw in the technology of lymphoma vaccines a clear path to a cure. The obstacles were only regulatory, not scientific, easier hurdles to jump when the time came.

• • •

Every night between Christmas and New Year's almost everybody we knew came over, as though to a wake for the still living: neighbors, relatives, and friends from as far back as the army, college, and even grade school—friends not seen in years, including those from the magazine and from the island, pilots, boaters, skiers, scuba divers, chess players, scientists. Beneath their cheer lay unambiguous tones of final goodbyes: reminiscences of interesting times shared, of a life lived well, whispered in past tense, final handshakes at the door held a moment longer than normal.

After each of these impromptu gatherings and one big party that Carol organized, we resumed our lymphoma studies. We read about other laboratories also developing cancer vaccines. Aside from Denney and another Levy protégé, Larry Kwak, who was similarly customizing vaccines at the National Cancer Institute, most of these labs were working on generic rather than personally tailored vaccines. UCLA's Jonsson Cancer Center was investigating a vaccine based on dendritic-cell replication and interleukin-4, a signaling protein that promotes proliferation of stem cells in the bone marrow. USC's Norris Cancer Center had one for melanoma. Johns Hopkins was developing a vaccine for prostate cancer. Progenics Pharmaceuticals, a biotech company working with Memorial Sloan-Kettering in New York, was conducting clinical trials on a vaccine for most cancers, including lymphoma, colorectal cancer, gastric cancer, small-cell lung cancer, sarcoma, and neuroblastoma. Sloan-Kettering also was experimenting with a melanoma vaccine using a "gene gun" to drive tiny gold particles coated with human DNA into the skin of affected mice. Biomira in Canada and New Jersey, together with Biovector Therapeutics in France, was conducting trials of a patented idiotypic vaccine against B-cell lymphoma. Germany's University of Göttingen was showing results with advanced kidney cancer. Vical was working with Ron Levy on DNA vaccines to prevent the recurrence of lymphoma.

Of great interest to me at the end of my story would become the research going on at Large Scale Biology Corporation, a biotech in New York that was deriving recombinant vaccines from plants instead of animals. Their scientists, collaborating with Levy, use tobacco plants into which they introduce lymphoma proteins carried by harmless viruses to the leaves. The proteins then are harvested, extracted, purified, and inserted into a patient's tumor cells. When the resulting personalized vaccine is readministered, the treatment stimulates the patient's immune system to attack the tumor. An advantage is that the proteins can be grown in weeks instead of the four to twelve months usually required using animal cultures. In 2003 the company completed phase one and was beginning phase-two clinical trials.

As this book goes to press, seventy vaccines are under development, not only for blood cancers, but also for breast, skin, and other organ malignancies.

The Levy lab continues working with Genitope, with other companies, and on its own. Recently Ron Levy revisited an earlier idea in vaccine research, using "dendritic cells" (so called because they branch like a tree). These cells of the lymph nodes, blood, and spleen function as a network trapping foreign proteins, but more important, they are distinguished by their powerful antigen-presenting capabilities. In other words, they present an antigen to the immune system as if from a special-delivery mailman, thereby enabling a diseased cell to be recognized by the immune fighters. Levy and colleagues segregated dendritic cells from a lymphoma patient's blood, mixed them with the idiotype protein, and returned them to his body. The method provokes a strong T-cell response that regresses most lymph tumors.

Levy also is working on streamlining the molecular fusion process. He adapted and refined a strategy involving the making of "transfectomas," originally devised by Sherie Morrison, a professor of molecular genetics at UCLA. In this procedure you first clone the lymphoma idiotype genes by polymerase chain reaction, or PCR (explained in chapter 16 and in the glossary). Next you transfer them into a mouse myeloma B-cell line, because this type of cell possesses the biochemical machinery to produce high levels of antibodies when it's provided with active immunoglobulin genes. Although the original cells were isolated from a mouse cancer, they are grown easily in the laboratory with simple nutrient broths. No mice required. Then the scientists mix the cells with those from a human cell line, using machinery for producing cancerous B-cell hybridomas. Finally they put the cells into a fermentation culture vat, and out come large quantities of pure iodiotype protein for immunization.

• • •

When I started my quest for research answers still in the laboratory, I had no idea there was so much progress in so many places. I could not have imagined, in a world filled with cancer victims, that so much of this activity has gone unreported in the popular media. Over the past twenty years perhaps as many as five hundred people with lymphoma and leukemia have been essentially *cured of their cancer* by participating in vaccine trials. I know that *cured* is a strong word, seldom whispered among conservative scientists who have seen their hopes dashed year after year. I know we won't be certain until a large number of vaccinated patients have lived out their lives cancer-free. I know all that. Yet there are some five hundred people alive today because they have had idiotype vaccines well after their cancers began. And I expect the number to increase dramatically over the next few years as a result of new trials.

There was plenty of hope in those numbers even in 1998—hope for the future, perhaps, but still meaningful. When I built my publishing company and later the Island for Science, I often visited the future before falling asleep at night, moving around in imagined surroundings, shaping it the way I wanted it to be, then returning to the present to plan the steps that would make it happen.

This latest challenge was different, unresponsive to direct action. The rules had changed. No longer could I innovate my own way out of crises to create my own destiny. Curing cancer was someone else's job; my role was passive, merely finding the most suitable of unproved therapies and trying to shortcut the long process of proof and approval to save my life.

I kept prodding myself to learn enough to devise a plan of action that would begin with today's biological agents, constantly cognizant of the "three-month" admonition. On the other hand, the pain of the surgery and of the cancer had subsided; my lymph nodes were deceasing in size, as shown every six weeks by CAT scan. Were it not for the useless warnings of the cancer physicians I had seen, I would have felt just about normal.

And less stressed, by far.

I was beyond the three-month limit; it had been more than a hundred days since my surgery, the busiest and most worrisome time of my life. Now, as the last day of the year arrived, David and his family and the Pejics assembled at our house for New Year's Eve. Although we sipped drinks, we weren't exactly partying but rather regarding each other pensively, my grand-sons, Ryan and Brandon, quiet as we stared into the flickering fireplace. I looked around at the things that used to occupy me: the office across the bridge from the house I designed, the furniture I'd made, the island memo-rialized in a model used as a chess table, a library on a balcony cantilevered over the living room containing books I had written that had absolutely nothing to do with medicine or cancer.

Finally the bells tolled and we celebrated the first moments of 1999 with laughter and kisses requisite for a new year, the bad year dead. There was cheerful conversation. But no one said anything about the future, which on that night, for one of us, might no longer exist.

Premature Results

ON NEW YEAR'S DAY SHAHID SIDDIQI CALLED, HIS LIQUID VOICE OVER-flowing with excitement. "Did you see the *Time* magazine story about the new vaccine at Duke?"

"No, but I do get *Time*. I'll look."

"It sounds like the closest thing to a cure I've seen yet. Want me to try for an appointment?"

"Absolutely."

The *Time* story showed a young man with dark hair in a white lab coat, Dr. H. Kim Lyerly, clinical director of Duke University's Gene and Thera-peutics Center. According to the story, Lyerly's team had "discovered how to prod mass quantities of the body's immune system white blood cells that tell all others to go into battle. They are now primed to use these new forces to fight lung, breast, and colorectal cancers."

The article explained that Lyerly, the oncology researcher Dr. Clayton Smith, and the molecular biologist Dr. Eli Gilboa—obviously resisting the Chemo Culture—planned to treat eighteen advanced cancer patients with their own dendritic immune cells in the first clinical trial of its kind approved by the FDA. These dendrites belong to the class of cells that Ron Levy in-vestigated for many years. They are nature's sentinels, presenting antigens to the immune system so that both the body's B-cell antibodies and aggres-sive T cells can recognize and kill them and the cancer cells they mark. *Time* recounted how an elderly woman with breast and liver cancer, having gone through several years of chemotherapy, including tamoxifen, had run out of options. The story also cited a small trial at Stanford (without mentioning Ronald Levy) that "cleared two patients of lymphoma" and "reduced tumor size in two others." The focus, however, was on Duke. "Lyerly and his colleagues achieve their results by infusing patients with their own dendritic cells," the article said, "after the cells have been encouraged to grow and have been altered in a way that enables them to stimulate a more-aggressive immune response. To do that, the cells now carry a protein on their surface that stimulates a specialized subtype of T cells to attack the tumors."

Time had been ingrained somewhere in my journalistic mind as a serious, in-depth interpretive magazine, such that I had ignored the gradual disintegration of its science coverage into a pop accumulation of "print bites" (except when it does special issues). Because *Time* reported that Lyerly and colleagues "achieve their results," Shahid and I assumed that they were achieving results. Referring to the Duke trial as "one of several vaccine tests approved by the FDA" implied that the research was in progress. And when *Time* said, "Last fall Duke opened a new 10,000-sq.-ft. laboratory . . . where cell cultures can be cultivated in sterile surroundings . . . paid for by pharmaceutical giant Rhone-Poulenc Rorer," we assumed the lab was in use.

Shahid won an immediate appointment. I flew Papa Whiskey to Newport News to pick him up, and together we landed at Durham, North Carolina, in time for a dinner meeting with Kim Lyerly and his colleagues, Eli Gilboa and a husband-wife scientist team, Cristina and Clay Smith. Lyerly and both Smiths were M.D.s. Gilboa, a Ph.D., turned out to be not only a biologist but the center's research director. The dinner was cordial, the conversation filled with descriptions of the tremendous potential of the Duke approach. Lyerly handed me a news release stating that Duke researchers had "taken a significant step forward in the laboratory in demonstrating that a person's own immune system may be the best weapon they have to fight cancer."

Despairing of getting into the Stanford vaccine program any time soon without accepting chemotherapy, I was eager to learn what the Duke researchers were doing. I still worried about exceeding my three-month "deadline" for therapy with no plan in place should my MCL turn aggressive. I was immensely heartened that chemo was not a requirement of the Duke program, as it had been both at Stanford and at Genitope.

Eli Gilboa is an intriguing man. His heavily accented English stems from his childhood in Romania and the many years he lived in Israel. Eli is bright, articulate, upbeat, and funny—he told us he originally came from Transylvania and "somehow remained in the blood business." Talking about his research, however, he was all business, exuding an aura of confidence. "The work we're doing on dendrites yields a more-powerful response compared to what has been seen in other cancer vaccines," Gilboa said.

We were having dinner near the university, in a stately mansion that had been converted into a restaurant. Eli barely touched his plate. You could read his personality in his physical features: slim because food is unimportant, eyes alert because he is aware of everything, hair unruly because it is of no consequence, soft-spoken because he is self-effacing, reserved but hardly diffident, using intense, passionate words. He is a man of accomplishment, past and future.

Our war within turned out to be more complex than I had learned to date. B cells and ordinary T cells weren't the whole story. Nature abounds in branched structures—rivers, trees, air vessels in lungs—and dendritic cells in the immune system are no exception. The sweeping structure of dendrites captures antigens from a foreign substance and presents them to our T cells, telling them, in effect what to seek out and destroy and what to leave alone. They help the macrophages (those "big eaters") in patrolling the lymphatic and blood systems and rushing the invaders to the lymph nodes, where they call for reinforcements. The dendrites then begin a kind of chemical warfare, spewing interleukin-12, a protein that enables communication among white blood cells.

The dendrites are professional soldiers, if you will, and scientists actu- ally call them "professional antigen-presenting cells," or APCs, because they possess a specialized ability to absorb the pathogens, change their structure, and send them to the targeted cell's surface as antigens. Nonprofessional (I wanted to call them "amateur") cells present antigens to nonspecific killer

T cells, or cells with the CD8 marker. But the professional APCs elicit support from yet another group of fighters, called "helper T cells."

Eli Gilboa's research plan flowed from that understanding: if you could boost the dendrites in just the right way, they could produce a cascade of all these immune-system warriors to kill tumor cells. And maybe, just maybe, the result would constitute a universal cancer vaccine.

• • •

The next day Eli showed us the Rhone-Poulenc lab, a modern one-story structure so new that the plaster was still wet in some rooms. Others contained crates with unpacked equipment. Contrary to *Time*'s implication, however, it was bereft of laboratory personnel. Eli then brought us to another, older building that was very much in use, this one near the hospital where bone-marrow and stem-cell transplants were being performed on lymphoma and leukemia patients, mostly children. Dr. Cristina Gasparetto Smith's lab was in that building, and when we arrived, Clay was visiting his wife. Clay—handsome, blue-eyed, neat, facial stubble betraying his long hours at work. Cristina—dark hair flowing well down her back, eyes shining out of an olive eloquence that carried from her native Italy. Eli explained that she would be the principal investigator on the project and that she had mastered the art of growing cell cultures like few others.

Indeed, Cristina was in the process of culturing cells, and she returned to them like a mother to her children. An art as well as a science.

"I really *love* cells," Cristina said, her long hair askew as she bent over her tubes, beakers, and incubators. "You have to keep them"—she searched for the right word in English—"*spirited*," a momentary embarrassment forgotten as she saw we took her seriously. Clay offered goodbyes before returning to his own lab, where he worked on identifying antigens unique to human mutations. He was beaming, proud of Cristina's abilities and of the fact that she was pregnant.

She looked more like a chef than a biologist as she nurtured her human dendritic cells. She enticed and lovingly persuaded a *single cell* in a wide culture (Petri) dish into begetting children—perhaps, I imagined, as only an expectant mother might be able to do. You could imagine the cells dividing again and again as she bathed the clones in human serum to make them *vivacious*. (Now she had me thinking of these cells as sentient beings!) They lay like clumps of whey at the bottom of her containers, but under the microscope you could see them squirming, exquisite living creatures, parts of us, essential parts that keep us healthy.

"In a few weeks we'll have cloned *billions* of these babies," she said exuberantly. "If we do not have contamination," she added, the artist giving way to the molecular biologist once again.

Vaccination against polio, measles, or diphtheria involves injecting a body with a weakened form of the virus or bacterium you're trying to prevent from causing disease so that the immune system will react as if it were a real infection and fight it. Cancer vaccines, as we had learned from Levy, invoke information from a patient's own tumors to coach the immune system to reverse the disease *after* you've already contracted it.

"The hypothesis involved," Cristina explained, "is that tumor cells are able to proliferate and expand freely because, somehow and somewhere, they have escaped control by the immune system. So if we are able to reinstruct the immune system to recognize the tumor cells, their growth must be blocked or at least suppressed . . . finally eliminated." She had begun talking while still maneuvering the Petri dishes containing the cells. She then placed them inside an incubator to keep them warm and happy—"perhaps blissful," she joked.

"The tumor antigens need to be presented to lymphocytes in APCs to make T cells function normally. The most potent APCs are the dendrites. They're found in many of our organs and they circulate freely in the blood outside the organs at a low percentage, less than a tenth of 1 percent of total white cells. There are lots of ways to design a dendritic-cell tumor vaccine, but the way we do it is by expanding the dendrites in vitro—in glass, or outside the body." Her words cascaded, a waterfall that stopped every few seconds to make sure we followed her accented English.

"We load—or pulse—these dendrites, or host cells, with a specific tumor antigen in glassware containing a patient's blood. The pulsed cells run around recognizing and killing the tumor cells, and so we reinfuse the treated dendrite cells *in vivo*, into the body of the patient. The antigen-loaded dendritic cells now should be able to reboost the immune system to attack the particular antigen. So far a few unique tumor antigens have been identified on several different kinds of malignancies. But most tumor antigens are still unknown."

As Cristina readily acknowledged, hers is only one of several ways to design a tumor vaccine. The Duke research thus complemented, rather than repeated, the work going on in the Levy lab at Stanford. For all the data scientists uncover, building on the mountain of knowledge their predecessors have amassed; for all the dry scientific papers they produce; for all the dedication of these doctors, who shun money and dedicate their lives to exploring the unknown—for all this, it is still the left-brain, right-brain combination of scientific method, art, experience, and intuition that produces the most breakthroughs.

• • •

In the coming months I returned again and again to the Durham campus of Duke, which was only a three-hour flight in Papa Whiskey. I was frustrated to learn that Eli Gilboa and the other accomplished scientists were not funded sufficiently by the National Cancer Institute—and that only 25 percent of cancer-research projects submitted to the NCI receive funding. These projects are not offhand ideas for research. They are well-thought-out projects that have passed lengthy peer reviews first at the university or cancer center, second at the NCI, and third in a long rereview process. The fact that 75 percent of worthwhile projects go begging to private foundations or to cancer victims themselves—or worse, never see the light of day—seemed unconscionable when fifteen hundred Americans are dying of cancer *every day*, when more than 12 million of us are taking the old standard chemo treatments instead of therapies based on new research.

At this stage of my disease, I was still afraid, less interested in funding a project than in my own survival. When Eli discovered that, he hastened to tell me the *Time* story was misleading, that the phase-one study they had performed on dendrite vaccines had proved only that the cloned dendritic cells were not toxic.

Eli Gilboa was a hard taskmaster, often criticizing his own results to reach beyond the research of the moment, using each project as a springboard to answer questions raised by the previous study. Like others investigating cancer, Eli and his team were besieged by lack of time and money, suffocated by the demands of writing proposals and raising funds, tremulously watching while precious time passed, seeing it wasted by the dearth of manpower on his project, suffering the deaths of patients who succumb every day of cancers that should have been cured years ago.

At one of our meetings he asked me a question, perhaps born of his contrasting former life in Israel, "Why do you think these funding problems exist in the United States, the richest nation in history that otherwise spends so heavily to defend its citizens?"

"Because, Eli, we are a nation of scientific illiterates." I answered without hesitation, having visited this subject for most of my life in different, nonmedical fields of science. "We elect nonscientific representatives in our own image. An informed Congress could easily change the federal establishment if its members understood what could be done: a massive recruitment of young men and women to enter molecular science."

"How about a cancer-research effort like the total commitment to winning World War II?"

"Why not?" I said. The thought hung in the air like a tangible object. I would revisit this subject often as the months and years progressed, but right then I had to focus on staying alive in order to be here during those years to come.

• • •

During those opening months of 1999, Eli Gilboa and another group at Duke began to immunize mice with dendritic-stimulated T cells to inhibit the growth of unrelated tumors of different genetic backgrounds. These T-cell preparations wiped out various cancer cells in test tubes, making a splash in the media, as had the earlier research. Eli Gilboa hastened to tell me on one of my visits, "Contrary to some statements in the lay press and despite my attempts to set the reporters straight, this work has no immediate clinical consequences."

I wondered, though, how soon it would. As Cristina had pointed out, most tumor antigens are still hiding from researchers. One way Eli's group is trying to circumvent the problem is to use "total tumor RNA" as a source of multiple antigens. RNA, or ribonucleic acid, constitutes a reservoir of genetic information in addition to DNA, which is deoxyribonucleic acid. Both are able to carry enormous amounts of information. The difference is that DNA is a super-long molecule. Because of its rather miraculous double helix configuration, if you were to extract DNA from the chromosomes of a single human cell and stretch it out, it would measure about seven feet! DNA's extreme length allows it to contain the information for all the genes in our bodies. RNA is a much shorter fragment that carries information about only one or a few genes that are important for the cell at a particular moment.

Gilboa's complex technique for extracting RNA from tumors requires the scientists first to isolate the tumor cells. Then they use phenol to render the tumor-cell membrane permeable and collect the RNA in a high-speed centrifuge. Finally, they transfect the dendrites, which means that they make the RNA play an active role in the cells' metabolism. Cristina is attempting to obtain a large number of dendrites by expanding them in the lab and injecting them in an animal using a growth factor called "Flt-3," a small molecule that not only helps T cells find foreign antigens but also stimulates production of natural killer (NK) cells that can kill tumor cells directly.

From Cristina I found that the biotech company Immunex (now part of Amgen) was making Flt-3 molecules and had begun human clinical trials to generate antitumor immune responses. In trials with mice Immunex was able to send skin tumors into remission in a large percentage of cases and reduce these sarcomas in the others. The results in humans were not yet in. Would this turn out to be just one more case in which "we can cure your cancer, provided you are a mouse"?

Whether these and hundreds of other promising leads such as Cristina

Gasparetto's and Eli Gilboa's eventually will result in the dendritic vaccine heralded in *Time* remains to be seen. Trials that don't see phase two are abundant in cancer research. As is true in acquiring knowledge in any field, we learn more from failure than success, more from tragedy than ecstasy. Émile Zola, the French "black novelist" of a doomed world going down to destruction in flame and smoke (who in 1902 met his demise from chimney-smoke asphyxiation), once said, "We rarely stop to analyze our lives when they are flying along successfully. . . . We only pause to see what has gone wrong." Zola's comment is especially pertinent to scientists, who even more than the rest of us rise from the flame and smoke of their failures, again and again.

Then they begin anew.

10

Co-stimulating T Cells

THE URGENCY IN FINDING AN ANSWER TO MY MANTLE-CELL LYM-
phoma paralleled the urgency of those first dark years with my magazine
company, which four decades earlier only *seemed* to be a matter of life or
death. I was convinced in both cases that effective answers existed, as determined now to cure my cancer, or at least hold it at bay for some years, as I
had been committed to solve the start-up crises of *Industrial Research,* and
in much the same way: using the ability to ask questions, the strength to
persevere, and a fierce tenacity.

Every few evenings Rade and Leslie Pejic came over to help me think
through alternatives. Sometimes we were joined by Mike Blend; by David,
who would drive up from Champaign; and by Shahid, who flew from Virginia in his old Mooney. Leslie, the director of a nonprofit mental-health
center and a neuroscientist, gave me a crash course in molecular biology.
Mike thought it would be difficult, yet barely possible, to receive a "compassionate exemption" for Zevalin or Bexxar, or maybe the newer Oncolym.
We would have to prove that chemotherapy doesn't work for mantle-cell
lymphoma, however, or show that it does more harm than good, a daunt-
ing, long-term project. I reviewed about a hundred papers that detailed the
histories of patients who had undergone aggressive chemo for MCL and
summarized the outcomes. Shahid put together a table listing authors, title,
date, and condensed the results in a wide last column. I kept those spread-

sheets ready like the shotgun you keep in the basement, oiled, accessible, hoping you never need it but standing by. The proof would be there in case we needed data to back up a request for compassionate exemption. Before applying for FDA permission to get a vaccine or a radioactive antibody without chemo, however, I wanted to make certain there wasn't something even better.

I continued to get CAT scans every six weeks to monitor the size of the lymph nodes. Fortunately, the scans showed the nodes remaining stable, like the cherry-blossom buds on the hospital ceiling I got to examine during each session. I lay on my back while the scanner shot X rays at my body. By now these scans were familiar, and I regarded them more in curiosity than dread, although the hot surge of iodine through my veins was not exactly fun.

After each session Rade would take Carol and me down to the room with the light boxes on the wall, where the radiologist would apply his calipers to the shadows representing lymph nodes and compare them to previous X rays. His interpretations were somewhat subjective, because each CAT scan produced images taken at angles slightly different from those of earlier films. In December I accused Rade of being an optimist when he said once more that the nodes looked to him as though they actually might be shrinking. Ron Levy at Stanford had said the opposite. But that was two months before. It was February 1999 now, and yet another CAT scan showed clearly that the lymph nodes had shrunk.

• • •

The following week my helpful copilot Shahid and I flew to Gaithersburg, Maryland, to see the Levy protégé Larry Kwak. The NCI facility there is another huge cancer-research center consisting of thirty-five hundred people, including principal investigators such as Kwak, postdoctoral fellows, and students who do basic and clinical research. The NCI is only one of the twenty-seven in the National Institutes of Health, which together spend some $23 billion annually—up somewhat from the original 1887 budget of $300. (No, not 300 million dollars. Just 300 dollars!) The national institutes employ thirteen thousand scientists, spread far beyond Gaithersburg and their home base in Bethesda. For all that, the entire NIH is only one of eight agencies that make up the U.S. Department of Health and Human Services.

We entered the building where Dr. Kwak worked and were surrounded by institutional sounds: the humming of elevators, a dropped book, the skidding of machinery being moved, background music testifying to the ordinariness of life despite the deadly topic under study. Larry Kwak's office was modest, like the man. He is thin, dark, quick, and curt, a youthful American of Korean descent. After what had become my standard allegation, my claim of shrinking lymph notes, he replied with the standard question: how did I know my lymph-node variations were anything other than waxing and waning?

"Maybe it's wishful thinking," I said and then lapsed into an electric quiet as if the vibrations from a long flight in Papa Whiskey were still murmuring in my bones.

Shahid inquired how the NCI idiotype vaccine differed from others. Kwak explained that his research in finding better ways to make lymphoma vaccines had flowed seamlessly from his time at Stanford. He used the same rescue-fusion method devised by Ron Levy—the lengthy, complex process in which cells from a patient's tumor are fused with a mouse-human cell line. The rescue-fusion method still limited the number of patients able to be treated, however, while the NCI vaccine employed a different adjuvant, or helper drug, to catalyze a generalized immune response. Whether the new adjuvant would prove better than Levy's or Denney's, or better for some lymphoma patients and not others, Kwak said, remained to be seen. He added that he was cooperating with a biotech company called Genzyme Transgenics.

Kwak then looked at me carefully, with empathy, as if seeing for the first time a patient in front of him instead of an investigator of his work. "First," he said, "make sure your lymph nodes are *really* shrinking. Continue what you're doing with the CAT scans. If the scans show that the lymph nodes are starting to grow, you'll know it."

"If they do, will you accept me in one of your clinical trials?"

"Absolutely."

"Do I have to take chemo first?" I asked, still hoping for a negative answer against FDA reality.

"Well . . . of course."

• • •

After leaving the NCI, we flew to Philadelphia to visit another big new cancer center, this one located on the campus of the University of Pennsylvania. Dan Longo, the erudite scientific director of one of the NIH institutes, had told me by phone that the university was doing some unique research into stimulating the body's own T cells to fight cancer, and we had made some appointments.

The University of Pennsylvania Cancer Center was created in 1997 by a $100 million gift from Leonard Abramson, the founder of U.S. Healthcare, (later sold to Aetna). A large portion of the Philadelphia Civic Center had been taken over to build the Abramson facility. Dozens of concrete and tan brick buildings rose from winter lawns dusted lightly by snow. We headed for the building on Curie Boulevard, where we were scheduled to see David Liebowitz, who with Craig Thompson had come from the University of Chicago. The T-cell team was newly assembled at the university; Thompson, a professor of medicine and molecular biology, had just arrived to head the oncology department. In turn he recruited Carl June, the M.D. who developed the T-cell process at the Naval Medical Research Institute, but at the time of our visit June had not yet arrived, and Liebowitz had been there only a few months.

The building where David Liebowitz worked carried the clean and antiseptic look of a hospital. The third-floor hallway was like a dry moat separating windowed offices from foot traffic that seemed unusually heavy. Liebowitz signaled to us from behind one of the window walls, and we stepped into his sparsely furnished temporary office. In his late thirties, with black hair and a devil's goatee, Dave wore an intense expression behind his glasses. Liebowitz, who holds both an M.D. and a Ph.D. in immunology, was quietly excited about his work. He explained that T cells—the most effective killers of organisms harmful to the body—blithely ignore cancer and allow it to grow and grow while the tremendous arsenal of our immune system stays quiet. I imagined thousands of warplanes loaded with 500-pound bombs ready to destroy an army of invaders but not using them because the pilots can't find the enemy.

While the body contains T cells that express millions of different T-cell receptors recognized by specific antigens, all T cells contain the CD3 receptor, or marker. It seems that CD3 *ought* to tell the T cells when cancer is massing and should set in motion a chain of events to make anti-CD3 antibodies. But CD3 stimulation is not sufficient to activate T cells, which play the central role in orchestrating most immune responses. Although the mechanism has been understood for many years, countless efforts to jump-start this portion of the immune system have failed—until Carl June learned not merely to stimulate T cells but to *co-stimulate* them.

According to Dave Liebowitz, Carl June started with a tremendous scientific curiosity and an equally tremendous incentive: his wife suffered for six years from ovarian cancer (she succumbed in 2001). Carl began by wondering how tumors evade detection. He kept coming back to the same question: why don't the T cells of cancer patients respond to stimuli that readily activate the T cells of healthy people?

He knew the answer lay somewhere in the way cancer cells evolve. After all, these cells have been multiplying at a faster rate than their human hosts and existed for at least a billion years before the era of mankind—that is, before mammals, reptiles, birds, dinosaurs, and fish, long before the vertebrates, before the worms. Over those enormous timeframes, cells that became environmentally mutated into cancer, perhaps starting first in protozoa and working their way up to humans, evolved mechanisms to prevent T cells from recognizing the signals that normally propel them into action against foreign invaders. If these cancer cells had been entrenched early in evolution, they'd had billions of years to perfect evasion techniques, so that the T cells ignore the antigen signals. June, Thompson, and later Liebowitz began looking for ways to help the body recognize them.

As his research progressed over the years, Carl June discovered that by prodding the immune system with two stimuli—using *both* anti-CD3 and anti-CD28 antibodies—he could activate the T cells in lymphoma patients, causing them to respond as they do against other diseases. Now the human defense system could drop those 500-pound bombs with precision!

Not only do the provoked T cells launch a vigorous immune-system attack, Dave explained, but they are so sensitive to the continuing co-stimulation that they also secrete chemical messengers, or cytokines, that excite the production of even more T cells. And in vast quantities! This self-amplifying cascade of responses is a key benefit of the University of Pennsylvania technique.

"While co-stimulation produces massive numbers of T cells, they don't belong to the same cell population," Dave said. "They're mostly helper T cells, so called because they coordinate and help the actions of the entire immune system."

Here was yet another sound scientific approach, one as basic as vaccines. Unlike vaccines, which primarily stimulate B-cell antibodies to fight the cancer, the Pennsylvania method invoked the more-powerful T cells to do the fighting. I wondered how long it would be before the FDA would allow trials using both techniques as a first treatment or a second treatment after Mabs.

"How far along are you?" I asked Dr. Dave Liebowitz.

"Far enough to know it works."

"Clinical trials soon?"

"We've done phase one," Dave said. "Out of twelve patients with aggressive lymphomas, six have stayed in complete remission for two years. So far. We'll be doing phase-two and -three trials next year."

"Without chemo?" The words seemed to stick in my throat, and I had the feeling that they stuck in his throat as well, as if we both sensed the futility of attempting a clinical trial any other way.

He looked at me intently as though recognizing the eternal discussion, the three-act tragicomedy conducted in FDA phases. "No," he said at length. "Unfortunately, the T-cell co-stimulation protocol had been formulated to begin with both the standards of chemo and stem-cell transplantation. But we *know* co-stimulation was the main factor—not chemo or transplant—

because antigens binding to T-cell receptors without co-stimulation don't activate the T cells. Instead, they lead to a state called anergy, in which the T cell becomes refractory to further activation."

I skimmed the scientific papers he gave me while still in his office, eager to read them later in full. Maybe it was his words, or my intuition, or both, but I felt as though I'd been hit with an electric current. My enthusiasm for co-stimulation sprang from its sound basis in Carl June's theory, yes, but also because the technique—as far as the science was concerned—involved no chemotherapy. Co-stimulation had achieved success in initial trials with both mice and men.

I was encouraged further when Dave told me that Craig Thompson and Carl June had founded Xcyte Therapies in 1996 to push this technology and that this Seattle company was headed by the biotech veteran Ron Berenson, the physician-scientist who had founded CellPro. These were stalwart cancer investigators with impeccable reputations, of whom I had read and whose basic findings now were being replicated by other labs. If they were ready to take the next step, the commercial leap, there could be a cure lurking here somewhere.

Dave Liebowitz asked for my financial help, and I wrote personal checks to both the University of Pennsylvania and Xcyte. (I would cover the checks by selling some securities when I got home.) Small potatoes as cancer funding goes, but it was a large amount for me. I saw it as the only way I could help advance a practical therapy, for the co-stimulation breakthrough had the potential to save countless lives, to cure not only blood cancer but *all* cancers, starting first with lymphoma and leukemia, then progressing through melanoma to kidney, prostate, and the other cancers.

The breathtaking originality of these scientists could transform the entire world as we know it. Who among us does not grieve for some family member or friend who has this disease, the "C word" so dreaded that its very name, like the devil in the Dark Ages, invokes fear, denial, and too often, surrender?

· · ·

I continued to find more information related to the University of Pennsylvania project. An e-mail sent to the MCL Group arrived from CellPro's chief operating officer, Rick Murdock, who related one of the more-astounding coincidences in the land of adversity. The story started in the 1980s when Ron Berenson found that an antibody discovered by his colleague Irv Bernstein could be chemically bound to biotin, a B vitamin existing in living cells.

Berenson, a highly intuitive inventor, was experienced in using the ability that molecules possess to bind together and create new compounds. He bound biotin to Bernstein's antibody and then introduced the "biotinated" antibody into a container of bone marrow where, as he hoped, it glued itself to stem cells. He passed the combination through a column filled with tiny plastic beads previously coated with "avidin" (a protein found in egg whites), because the remarkable fusion between biotin and avidin is one of the strongest bonds known in biochemistry. The biotin and avidin stuck together, carrying with it the antibody and the stem cells. What he accomplished was nothing less than the separation of stem cells from cancerous blood!

After this initial success, Berenson and his team spent years conducting thousands of experiments until they came up with a mechanical instrument that they called "Ceprate" (after *separate*). The device allowed them to isolate one of a hundred thousand stem cells from your blood *in vitro* (in glass, or in the laboratory). You then could tolerate a stem-cell transplant of your own blood, an "autologous" transplant, which would eliminate any danger of the graft-versus-host hazard often encountered in "allogenic" transplants—that is, when a donor's blood is used, no matter how close the match. Before the advent of this technique, many patients who received autologous transplants eventually died because their "dirty" reinfused stem cells generated additional cancer as well as normal cells.

MCL Group members were vigilant for advances in bone-marrow and stem-cell transplants because most of their oncologists recommend them at some point. An ironic coincidence menaced group member Rick Murdock when he himself was diagnosed with mantle-cell lymphoma and desperately needed the separation system under development at his own company. Talk about dedication to a new product—the product that could save his life was his own! Among group members, Rick's outcome became a contagious, almost ecumenical force for hope. CellPro researchers worked day and night to perfect Ron Berenson's first tumor-purging Ceprate system and used it to save Rick Murdock's life. That was in 1996, and to this day he remains well. The rest of the story was less auspicious: CellPro was forced out of business by a larger company's patent-infringement suit. Before other companies were able to come up with similar cell-purging devices, I learned of the deaths of some transplanted patients, including some in the MCL Group, who might have lived had that company stayed in business.

Ron Berenson went on to become president of Xcyte Therapies, and both Xcyte and the University of Pennsylvania began conducting human T-cell co-stimulation trials without invasive stem-cell transplants and chemotherapy.

• • •

Soon afterwards Carol and I flew to Seattle (on a commercial airplane for a change) to see firsthand what Dr. Berenson and his team were doing. After the unfortunate outcome of CellPro, Berenson retreated to the laboratory with his colleagues, started a discovery research group, and then merged it with another company in 1996 to create Xcyte Therapies. The focus of this biotech company had shifted from chemistry to cell therapy.

The change transformed Xcyte into—well, an exciting company. It is busy translating the basic co-stimulation discoveries of Carl June and Craig Thompson into a universal process. One of the company's goals is to improve the jump-starting of T cells to fight cancer, and one of their methods uses tiny metal beads to create artificial APCs, the antigen-presenting cells that were under scrutiny at the Duke University laboratories (and many others around the country).

In the Xcyte procedure, a doctor draws blood from the patient and mixes it outside the body with the beads, which are coated with monoclonal antibodies specifically targeted to lock into the cell-surface markers CD3 and CD28. The process stimulates T cells to proliferate by the billions. Later the beads are extracted magnetically, and the T-cell-stimulated blood is reinfused into the patient. The billions of new T cells then cascade throughout the system, not like a waterfall, but like a vast army of highly trained commandos who choose which cells shall live and which shall die. Called "Xcellerate," the method improves earlier attempts to activate T cells by halving the time required to refine the cancerous blood outside the body, so that it now takes only about a week. It is not the only method Xcyte Therapies is testing in clinical trials of patients with leukemia, lymphoma, and ovarian and breast cancers—as well as the autoimmune disease AIDS, a natural candidate for an immune-system enhancer. Some of the other techniques use more than two stimulators of T cells.

Ron Berenson himself is as cutting edge as Xcyte, having earned some of the dozen patents held by his company. In his early fifties, he is tall and well-built, with dark hair, high forehead, and a quick smile—a phenotype matched exactly by his twin brother, Jim, also an M.D. and also doing cancer research, although at Cedars-Sinai, in Los Angeles. The Berenson brothers became scientists dedicated to conquering cancer after the disease killed their father. Their similarities are easily explained: they are identical twins.

• • •

A few weeks later someone at the William H. Gates Foundation called me at my office. What did I know about the co-stimulation T-cell research at the University of Pennsylvania? What did I think of the scientists doing the work? Why had I decided to help fund the project? Perhaps in response to my positive and enthusiastic answers, or perhaps only to verify their foregone conclusion, the Gates foundation awarded the university a grant for the June-Liebowitz research. This grant was significantly larger than mine, however: $4.5 million.

Today, during a dozen clinical trials devised by both the University of Pennsylvania and Xcyte Therapies, about sixty patients with renal, lung, and other organ cancers, as well as with lymphoma and leukemia, have had their T cells co-stimulated. These were highly refractory patients who had suffered many rounds of chemotherapy, which weakens the immune system. Despite that obstacle, twelve of seventeen, or 71 percent of those who entered the lymphoma trial, have gone into remission—41 percent partial and about 30 percent complete remission, as determined by clinical exams and scans. It will be years before we know whether these patients remain cancer-free, but the beauty of the method is that, unlike patients facing chemotherapy, they can be treated again and again, if necessary.

As I finished reading the latest co-stimulation paper, I gazed out my living-room window at the metallic winter colors of Lake Michigan, sweeping up to the fine line of horizon between water and sky. I had been reading all night, and the lake and air merged like science and cancer, producing a blinding flash of dawn . . . but more than that, a pure passion such as I once had taken into my veins when working on the scientific colonization of the moon. The dawn spread across the lake like a wave of expanded life: a realization that if these researchers could pull it off, the T-cell co-stimulation dream, now fully funded by Gates, would be more universal than even the Denney vaccine.

The Carl June and Xcyte Therapies goal ran like this: Oncologists anywhere on the planet extract a unit of blood from a cancer patient. There is no pain, merely the prick of a needle, as in that time before your cancer when you were privileged to donate blood. Your physician or even a nurse or technician packages your blood in a bed of ice and sends it express to an Xcyte-authorized laboratory. The lab then processes the blood to boost an enormous production of T cells—cells that cannot be rejected because they are your own. After T-cell expansion by multiple interactions, the lab returns your blood to wherever you are, in Philadelphia or Nairobi or even a small town like Michigan City, where your family doctor gives you a simple blood transfusion, actually a reinfusion of your own stimulated blood.

And your own T cells cure you of your cancer.

• • •

The co-stimulation lead and a host of other recommendations emerged from my myriad phone calls to Dan Longo, the scientific director of the National Institute on Aging (NIA), another one of the National Institutes of Health but far smaller than the NCI. I had been wanting to meet Dan, who directed scientists working on age-related diseases, not only because a preponderance of lymphomas begin when you are older—victims typically are diagnosed in their midfifties—but because he had his fingers on the pulse of the worldwide cancer-research community.

I picked up Shahid in Virginia and flew to Baltimore, home of the Johns Hopkins Bayview Medical Center, which houses part of the NIA. Founded in 1773 as an insane asylum, Bayview today accommodates twenty-five hundred physicians in forty buildings.

We found Dan Longo in an office quite spacious as government offices go, with a good view of the campus, now in February wet and sticky with melting snow. Longo is a handsome man in his fifties. Graying dark brown hair. Medium build. Relaxing behind his desk, he answered my incessant questions in detail, replying in a self-confident voice, low and even. He explained that even in aggressive cancers only a minority of cells grow at any one time and that the majority of cancers—if you could take a snapshot of them at a given moment—are indolent.

"Mine is, too," I said.

"Any symptoms?"

"Not any more. They have stopped."

"And your lymph nodes are stable?"

"Yes, they definitely are not growing. If anything, they've shrunk a little. Only a few are three centimeters; most are one or two."

"Sounds like indolent to me." That word of choice again for a so-far lazy kind of cancer, like a sleeping lion.

"I hope so, but . . ."

"What?"

"Dan, it's been five months since my splenectomy and diagnosis, and I've been warned at two medical centers in Chicago and again at M. D. Anderson and Stanford to get into therapy within three months. What do these cancer doctors know that I don't?"

A ruminative pause. Dan apparently was trying to reconcile the unanimous opinions I had received from the renowned cancer centers in the face of his own. When at last he spoke, he chose his words carefully, and they landed hard as cannonballs. "Here's my advice: don't attack your lymphoma until it starts growing. Don't disrupt whatever equilibrium you have achieved—even with immunology, even with a vaccine. I have one patient with mantle-cell lymphoma like yours who has been in remission for sixteen years!"

I was incredulous. Everything I read described MCL as the most aggressive of lymphomas.

"One patient out of how many?" I said.

"Well, hundreds, of course. Yet some remain indolent despite tests that show they still have MCL. I have been tracking four patients like that whose diseases have never turned aggressive."

"I will be the fifth," I said out of a conviction suddenly felt. I walked over to the window and saw normal people moving normally along spacious normal walkways, leading normal lives, thinking normal thoughts. "Watch and worry, right?"

"Watch and *wait*—without the worry. Just having your spleen excised was the smartest thing you could have done. You've had a tremendous tumor burden removed—your spleen was five times normal size, wasn't it?"

"Yes," I said, impressed that he had remembered my spleen from one of our phone conversations.

"That's two pounds of diseased lymph system gone. Now your immune system can concentrate on fighting the tumor cells. Look at it another way: all those enlarged lymph-node tumors produce growth factors that trigger other sites to grow. You remove the biggest of them—the gigantic lymph node we call the spleen—and there is less triggering."

"Did your four MCL patients have splenectomies?"

"Yes."

The transformation from a lifelong disregard for my health into the opposite after contracting lymphoma had led me to paraphrase a famous remark: "Even paranoids get cancer." This year, though, I'd begun the return trip into a psyche that was reasonably normal given the uncertainty of my life. Dan Longo's words accelerated my normalcy, providing me with more hope than I had received from any of the cancer doctors seen so far.

"I don't have anyone I could call my oncologist," I said slowly. "Do you take patients?"

"I do, and I'd be happy to accept you as one. But won't it be difficult to see me, with you near Chicago and me in Baltimore?"

"It would be a problem coming here. Who do you recommend in Chicago?"

"Dr. John Ultmann, at the University of Chicago," he said without hesitation. "He's quite famous, really . . . born in Vienna, escaped the Nazis, served in U.S. Army intelligence in Italy . . . then after his mother died of cancer, he went to medical school and started the idea of a multidisciplinary approach to lymphoma. He's one of the few oncologists steeped in research. In fact, he was David Liebowitz's mentor before Dave moved to U. Penn. Ultmann, of course, was a lot older and head of his department, so he was one of the few to stay in Chicago."

Dan rose to his feet and extended his hand, but I didn't shake it just yet. My intuition was clearly focused on the subject I was going to bring up, and I had been saving it for the end. Throughout my life, my curiosity had seemed to expand year by year. Maybe the years of living enlarge the base of experience on which you make certain assumptions, giving rise to more-accurate hunches. The one concerning Celebrex ran strong within me.

"Dan, as scientific director of aging, you must be intimately familiar with Celebrex. What do you think of it?"

He sat down again and a fan of small laugh lines radiated from the corners of his eyes. "I think we ought to put it in the water!"

"Really?" asked Shahid, looking up from taking notes.

"Well, not really, but Celebrex prevents the formation of cyclooxygenase-2—Cox-2. It is truly a great idea, not only to reduce the inflammation of arthritis, but also for Alzheimer's, heart problems . . . all kinds of afflictions. How much are you taking, Neil?"

"Two hundred milligrams a day."

"You could increase it to four hundred."

Here was a man whose judgment I trusted, and I was convinced it was not because he had told me what I wanted to hear. His watch-and-wait recommendation had been based on an in-depth knowledge of the science of lymphoma and the art of medicine that I would never have.

"Is there any evidence that Celebrex or other Cox-2 inhibitors could be doing something specific for lymphoma?" The relationship between arthritis and lymphoma, both systemic and both involving maverick B cells, still seemed mysterious to me, but I felt that this arthritis drug was relieving more than joint pain.

"I think there *is* a connection," Dan said. "When tissues are inflamed, the Cox-2 enzyme is found in all the white blood cells—lymphocytes, monocytes, neutrophils, and macrophages. Tissue inflammation involves the arachidonic pathway."

Arachidonic acid is one of the essential fatty acids, and its metabolic pathway branches throughout the body. "This particular pathway is common to arthritis, arteriosclerosis—and probably cancer," Dan said. "Celebrex must have some anti-angiogenic effect." In other words, Celebrex might be killing the tiny capillaries that were trying to feed my lymph-node tumors, effectively starving them. "A lot of this research has begun only recently," he added.

Back home that Sunday, I started taking the higher dosage. It was the last day of February 1999. As it turned out, it was a date to remember.

11

Do They Have to Die?

EIGHTEEN PARTICIPANTS IN THE MCL GROUP HAVE DIED IN THE SIX months since I became part of this mutual-support club. All had suffered megacourses of chemotherapy; many received bone-marrow transplants or the newer stem-cell transplants that were coming into widespread practice.

. . . I am so sorry to report that Donna, my wife of twenty-seven years, succumbed to the effects of an opportunistic liver infection only a year after engraftment of her allo transplant. . . . My Dad discovered his lymphoma had spread to his brain and the chemo that the doctors gave him seemed to work but it lowered his white count; they gave him more chemo to try to reduce the tumors in the rest of his body and it killed him. . . . My husband is still alive but he thinks he is of no value to anyone any longer. . . . It is with a heavy heart that I tell you my mother lost her fight to MCL after chemo that was of no help. . . . My Dad was diagnosed with MCL exactly three years ago and lost his long hard struggle, never having had a response to the stem-cell transplant or other treatments. . . . I'm truly pissed that Jeff lost his battle with MCL while he was getting Rituxan too late after chemo. . . . My Dad died today after fighting for three years, and I am a mess, searching for a cure so long that I'm burned out. . . . If there's one thing I've come to believe it is that harsh treatment of aggressive chemo, especially when repeated, weakens one to the point of losing the battle to recover from any type of infection. . . . After his transplant, my son developed a fungus infection in the lungs and it caused pneumonia. . . .

Radiation-induced fibrosis was the main factor in the death of my husband, setting the stage for pneumonia and other infections—so we won the battle with MCL and lost the war to treatment complications, ignorance, and mismanagement. Good night my darling Alan, my husband of twenty-eight years who died this morning at 7:15. . . .

Death following death, like steps down an endless stairway. Friends, comrades in cancer, lost in battle—most of them from the "friendly fire" of chemotherapy or radiation. Having taken these drastic measures for years, their periods of regression diminished until stronger and stronger combinations of toxins failed to save them.

Seven of my best friends at various times in my life died young. As tragic as it is to die in your thirties or forties, as deeply felt by the survivors, there is a difference between those deaths caused by accidents or heart attacks and the deaths of the MCL Group members. Cancer, especially lymphoma and leukemia, grinds you down over a long period, and you have all you can do to preserve your identity and not replace it with the name of your disease: *"This patient is an MCL. Over there is a CLL awaiting transplant."* Mantle-cell lymphoma is particularly likely to steal your identity. You die more than once. You die with immense fatigue, with pain or the narcotics that relieve it, and then for a while you are resurrected to life and hope as your lymph nodes retract, only to die some more when it returns or when you suffer the rigors of chemotherapy. You have to survive every one of these battles, as in Russian roulette. When you don't, the cosmic game is over; your identity is finally and completely erased from this earth.

E-mails from surviving family members are brief when they tell about their last battles in the war we are waging together. Messages from those still on the front lines run page after page discussing options and hard-to-get treatment. Over the years the MCL Group has grown from its modest function of providing support to become a veritable worldwide intelligence agency. Among the six hundred members of the group, about thirty or forty are eloquent in their invisibility. We get to know one another well, by the way we seek and impart information, by revealing our innermost thoughts of life and death, and then suddenly realize, in most cases, that we have never met.

There is no trivia in the MCL Group's messages on the internet. No whining. No desperate pleas for sympathy despite the agonies endured. That doesn't mean the group is not sympathetic; it means the members are busy learning what they can to stay alive. As I came to know quite a few of them, first by e-mail, then by phone, and then in person, my own identity was restored in a way more complete than had been done with family and friends. The group helped me achieve emotional stability not only by substituting learning for self-pity but also by letting me know I was not alone in the strange land of lymphoma, where doctors are witches and patients are doctors.

Regrettably, the group is growing. For every death, two more victims with newly diagnosed mantle-cell lymphomas join.

• • •

The MCL Group was founded by David Granet, among the most altruistic in an altruistic profession. A young pediatric ophthalmologist, David established the internet group as a tribute to his father, Irving, who died from MCL in 1996. Few projects he could have started would have helped as much. Irving Granet, a physicist, had wanted a radioactive monoclonal antibody—preferably the one containing yttrium-90 (later named Zevalin and not approved until 2002)—but his efforts to enroll in a clinical trial were undermined by his chemotherapist, who was afraid of anything experimental. The Chemo Culture at work.

Here is one of David Granet's messages to the group in September 1999:

> Today is Yom Kippur, a difficult day for me because it is the anniversary of my Dad's passing from complications relating to his treatment for mantle-cell lymphoma. I continue to miss him and his impact on my life and family. What's changed in those six years? The approved treatment choices still remain various cocktails of chemotherapy. Monoclonal antibody treatments, with or without radiation attached, that we were feverishly trying to get for my Dad now are available and appear exciting. The transplant options we considered may be better now, but many lives have been lost. I remember my father's anguish in living with this disease and the havoc it brought to our lives, the life-altering decisions we had to make, the future we saw slip-

ping away. I know the difficulty of getting through each day. Failure for us would have been *not to try.* Cancer wasn't the end of my Dad; look how much good has come in his name. How many of you learned more about your choices and found support in the Group? Cancer can never eradicate the dignity with which you lead your life. It can never take away control of your own actions. Do something to help yourself. Failure is not an option.

Such messages to the group are rare. There is little time for inspiration. Instead, scores of queries and suggestions fly back and forth every day, with members throughout the world exchanging information about new therapies, detailing the effects of an experimental or other drug, and comparing widely varying experiences with a disease that comes in almost as many varieties as there are sufferers. Members also compare their chemotherapists and the problems encountered in convincing them to let patients enter a clinical trial for a promising new therapy. Countless cases of horses leading their drivers.

Like many of those engaged in this fight for knowledge, I find there isn't enough time to digest the mass of data pouring out of the world's laboratories. Carol helps by reading the group's messages, as well as accessing various medical information services on-line, and then giving me those of most interest. As I travel, I make it a point to meet as many of the members as possible, and quite a few come here to see me. I now count among my friends about twenty group members.

The most frequent writer, Ron Edwards ("Papy Ronnie"), became a bright light of information to those in the group. In addition, Ron, a retired children's-book author, worked full time putting together and constantly updating an extensive Web site on the subject. The site contains case histories and information on possible causes, complementary therapies, hospitals, diagnoses, symptoms, immunology, genetics, treatments, and emerging research, including extracts from recent scientific papers on changes to the blood caused by MCL. Ron suffered from a particularly sinister subset of mantle-cell lymphoma that produces sheets of polyps throughout the gastrointestinal tract, making it painful and difficult to metabolize food properly, causing him to lose weight. Here is a typical exchange:

Ron: I had a long meeting with my Dr. Andy Haynes this morning, Neil, and he was quite adamant that high-dose Rituxan would be dangerous for an MCL patient since the CD20 antigen is so dense. In the paper you sent me, however, the M.D. Anderson team (as far as their rather muddled language could be deciphered) recognized a lack of toxicity at six times the normal dosage. Too bad it wasn't tried on MCL patients. I'm at wit's end, ready to attempt anything.

Neil: I talked to Mike Blend about you. He's finishing a round of clinical trials on Bexxar and Zevalin, and found they haven't helped much for your kind of MCL. Why not get someone else to give you high-dose Rituxan? You could always stop if you have adverse affects.

Ron: Someone else? In merry old England, we are united by our love of waiting three years for a hernia operation; it's the price we pay for our "free medicine." Haynes wasn't very optimistic regarding my future as I appear to be a particularly refractory case. He'd like to try Bexxar but I don't qualify for any of the clinical trials in this country. Now he's talking to his colleagues about pelvic radiotherapy and maybe thalidomide as an anti-angiogenic. So far it's just talk.

The infamous thalidomide, once banned because it caused children to be born with deformed limbs, had recently undergone a revival as a drug to inhibit angiogenesis, and at that point Ron was considering everything— except my suggestion that I send him an airplane ticket to come to the United States for treatment. Although we never met in person, Ron and I corresponded for so long that we came to know each other. I had no idea what he looked like—not that it mattered. Knowing a mind is the important part of friendship, especially when discussing matters of life and death.

• • •

Following Dan Longo's suggestion, I called to make an appointment with John Ultmann and was agreeably surprised when he answered the phone himself and proceeded to tell me that he, too, accessed the MCL Group's e-mails. It made perfect sense to me that an oncologist would tune in on one if not all cancer-information groups.

David, Carol, and I drove to see Ultmann at the University of Chicago, where I had been only a few times since my brother graduated from its medical school almost a half-century before. The gray stone buildings, some of them hospitals, looked the same as they had then, clustered on the north side of the Midway Plaisance. Named for an arcade at the 1893 Columbian Exposition, from whose site the road had started in the early 1930s, the Plaisance consisted of a long, narrow parkway depressed some six feet below the parallel streets on either side so it could be flooded in the winter for ice-skating. Students were darting around on it like random molecules. We walked from the parking garage to Ultmann's building while large snowflakes hurled off the lake with the plangent and confident Chicago wind.

"Dog-tor Ruzic!" exclaimed the renowned Dr. John Ultmann in his thick Austrian accent, rising from his desk as we entered.

"I'm not a doctor," I said. "Please call me Neil. David's a Ph.D., but call him David."

"Then you must call me John."

Younger doctors call you by your first name and expect you to address them obsequiously as "doctor," just as you call priests "father" even when they are half your age. John Ultmann was different. In his midseventies yet bearing a ramrod-straight posture, he was the epitome of Viennese courtesy and aristocracy. My first impression was of a strong personality. Posture, ramrod straight. White hair, rimless glasses. The grin of a cat. As he talked, though, he morphed into a wide-eyed deer, alert, unhurried, speaking with droll humor and an uncommon compassion that suggested a personal commitment, as though someone close to him had lymphoma. He let me know that he never gave up on a patient. It made me wish I could get Ron Edwards here to see him.

"So, Neil, what have you been doing for your lymphoma?"

"Learning, visiting research labs. I met your protégé Dave Liebowitz at U. Penn."

"And so . . . ? Liebowitz is a scientist. Do you visit your barber when you need surgery?"

I laughed. "Not anymore," I said. "Surgery seems to have split off from haircutting in the last few years."

"As chemotherapy will from oncology some day!" he said with a flourish, utterly amazing me. His suit coat was off, hanging on a peg, and a coffee pot steamed enthusiastically. He poured a cup for Carol, who declined, and queried David with a raised eyebrow; when David said no, he gave the cup to me and poured another for himself. "Who is your oncologist?" he asked.

I followed my intuition. "You are," I said, matching his enthusiasm.

He smiled his noble yet benevolent smile, showing strong teeth, like an herbivore's.

To verify the soundness of my decision, I asked my standard question: "How much time do I have before I need to get into therapy?"

"Who knows?"

"Not three months?"

"Good gracious, no. What we must do is watch and wait. You could go a year or two doing that. In the meantime learn everything you can."

He gave me not only advice but a thorough physical examination, the old-fashioned way—no machines—and wanted to know my complete medical history, preparing to treat the patient, not the disease. He explained about lymphoma, adding infections to the list of the usual symptoms of fatigue, pain, night sweats, and fever and telling me to keep my penicillin handy because without a spleen I was vulnerable. He handed me a note with a number on it. "This is my home phone," he said. "Call me anytime, even in the middle of the night if you start having symptoms."

I had the rare feeling that I was talking not only to an oncologist, not only to a scientist, but to someone with a patient's view as well.

And then he told me.

"I have lymphoma," he said simply. "I've had it for many years. I have learned to live with it . . . as you also will learn."

I was shocked. Doctors don't have the disease they treat you for, do they? Considering John Ultmann, the ultimate man, as the archetype for oncologists, maybe having cancer should be a prerequisite for that profession. He told me how he had suffered the T-cell destroying ravages of chemo back when there wasn't anything else. "You know about the co-stimulation research that Carl June started?" he asked. "Well, Dave Liebowitz began investigating it here with Craig Thompson before they left and took half my laboratory people to Pennsylvania." The way he said it, you could tell he was proud of his protégés, despite their having left his nest.

I nodded yes to his question and asked him why oncologists were still giving chemo as first treatment for lymphoma.

He paused, organizing his answer. "I'm sure you know that it is effective on some kinds of cancers, for instance, large B-cell lymphoma."

"But not for mantle-cell lymphoma," I said.

"No," he replied thoughtfully, "not for mantle-cell."

• • •

Two other members of the MCL Group who began e-mailing and then phoning me at about the same time were women actively trying to help loved ones afflicted with mantle-cell lymphoma, men who were in no shape emotionally or physically to help themselves. Judy Cardin called from St. Louis to tell me that her biochemist husband, David, was despondent, fatigued, and fevered with MCL that had pervaded 95 percent of his bone marrow. The Cardins were in their sixties. The other woman, Michele McKenna, in her early forties, phoned me on behalf of her brother John, a young lawyer in New Jersey. Neither woman knew the other. Both worked full time: Michele traveled the globe for Western Union, and Judy worked at her own publicity company. They had dedicated themselves to saving the lives of these men. Both David Cardin and John McKenna bore the burden of grossly enlarged spleens, twice the size of mine, ten times bigger than normal.

Judy and Michele questioned me extensively about my splenectomy, asking why it was done and what the results had been. As in my case, their physicians had suggested radiation, chemotherapy, and everything else they could think of except surgery. Rade Pejic had told me that if you ask a physician what to do about most serious diseases, he'll routinely try anything but surgery. Ask a surgeon and he'll drive you on a gurney to the operating room.

• • •

One day in early spring I flew Papa Whiskey to Teterboro, New Jersey, and had lunch with John and Michele McKenna. John had surmounted his initial phase of denial and was ready to take charge of his life again.

"The problem for most of us," John said, "is that we don't have an airplane or the time to visit all these laboratories . . . and we don't have your scientific background."

Judy and her husband, who had driven to northern Indiana to see me on their way to the Mayo Clinic, also had spoken of a lack of resources. In fact, it was typical of conversations I'd had with some group members, many of whom sought to shortcut understanding of their cancers by seeking cures in herbal medicine, acupuncture, and other "alternative" treatments.

"Flying gives me a chance to retain a portion of my former life," I explained, "kind of a hobby combining travel. But commercial flights are cheaper and faster. And believe me, I'm acutely aware of the time and money restrictions of most cancer victims. Too many, though, resign themselves to their fate, helpless to do anything except the most difficult job of all: nothing."

"All right, what can we do?" John asked.

"Read the scientific papers, or at least the abstracts. Pick your targets, for instance, a vaccine or other nontoxic therapy—what you want first, second, and third in case the previous ones aren't effective. Be tenacious. Remember, if you can't sell them—for instance, into a clinical trial—then they have sold you."

John looked thoughtful and said nothing. As an attorney, he was used to competitive salesmanship. He had swallowed his despondency and started his own search for a cure. "I'll try," he said, and he meant it. "It's my life. As you have said, 'curing cancer is too important to leave to the generals.'"

"What do you think could have caused you and John to have MCL?" Michele asked, as if waiting her turn. It was another typical question, as if by knowing the answer a cancer victim could somehow reverse the chain of events that had taken place.

I mentioned that in my case it could have been darkroom chemicals earlier in life or diesel fumes from the machinery on the Island for Science, and then I added, "Northwest Indiana, from the Calumet area to Michigan City, is to Chicago as northern New Jersey is to New York City." Through the restaurant window where we sat in Teterboro you could see the Manhattan skyline—as you can see downtown Chicago across the lake from my home—similar proximities to big cities and their oil refineries.

"What do these areas have in common?" Michelle said. "Hydrocarbon burning?"

"Sure," I said. "But you can't blame it only on that. After all, most people in northern Jersey and northern Indiana do not get cancer."

"Don't scientists know what causes cancer? Especially lymphoma?"

"Cancer is caused by mutated genes. An accumulation of cells and genes mutate, or change, over time. Until civilization, human beings existed for hundreds of thousands of years with an average lifespan of only eighteen years. Few people lived long enough to develop cancer."

"Here's what puzzles me," Michele said. "I've got pretty much the same genes as my brother, we're only a year apart in age, and we've lived pretty much in the same places. Why does one of us get cancer and not the other?"

"Don't forget that in mantle-cell lymphoma there's a male-female ratio of about six to one. There's got to be some relationship between the X chromosome and protection from MCL."

"Because males have only one X chromosome?"

"Well, if an X chromosome is relatively quiescent for MCL, and as a female you have two of them, your chances of avoiding MCL are increased." I realized I wasn't saying much, so I added, "Nobody seems to know *why* X chromosomes are implicated."

"Senator Paul Tsongas of Massachusetts died of MCL," she said. "He was the son of a dry cleaner." She told me how, when they were kids, she and her brother had spent their summers at a lake in Italy that had been contaminated with nitrates from fertilizer runoff, or worse.

• • •

At home after that trip, I began reading about causes. Environmental events doubtless contribute to lymphoma, but the links aren't as evident as, say, the one between smoking and lung cancer. Scientists lean more toward an evolutionary explanation. Cancer started well before *Homo sapiens* appeared. If it weren't for DNA mutations, we wouldn't be here. It's a double agent, though, because most mutations, being random, are harmful, offering no adaptive advantage. One authority on the subject is Mel Greaves, a Ph.D. in England who says that unlike other animals, we evolved to survive long after our reproductive period. That's fine, but living longer allows more time for mutations to take place. After we came down from the trees, we developed agriculture and started eating fewer varieties of plants. Greaves says that led to our ingesting fewer antioxidants, which stave off cancer. At the same time, we began to eat more animal products, made worse by being cooked at high temperatures. The combination of these practices results in more nicks to our DNA. Some of these mutant cells survive as the reproductively fittest of the lot and thus proliferate; we call this cancer.

The cause of lymphoma and other cancers, according to Greaves, is nothing less than the historically recent change in human lifestyle: overeating, physical inactivity, and recreational sex. Everything we do interacts with our genes—not only the defective genes we inherited but also the genes that began as healthy and were damaged by too much sunshine, X rays, cosmic rays, viruses, insecticides, tobacco smoke, other carcinogens, too much food . . . everything. The random combinations lead to random mutations. The older we get, the more exposure we have to hostile environments, and the more our chances that hit-or-miss events ultimately will trigger cancer.

One MCL Group member posted a report from the National Cancer Institute showing no connection between DDT and lymphoma. Nevertheless, the NCI investigators did discover unexpectedly that people whose blood contained PCB concentrations of 1,000 parts per billion contracted lymphomas four times more often than did those with only 650 ppb or less. PCBs are polychlorinated biphenyls, a family of toxic resins used as lubricants, adhesives, and coatings for paper, wood, and concrete. For years they've been known to be toxic to fish and to cause skin diseases in humans. In 2002 a study at the Baylor College of Medicine established yet another link, this one between human lymphomas and a monkey virus present in 43 percent of B-cell lymphoma patients; this virus appears in no more than 6 percent of healthy subjects and those with other types of cancer. The virus, SV40, was traced to contaminated batches of polio vaccine administered to some thirty million people between 1955 and 1963.

Everybody wants to know what caused his or her cancer when it isn't obvious. A cartoon in Mel Greaves's book on cancer and evolution shows a caveman and cavewoman in their grotto surrounded by children. The woman says, "How can we *prevent* pregnancy? We don't even know what *causes* it!"

· · ·

When you have cancer, its cause becomes of secondary importance; your mind is totally and wonderfully focused on the hangman's noose, and you concentrate on getting rid of it. When you do *not* have cancer, you tend to ignore the advice of people like Samuel Epstein, the outspoken M.D. at the University of Illinois at Chicago, who feels the government should favor prevention over research. Crusades against lead, asbestos, and other known carcinogens, especially tobacco smoke, have diminished only slightly the incidence of organ cancers in recent years. Yet lymphoma and melanoma are epidemic. Since 1950 non-Hodgkin's lymphoma (NHL) has increased about 4 percent per year, resulting in some sixty thousand new cases annually in the United States and about three hundred thousand new cases worldwide.

Reading that, I thought that someone—maybe the United Nations World Health Organization—could conduct a global epidemiological study to highlight the world's lymphoma belts and then correlate the environmental differences among them. One German review of sixty-four regional studies confirmed a strong trend toward non-Hodgkin's lymphoma epidemics in industrialized countries. However, the numerous diseases associated with an impaired immune system, such as HIV and other viral infections that may turn into lymphomas, explained only a small percentage of the upsurge in NHL. Nor did smoking or nutritional factors have much to do with it.

Another study blamed not the smoke and pollution of industrialization but simply the higher socioeconomic regions of Western societies. Why? One hypothesis is that children raised in poor places develop immunity to diseases because they are exposed to infectious organisms at a young age, whereas more-affluent kids grow up in hygienic conditions and don't develop as great a defense. Immunologists point out that, if it weren't for the hundred trillion bacteria and countless viruses terrorizing our systems, no soldiers of our immune system would be recruited and cloned for defense against the really harmful pathogens that invade us from time to time.

I have had so many strep throats throughout my life that I sometimes feel like a heroin addict until I get my shot—in my case, penicillin. At one of our Saturday night dinners with the Pejics, Leslie told of her own lifetime annoyance with strep throats. She wondered with me whether infections can trigger the complex chain of genetic events that lead to cancer—or maybe the opposite.

There is one infection known to contribute to cancer. Some 90 percent of "mucosa-associated lymphoid tissue" (MALT) lymphomas are caused by the bacterium *Helicobacter pylori,* and antibiotics cure about 50 percent of the cases. *H. pylori* lives in the guts of half the world's population. By comparison, Leslie's and my nemesis of *Streptococcus* was rather benign—not leading to cancer but merely standing by to stab us in our throats whenever our defenses are lowered, for instance, by a missed night's sleep.

"We're both lucky we haven't become antibiotic resistant," I said.

"Well, luck is relative," she said. "Like the scientist who discovers a disease by catching it."

Leslie smiled her intelligent smile and added another ingredient to the stew of prevention. "Lots of studies have shown recently that sleep deprivation is much more dangerous than previously believed," she said. "Even one night of missed sleep lowers levels of natural killer white blood cells. Although they are replenished with additional sleep, continual lack of sleep can lead to illness."

I thought of the mindset of those who conducted these studies and recalled the mathematician and philosopher Alfred North Whitehead's famous and not entirely tongue-in-cheek comment: *It requires a very unusual mind to undertake the analysis of the obvious.* It does. I remembered our Island for Science marine biologists telling me that shrimp grow faster in the longer light of summer than in winter and especially longer than in winters of higher latitudes. The research led to the discovery that white-blood-cell counts of shrimp and fish decrease when their sleep cycles are interrupted by artificially changed patterns of light and dark. Now separate evidence from sleep researchers at the University of Chicago, Northwestern University, Washington State University, and elsewhere shows that insufficient sleep in humans causes the malfunction of hormones important for repairing tissue and fighting cancer as well as infections.

Neurobiologists at Northwestern's Sleep Center believe sleep allows cells time to process information both in the brain and in other organs, including the immune system. So far they have discovered nine genes responsible for the circadian rhythm—the biological cycles recurring each day—genes that exist throughout the body, not just in the brain. They believe that sleep dysfunction should be included in the growing list of factors that may lead to the onset or proliferation of cancer. Because most cancer patients have difficulty sleeping well, effective sleeping aids without hangover or addiction ought to be added to the cancer fighter's arsenal.

Insufficient sleep, solar and other radiation, longevity, and everything involved in the modern lifestyle interact in complex ways to mutate our genes. The result is the expansion of cancer: unnatural death.

The bizarre acceptance of cancer in our society, however—the acquiescence of being condemned to the gallows with no crime, no trial, no jury, and no defense lawyers, yet sentenced to cruel and unusual punishment ending in certain death—is another story. It is one that can be told in the context of alternative medicines, the desperation felt by cancer patients to try anything, even therapies based on superstition.

12

Alternative Magic

MY BROTHER AND I DID NOT GROW UP IN A SUPERSTITIOUS HOUSE-
hold. It became that way after I left. It was Jay who began to embrace astrology and numerology well after I had graduated from college, married, and
moved to Indiana. Carol and I stayed in close touch with him; Chicago is
little more than an hour away.

Jay's superstition began in his attempts to stop a constant, brutal headache, far worse than a migraine because it became permanent. The headache, which he described as "an axe buried in my skull," had descended upon
him like a malevolent and turbulent cloud after the rigors of the University
of Chicago Medical School and two residencies, one in general surgery and
the other in orthopedics. For ten years this relentless pain left him depressed
and incapable of work. He tried prescription drugs, including psychophar-
maceuticals, as well as psychotherapy; he visited physicians in many branches
of medicine, considered and rejected suicide, and went to India to spend a
few months among swamies and acupuncturists. He never visited medical
research laboratories, though, despite my urgings to do so.

"There are things in this world undreamed of by modern science!" he
would tell me, his younger brother, in defense. The swami influence.

Toward the end of those long and painful years, he came to eschew both
talk therapy and psychodrugs, experimenting instead with various "alternative" therapies such as eating organic vegetables and herbal extracts that

he believed would alter the balance of the neurotransmitters in his brain. During his thirties and early forties—completely isolated from medical colleagues, friends, and his family except for Mother—he read extensively about astrology and numerology.

Jay became an allergist, with himself as his only patient. He abandoned the usual foods and ate collards, kale, soybeans, breadfruit, loquats, tamarinds, pomegranates, macadamias, lychee nuts, and whatever other vegetables and fruits he could find, taking them one at a time. If a specific food made him feel slightly better, he would note the time and date and look for the concordance of planets or a pattern of time-date numbers, applying those findings to a regimen of exercise, eating, sleeping, reading, and eating again. Gradually the axelike pain cleaving his head diminished. After a few years the pain stopped completely. It was hard to argue with success, for he was no longer in pain, and his depression was only a dark memory.

Unfortunately, the constant diet of raw food produced severe colitis, which he refused to heed, trying other leafy vegetables instead but constantly losing weight. Finally, when his six-foot-two body dropped to 110 pounds, he became so weak that my father carried him against his will to the University of Chicago hospital. Two surgeons spent eight hours picking out his disintegrated colon with tweezers. They emerged from the operating room, mad as hell, and told us that there was no reason not to have treated his colitis earlier, no reason to have waited so long, and that now, despite his having had no cancer, he would have to wear a colostomy bag for the rest of his life.

As an allergist, though, Jay reveled in his colostomy, claiming it was a gift from God. He regained his weight and became an enthusiastic eater, for now he could see the results of digesting various foods before they were churned beyond recognition in the usual way through the intestinal tract. In explaining digestion, he resorted increasingly to numerology. Those experiments on himself extended to treating our mother, using nutritional approaches to relieve her symptoms of arthritis and macular degeneration.

Finally, in his midforties, Jay began to work again. The patients he attracted were middle-aged men and women who had found no relief from standard treatments for their cancers, heart fibrillations, kidney disease, diabetes, or back pains. In this country, according to one study, oncologists spend less than two minutes with their patients during an office visit (although the patients believe that they spend ten minutes). Jay would spend *hours,* sometimes all day, with one patient, taking a medical history and examining complaints in minute detail. For all his work, Jay charged nothing. His patients, oblivious to the placebo effect, regularly announced themselves cured. They revered him, and they reinforced his belief in his methods. Jay was never happier than when a patient responded favorably to his treatments, whatever the reason. His eyes would light up, and he would smile with an inner glow, delighted that there were doctors in the world who cared and that he was one of them.

Carol and I drove from northern Indiana every few months during the last half of the century to visit my parents and Jay in the old three-story colonial house they shared on Chicago's South Side. If the lights were on, we would stop first at my father's dental office, which he had built himself, an annex to the garage, where he would be casting gold inlays or organizing X rays after a day's work. He would complain about Jay's not charging patients, the waste of Jay's brilliant mind and M.D. degree, and the way Mother and Jay increasingly excluded him from their lives. Afterward the three of us would enter the house to find Jay's evening patients (he worked mostly at night) strewn like corpses on the floor of the living room while Jay, the only one standing, surveyed the scene. Now and then Dr. Jay would bend over a horizontal body, extract a drop of blood from a right ear, and insert a suspected allergen in the patient's mouth. The allergens, tried one at a time, might be a piece of white bread, a bit of hamburger meat, or a sip of whiskey or coffee—substances the patient had said were prominent in his diet.

Seeing us, Jay would smile in recognition and then adjourn briefly to his laboratory, which he had set up in an adjacent wing of the house. There, amid tubes and glassware, he would analyze, or titrate, the blood, much as you measure the hardness or chlorine content in a swimming pool, by adding known amounts of reagents until a certain color is achieved. After the suspected allergen had been digested by a patient, in about an hour, Jay would take a blood drop from the left ear and titrate the second sample. In this way he sought to determine foods or other substances to which these people were allergic. Jay believed he had discovered a previously unknown yin-yang process in which an allergen that relieved one set of symptoms would initiate others.

So far, so good, although as I came to know some of these patients, I noticed that they shared his belief in alien UFOs, astrology, and various psychic phenomena. The patients, given short shrift by orthodox physicians, were delighted with this doctor's lengthy and free attentions.

• • •

After David received his Ph.D. from Princeton and began teaching at the University of Illinois, the whole family would get together on holidays. Jay—introverted yet garrulous at times, clutching a cup of rose-hip tea—would corner David and me to explain his latest theory. In excruciating detail. Afterwards we would urge him to consult with his peers, publish his results, and proceed along the lines of normal scientific investigation. Jay always demurred, answering that the orthodox medical establishment would never accept his findings.

One day Carol and I found out why.

We entered the usual scene of supine bodies distributed about the living room, with Jay stepping among them, tending to one and then another like a battlefield surgeon. This time we noticed that, after taking a drop of a patient's blood, he went not to his lab, as he usually did, but upstairs, where Mother was reading in her bedroom. He hurried back down and jotted something in the journal he kept on the patient. After the last of his disciples had gone home, I asked him what was going on. Jay took me upstairs into his office, which had been my bedroom for the few months after Dad bought the house and before I started college.

He glanced briefly around, as though making sure that no one was eavesdropping, grinned puckishly, and said, "Don't tell anyone what I'm about to tell you, except maybe Carol and David, because I could lose my license, but . . . well . . . you *know* our mother is psychic . . ."

"She's about as psychic as my cat," I said with as ingratiating a smile as I could manage.

"I don't know how psychic your cat is, but Mother definitely is psychic. She is an *unknowing savant!*"

"Isn't that *idiot* savant? As in this idea of yours?" I knew what was coming.

"There's *no doubt* that she is psychic!" Jay said.

Superstitious, I thought, not psychic.

Jay regarded me closely, as if reading my negative thought. "I'll convince you later," he said. "What I've been doing for the last six months is compiling a list of eight suspected allergens that I identify when I do a workup of each patient's medical history. Then, instead of the laborious process of trying each allergen and titrating his blood, I ask Mother for a number from one to eight."

"Why not one to nine? Or one to ten—a nice round number?"

His nostrils flared, and he wrinkled his forehead. "There's a . . . problem with the number nine." He saw me take a brief look at the door, like a boxer craving his corner. "Look, Neil, I know this sounds crazy to you," he said while I shook my head in agreement. He had been eating garlic cloves, which may have been healthful as he claimed, but as I moved away from the odor, he unconsciously pursued me step by step until my back was against a wall of books. "But *it works!*" he said, referring not to the garlic, of which he was oblivious, but to his numerological strategies. "If you don't think so, ask these patients! I'm *curing* them, of all kinds of things—*including cancer!*"

"Well, you ought to publish a scientific paper on it," I said.

I stole a look around his office, which was lined to the ceiling with bookshelves containing medical texts and journals. Interspersed among them various titles leapt out like dark and dangerous panthers: *Spiritual Scientists, Reincarnation and Immortality, Alchemy through the Ages, A Guide to Psychic Awareness, The Rosicrucian Supply Bureau, What Occurs after Death.* Many of his books discussed "Gemini" because that was his astrological sign (Jay was born between May 21 and June 21) and—especially—numerology. Disconnected from peers, from the world, he was drowning in a sea of numbers. He weighed everything he and Mother ate and filled hundreds of journals with numbers gleaned from patients: numbers for grams of certain foods, numbers for the times of ingestion, and numbers for dosages, drugs administered, moods, emotions, and physical abilities. Numerology, the study of the occult meanings of numbers and their supposed influence on human life, became his fountainhead, his sacred machine.

Numerology springs from seemingly significant coincidences. For instance, consider the attack on the World Trade Center: not only do the date's digits coincide with those of the 911 emergency number, but if you add these three digits together, you get 11, which mimics the shape of the towers. Nor is that all: September 11 is the 254th day of the year, which digits also add up to 11, New York is the 11th state in the union, and so on. "Spooky stuff!" say numerologists. Of course, you can manipulate numbers to come up with just about anything—*provided you are unrestricted as to what you reveal.* Type anything into your computer and play around with it until you find something weird. Someone did that using Microsoft Word, entering "Q33 NY" (ostensibly the flight number of the second plane to hit the World Trade Center), changing the type size to twenty-six points, and accessing the first set of Wingdings, for no other reason than such contrivances result in these creepy symbols:

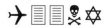

. . .

The way my brother, a member of Phi Beta Kappa, an educated man, descended from orthodox medicine to the dungeon of nonsense was not far different from the way desperate people with cancer and other incurable diseases have ignored the lessons of the last five hundred years and fall for magnet therapy, energy fields and auras, therapeutic nontouch, astrology, and other myths. One of the problems is faulty logic. Like Jay, cancer patients often confuse a hypothesis with a result or a conditional with its converse. If a true believer moves her hands close to your head and feels a tingling sensation, she assumes she is "interrupting your energy flow," a gush whose existence biology denies. Because serotonin helped Jay sleep, he believed a dearth of serotonin in the body must *cause* insomnia. Cause confused with effect. It's an easy mistake to make. Because whiskey lowers blood pressure, does a lack of alcohol in the bloodstream cause hypertension?

Mother's entry into Jay's superstitions was easy to trace. She was "sensitive," as the hypnotists put it. Gullible. Carol, Dad, Mother, and I once attended a demonstration of hypnotism. The hypnotist requested that the entire audience of about five hundred smiling people stand up, reach as high as possible, and clasp both hands together tightly. He talked softly, telling us that we could not retract our arms until he used the word *now*. At length he said, "Those who can, put your arms down and be seated."

We took our seats as Mother continued to stand, transfixed, her face contorted, arms extended, hands clasped. "Neil," she said over her shoulder, "I can't move my arms!" I looked around the audience. Here and there a dozen people stood in similar straits until the hypnotist uttered his planted word: *now*!

Over time Jay had convinced Mother that she was psychic. My father's seething censure served only to drive her and Jay closer together and away from him. If each unhappy family is unhappy in its own way, as Tolstoy tells us, the unhappiness in this family gave a new meaning to the word *unique.* Long arguments over almost everything, especially astrology, ensued between my father on one side and Mother and Jay on the other. Dad would argue that astrology is baloney, an argument from ignorance, the opposite of science, making predictions sufficiently vague that believers simply modify the facts to fit their beliefs.

Astrologer Jay would repeat variations on the theme that "it works for us!"

One day Jay told me he had discovered a new system in the body, born coincidentally, I remembered, though he must have forgotten, of a conversation we'd had when transistors first were developed. Jay then had asked me to explain to him the plus-negative-plus junctions in diodes. That explanation contributed to his "discovery" of an unknown semiconductor system in the body, beyond the electron flow of cells, an eerie kind of biological alternating-current flow with low resistance in one direction and high resistance in the other—the human body as radio.

Jay quacked his way through life, predictably refusing to share his "research" with medical colleagues. After Dad died at age 83, and before Mother died at 93, she and Jay had seven years without interference. During that time they were in constant consultation with each other, filling hundreds of notebooks with numbers that applied to themselves, to Jay's growing number of patients, and to trading stock futures.

When Mother died, Jay was left with no supplier of "psychic numbers," and he had lost almost all his inheritance to stockbrokers. He solved the first problem by spending as much as $5,000 a month on "telephone psychics." He would phone a dozen times a day to ask these pretenders to pick a number from one to eight, which he would apply to the foods he ate and the order in which he ate them. He solved the second problem by letting Carol and me sell the house for him and find him an apartment near a hospital.

When I urged him to stop the costly psychic phoning, he said, "It's my only expense other than a little food. The psychics help me live." He then added, "You don't think that I *like* being like this, not being able to eat, not going out, meeting women, marrying, having a family?"

He had never said anything like that to me before, and it made me see this life, the life of my only brother, from a new perspective. A sad perception. Jay could not enjoy the simple pleasures—companionship other than a medical relationship, parties, or the sports he used to love. He had been a skier and once ran a marathon. Even in his sixties he still jogged two or three miles each night. Jay had relinquished normalcy not because of some religious shame or guilt but because the experiments he had performed on himself over the years had been successful. He had cured himself of his severe headaches, and according to his faithful patients, he had cured many of their cancers and other incurable diseases. The numbers suggested to him that he could absorb his food better after exercise and when lying on his side, but his vegetarian meals, though large and varied, failed to provide sufficient protein to his ravaged, colonless digestion. He had disintegrated to the point where he could eat only by numerology.

Jay began a long series of hospitalizations, demanding intravenous feeding, being discharged when his welcome wore thin, returning to his apartment for a few weeks, then trying another hospital and another sympathetic doctor, usually one whom he'd known in medical school. A year later, in October 1997, my emaciated and haggard sixty-nine-year-old brother was admitted to the University of Chicago hospital for the last time. Carol, David, and I were with him at the end, urging him to try harder. I talked to Jay about some of the fun we'd had together as children, hiding my sadness that his once-promising life had come to this, that he hadn't known much happiness. Toward evening he smiled at us, glanced heavenward, and said goodbye. The hospital certificate listed pneumonia as the cause of death, but that was only his final disease. My brother died of superstition.

• • •

Before cancer disrupted my life, I had tried in a small way, by writing magazine articles and books, to stem the flood of belief in UFOs and magic. Superstitions have become epidemic in our society, despite scientific marvels such as reaching the moon and understanding the complexities of the human body. I also joined a remarkable organization working to restore rationality to a world tilting dangerously backward to beliefs in magic. Called the Committee for the Scientific Investigation of Claims of the Paranormal, or CSICOP, it was started in 1976 by my friend Isaac Asimov and various science writers and included among its principals the famous magician James Randi, author Martin Gardner, Nobel physics laureate Murray Gell-Mann, Carl Sagan, and other men and women of science.

One day in 1998, a few months before my lymphoma struck, I had lunch in Ft. Lauderdale with James Randi, who, while he was talking to divert my attention—even *telling* me he was diverting my attention—casually dropped his napkin over a large saltshaker, fondled it a little, and placed his hands on his lap. The napkin slowly floated flat; the saltshaker holding it up had disappeared. "The Amazing Randi"—humorous, dexterous, white-bearded like a balding Santa Claus—runs a foundation that uncovers the frauds of the clairvoyant, the communicators with the dead, and the spoon benders and other "telekinetics," to whom he offers a million-dollar prize if they can prove their paranormalcy under controlled conditions. Despite repeated attempts, no one has won the prize, which rests in escrow in a New York bank, earning interest.

In one of his repeated experiments, Jim Randi has a high-school teacher announce to a class that this man in the white beard is a highly accurate astrologer. The teacher already has had the students write down their places and dates of birth, and Jim then takes from his briefcase a bunch of envelopes, each envelope containing an individual's "astrological documentation" as well as the horoscope he has prepared for that student. The students read their horoscopes. "You are intense, you strive for attention, you have a sound if not analytical mind." Almost all tell the white-bearded "astrologer" that the horoscope is accurate for them. Then Randi has the students pass their horoscopes to the person seated behind them.

The students are stunned. Randi reveals who he really is, a stage magician turned debunker of the pseudosciences. No amount of argument could be more effective than this stunt, for he had placed the exact same horoscope in each envelope!

We don't have enough James Randis to visit all the schools. And we don't have enough teachers who take the time to explain to their young students how superstition started with early man's ignorance as a way to explain the world and how it continues not because everyday phenomena still can't be explained but because the superstitious don't take the considerable time and effort required to understand what is known, what is real. Science works. Astrology, numerology, other superstitions do not work.

The first time you walk beneath a ladder and an automobile breaks your leg, you might not connect the two, but if an accident occurs every time you walk under a ladder—or if you were ladder-conditioned by your parents—you begin to blame the ladder for your misfortune. It's called conditioning and involves reinforcement. Superstitions are reinforced daily by stories repeated on television and other mass media until they become embedded in our culture, despite the progress of science, despite our pervasive technology, despite our easy access to information.

• • •

Since 1998, as I began searching medical laboratories for experimental lymphoma cures, I was battered from two equally unscientific sides. On one side were chemotherapists refusing to try harmless biological therapies, apparently happy with only short-term results. On the other were patients who, hearing of the horrors of chemo and despairing of orthodox medicine, were willing to try anything else to rid themselves of cancer, including "alternative medicines"—a rather distinguished term for a hodgepodge of mostly nonsense. Four of ten Americans use an alternative therapy today, up from one out of three a decade ago. In what has become a growth industry, Americans spend some $23 billion annually on lymphatic massage, replacements for mercury amalgam fillings, breathing exercises, holistic medicine, chelation therapy, and such quackery as unblocking the energy flow of "meridians" unknown to physiologists.

Maybe we should call this field "alternatoid" medicine to distinguish it from monoclonal antibodies, gene therapies, and other leading-edge technologies that are becoming alternatives to chemotherapy and radiation for cancer. In 1998 our truly representative Congress established the National Center for Complementary and Alternative Medicine, giving it $78 million a year to study the efficacy of alternatoid claims. So far fewer than a dozen controlled studies have been conducted, although recruiting patients for sixty clinical trials is underway. These studies include comparisons of shark cartilage to chemotherapy for lung cancer, megadoses of vitamins in the prevention of recurrent bladder carcinomas, and the effect of herbs, meditation, spiritual healing, and massage for woman at high risk for breast cancer. The results, when they come, will be instructive either way—making public which "alternatives" prove efficacious or worthless.

Herbal medicines, better diets, and vitamins often are lumped together into "alternative medicines," which skews the issue, for these are sensible treatments pursued by 70 percent of adults with cancer and are far from magic. A majority of compounds used in orthodox medicines were discovered in plants, and many herbal preventatives should not be thought of as quack treatments, such as blowing ozone into the rectum or eating ground-up tortoise shells. Sure, there are a few harmful herbs, such as kava, which has been linked to liver damage. Most herbs are safe, however, and some, such as saw palmetto (which relieves the advance of benign enlarged prostates) and antioxidants (which help prevent macular and other degenerations), are entering mainstream medicine. If you can determine that an herbal medicine will do no harm and that it has some basis in science, why not try it for prevention? The safety and scientific evidence for specific herbs eventually will emerge from clinical trials, but there seems no compelling reason to wait. The questionable alternatoid practices based on magic, however, are screaming to be resolved for a gullible public.

If we as a society are going to cure cancer, live healthier lives, and stop the ignorance and zealotry that give rise to terrorism—if we are going to move truly into the twenty-first century—we are going to have to educate the world, starting at home. A recent National Science Foundation poll revealed that 70 percent of American adults, including parents and teachers, do not understand the scientific process, 60 percent think that some people possess extrasensory perception, and 43 percent believe that UFOs come to earth bearing aliens. It is not sufficient to point out the illogic of magic. We have to educate the purveyors of those who have taken charge of our primary mechanism of adult education in this country: the media. We have to start objecting and laugh them out of business.

At a time when our technological civilization depends upon truth, when terrorists are turning their superstitions about paradise into warfare, how can we afford to regard *any* superstitions as harmless? How can we afford not to understand science? Aristotle's admonition was never truer than in our time, that "the educated differ from the uneducated as much as the living from the dead."

You need only to glance at television to realize that superstition is a preoccupation of American media and talk shows. They treat scientific and quackpot theories equally. It is the democratic way, politically correct. They believe there must be something to astrology, for instance, since it has lasted for three thousand years. (They could make the same claim for rhinoceros horns restoring male potency.) Almost every newspaper in the country carries a horoscope column; few run science columns. Horoscopes are just harmless diversions, aren't they? Like someone's asking your sign of the zodiac at a party? Like avoiding the number thirteen? Like Jay's receiving numbers from a psychic hotline?

Many big newspapers, especially the *Wall Street Journal* and the *New York Times,* do a superb job in reporting health science and technology. Those are exceptions. Most mass media, especially the ones from which the majority of Americans receive their continuing education—television and the movies—fail to distinguish between science and quackery. One day you'll see a story about cancer vaccines; the next day there's one about an exorcism. Television and movies are obsessed with ghosts, vampires, extraterrestrial abductions, alien-built pyramids, spirits, past-life regressions . . . there's no end to the nonsense. Phil Donahue holds the title for promoting medical and nutritional quackery. Oprah did a show on a dentist who has done thousands of past-life regressions. Sally Jessy Raphael loved to interview "unusual guests," such as "psychic surgery" experts. Today television brings us séances, ghosts in Gettysburg, psychic lectures in California, and a weekly feature called *Beyond,* whose host brags, "When the dead speak, I listen."

Energetically knowledgeable of things political, historical, and cultural, most TV hosts, writers, producers, and journalists blithely accept pseudoscience. Yet these are the predominant teachers of our society. They grab audience attention more effectively than does any high school or university educator on earth, using fabulous imagery and programming, the best that technology offers. Who is to blame for their lack of knowledge about the way the world works, for their promulgation of our culture of superstition? I blame the universities that allow journalism and humanities students to avoid "difficult" science, because these schools of advanced learning could change things. Universities *could* insist that humanities students enroll in not just one or two science classes but special courses specifically designed to combat superstitions, teaching the hard-won truths that have replaced pseudosciences over the centuries. Nothing like that is done today. Departments of journalism populate the media with intelligent, sharp, penetrating reporters, writers, and editors—who at the same time are scientific morons.

Too strong a term?

It may be too weak. On the intelligence-quotient scale, 100 is the norm; a genius is defined as having an IQ above 140. The earlier days of IQ testing added the following categories: moron (51–70), imbecile (26–50), and idiot (0–25). In an attempt to measure the lack of science education among those who will shape the primary adult educational process of most people in the United States, I asked a professor at Northwestern University's Medill School of Journalism to give to juniors and seniors a simple high-school-level science quiz. I chose Northwestern, my alma matter, because its journalism school continues to maintain a valuable premise: even the best writer needs something to write about, so students are required to take a second major. Mine was science. Most other j-school students studied political "science," history, or government, which continue to be favored by journalism students throughout the country.

Here are the questions David and I chose to represent various branches of science. The quiz was given to journalism students at both Northwestern and the University of Illinois (see the notes for answers):

1. What is the name of the molecule consisting of two atoms of hydrogen and one of oxygen?
2. What is the most common element?
3. What is the significance of the number pi (3.14)?
4. Why is the sun at sunset reddish orange and at noon relatively white?
5. How far is the moon from earth?
6. Where do legumes get their nitrogen?
7. How old is the solar system?
8. Which is larger, a bacterium or a virus?
9. What are the two major gases in the air and their percentages?
10. How is lift created by an airplane's wings?
11. Name the four states of matter.
12. Which is geologically older, sand or rock?

13. Define a mammal by listing the four characteristics all mammals have.
14. What is the approximate air pressure at sea level?
15. What is the closest star to the moon?

Admittedly, the quiz doesn't yield a precise evaluation of scientific literacy, but it gives a rough indication. On the science-IQ equivalence scale, journalism students fall into the range of scientific morons—just barely. These budding journalists averaged only 5.08 correct out of 15, scoring just above the imbecile level, if it were a standard intelligence test. I doubt that career journalists, further in years from school, know much more about how the world works.

But I have no doubt whatsoever that these senior journalists, talk-show hosts, and scriptwriters know their astrological signs.

13

Allies in the Quest

SO FAR I HAD LEARNED ABOUT MONOCLONAL ANTIBODIES, THE ROLE of cyclin D1 in regulating cancer progression, lymphoma vaccines to be taken *after* cancer lays claim to your body, dendrites, co-stimulation of T cells, anti-angiogenesis (at least a little), and the possible causes of lymphoma. If there were cures for me in this collection of theories and biotherapies, vetted in countless experiments, I would have to dig for them like diamonds lost under a snowdrift.

The Mabs continued to intrigue me because several already were FDA approved, and I regarded them as a currency with which to buy time without destroying my immune system until a truly curative molecular-targeted therapy came along. Mabs were being made throughout the United States and Europe for diverse cancers, an inchoate but definitely strengthening force. Unfortunately, clinical oncologists at the time thought that Rituxan offered no hope for mantle-cell lymphoma patients. Yet because this one Mab had been approved for use against lymphoma, I reasoned that there must be dozens more in the pipelines of the nation's pharmaceutical companies.

The creators of monoclonal antibodies were not the big drug companies. The Mab makers lay embedded among the thirteen hundred biotech companies in the United States. We visited one of these in April 1999, Peregrine Pharmaceuticals, in California's Orange County. Named after the patron saint of cancer sufferers, the company had developed Oncolym, a radioactive antibody that could prove effective against my lymphoma.

Originally created by Alan Epstein, an M.D. and Ph.D. at the University of Southern California (USC), Oncolym also is called "Lym-1" because Epstein also has been researching a related antibody called "Lym-2." Both are named after lymphoma. Like all Mabs, these "lyms" attach to specific markers on the surfaces of cells. Unlike many others, Oncolym attaches not to the CD20 cell marker but to a marker called "HLA-DR10" (human lymphocyte antigen, subclass D for receptor number 10). While anti-CD20 agents such as the radioactive Zevalin and Bexxar are directed specifically to the sites of lymphoma, they still destroy many normal B cells as they go about their work annihilating cancer cells. The beauty of Oncolym is that it binds to cells found almost exclusively in cancerous tissue and targets many closely related HLA-DRs in addition to number 10. It seemed more harmless than the other radio-Mabs and ought to be useful against a broad range of lymphomas.

Among the scientists Carol and I met at Peregrine was Missag Hagop Parseghian, an eager young Ph.D. molecular biologist of Armenian heritage who became a close ally in my quest for treatment. Tall, thin, and fair-skinned, Missag was unusually cordial and devoted to his research, which is primarily directing Peregrine's research department to turn Epstein's original Mab into a marketable and approved pharmaceutical. Unfortunately, everyone's lymphoma is unique, and none of these Mabs comes close to being a universal therapy. Missag told us that investigators at UC San Francisco had developed a blood test to reveal whether any one person's lymphoma would respond to Oncolym. He gave me the name of the designated scientist there, Larry Rose, so I could send him a sample of my blood.

Missag also described another radioactive Mab they were developing at Peregrine called "Cotara," which sounded quite amazing. Unlike other monoclonal antibodies that attach to cells via their surface markers, this one targets *the dead cells found in the center of any growing tumor.*

"These dead, or necrotic, cells are invariably ruptured," Missag explained with contagious enthusiasm. "So they allow easy access of the antibodies to their nuclei. Once inside the dead center of the tumors, radioactive antibodies bombard nearby living cancer cells without harming healthy tissue. The cancer cells then die off from the radiation."

He paused to take three cans of soda from a tiny refrigerator and handed one to each of us. Taking quick sips, he added, "But that's not all! When the cancer cells die, they also become future targets for the Cotara antibodies. In other words, the newly dead cells *let the antibodies in*—and then the whole process starts over again. Thus a tumor, regardless of origin, can be destroyed from the inside out, in a kind of cellular guerrilla warfare!"

By 2002 Cotara, initially for brain cancer, had progressed into phase-three clinical trials.

The "tumor-necrosis therapy" of Cotara and Oncolym aren't Peregrine's only ideas, Missag told us. Working with Philip Thorpe, a professor at the University of Texas at Dallas, the biotech company is also developing vascular-targeting agents. These are antibodies fused to compounds that cut off the blood supply to tumors by selectively forming blood clots in the tumor's blood vessels, thereby making it impossible for the vessels to provide oxygen and nutrients to the tumors themselves. The result would parallel anti-angiogenesis—denying the tumor any blood—but would be produced in a different way.

• • •

California seemed to me to be the country's most advanced state in both cancer research and patient activism. In fact, our primary purpose of this trip was to meet an outstanding woman, Ellen Glesby Cohen, the founder and president of the Lymphoma Research Foundation of America, based in Los Angeles. She had called me a dozen times after David Granet, the originator of the MCL Group, had told her about my travels to research laboratories, finally asking me to join her board of directors. She explained that, like other foundations, hers lacked "talent scouts" to find research projects to fund, primarily those with short time horizons.

Carol and I met Ellen at her home on the west side of Los Angeles, a graceful two-story house surrounded at the time by workmen and trucks bearing plants. We drove up in our rented car to find her barefoot, wearing jeans, coming in from her new garden, where she had been planting bushes. Her brown hair tousled and her face free of makeup, Ellen was in her late forties. Unpretentious. Attractive in her naturalness. Talking to her, it was easy to see how she had been successful in transferring her enthusiasm for the foundation to others. The idea for the foundation, she said, came fourteen years ago when, pregnant with her second child, she was diagnosed as having lymphoma. The original diagnosis was inaccurate—as is usually the case. She was told initially that she had small-cell lymphoma.

"That was my oncologist's first guess too," I said.

She smiled knowingly. "My son, Josh, was born healthy," she told us, "and I was so happy with him and with my eighteen-month daughter, I couldn't believe I had a serious disease. After all, small-cell lymphoma stays indolent, right?"

"Sure, until they tell you it's something worse," Carol said.

"I really felt strange at that time," Ellen continued. "I'll never forget being unable to stop my hand from touching my neck, checking to see if there were even more swollen lymph nodes. My husband, Mitch, is a physician—internal medicine—and he dragged me to an oncologist. 'Oh, my God!' said the oncologist, 'you've got swollen lymph nodes everywhere!' Well, after more tests they told me I had CLL, chronic lymphocytic leukemia, which is classified sometimes as lymphoma, sometimes as leukemia."

Carol's pained expression reflected our similar ordeal. Like me, Ellen Cohen had taken an active role in fighting lymphoma, though one quite different from mine. Talking to her reduced the sense of isolation that Carol and I still felt, and that all cancer patients feel, of being hit with a spotlight, singled out on the stage of life disruption. I could feel the despair retreating from Carol's heart as she heard Ellen's tale of tenacity.

"I didn't know enough not to take chemotherapy for CLL," Ellen said, "like you did for MCL, Neil. No one did then. The first chemo course gave me a high fever, and I landed in the hospital with a collapsed immune system. I developed 'neutropenia,' lack of sufficient white blood cells, so severe there were hardly any left in my body. . . . Anyway, I recovered, but only to take more and more chemo every few years afterwards."

Ellen told us that some hundred thousand Americans get lymphoid malignancies every year, with a 50 percent mortality rate, yet no new treatment options had appeared in the twenty years before she started the foundation. "The very idea made me mad as hell. So I started calling friends and acquaintances, and the next thing you know we incorporated the Lymphoma Research Foundation of America."

Ellen Cohen's startup of the foundation was a story of perseverance. Almost single-handedly she raised money and eventually achieved recognition for the foundation, which helped countless lymphoma patients learn about their disease, lobbied Congress, and awarded grants to postdoctoral fellows at universities. (In 2002 it doubled in size by combining with another nonprofit foundation in New York, dropped the words "of America," and now raises about $5 million a year, mostly for educational purposes.)

That evening Ellen took us to a gathering at the home of one of her directors, who was a helpful psychiatrist, knowledgeable about lymphoma. Behind his floor-to-ceiling windows overlooking a deep, lighted canyon, we had dinner with a half-dozen medical scientists, including Oncolym's inventor Alan Epstein and his USC colleague Ann Mohrbacher. Both M.D.s, they were now working on a cousin of the "lyms" that would specifically target CLL.

"Like Bexxar and Zevalin, our 'lyms' are radiolabeled," Ann explained. That is, the antibodies are coupled to radioisotopes because, I had found, they are not sufficiently effective alone. "So there is some concern that you can injure surrounding white blood cells or their precursors in the bone marrow. Not as indiscriminate as chemotherapy, but still not perfect."

Alan Epstein—a big, powerful-looking man, gray-haired, older than his slender, brunet colleague Ann—said his newer versions of these antibodies might work well as immune-system enhancers even without radioactivity. These naked Mabs were similar in their nonradioactivity to Rituxan but better, he thought, because he had shown them to be extremely active against lymphoma cells, including MCL—at least in Petri dishes. "We're testing them in clinical trials in China," he said.

"Why China?" I asked.

"The Chinese are interested; they've offered funding," Dr. Epstein said.

That dinner was also where I met UCLA's Jon Braun, who looked the way I imagined a medical scientist ought to look. Slight, thin, eyes bristling with the excitement of his work, he wore his facial hair somewhere between stubble and a short beard. Jon is an unassuming, brilliant M.D. and Ph.D. in molecular engineering. He uses a high degree of eye contact, is joyful without being lighthearted, and his voice holds a rich tone. He later became a close friend.

It was an interesting, highly intellectual party, made all the more enjoyable because the day was Carol's and my wedding anniversary.

A few days afterwards I attended one of the foundation's board meetings, held at night so that the directors who lived in southern California wouldn't have to miss work. Most of the directors were middle-aged lawyers, brokers, or businessmen. One psychiatrist. One oncologist, who functioned as the scientific review committee. No other scientists. I was elected to the board with some misgivings on my part, for the quarterly meetings were devoted exclusively to fund-raising and other commercial problems of running a foundation, whereas my private agenda involved investigating new cancer research. During the following months, however, Ellen and I talked almost daily by phone, and the subject invariably centered on emerging research that could benefit lymphoma victims.

"We have never funded a research project as such," she said during one of these conversations.

I was astounded. "But the Lymphoma *Research* Founda—"

"Oh, we fund research all right, but only by backing the studies of young M.D.s or Ph.D.s starting out. I think now we're ready to extend our efforts to actual projects of senior scientists that could lead to more-immediate therapies, which is why I wanted you on board."

"I notice you never use the word *cure*," I said.

"They'd tar and feather me," she said. "If we've learned anything in this business it's that you're *never* cured. I guess it's like being a drunk who goes without a drink for twenty years but is still supposed to consider himself an alcoholic."

"There must be some test for residual cancer cells that can tell you when they're gone," I said.

"There must be," she said. "Maybe you can find out about that as you look for promising projects we can fund."

. . .

Finding out was more than a full-time job, and I soon began hiring others to help. The best of them was Robin Cook, a woman we had met in San Diego whose husband suffered from both denial and the chemotherapy given for his mantle-cell lymphoma. For her husband and also for her best friend, who was dying of cancer, Robin taught herself to become an expert in various malignancies. A whiz at the computer, she darted e-mails at Carol, Ellen, and me almost daily. One day, seeking to extend our efforts, I asked Robin to interview the famous John Reed, an M.D. and Ph.D. who then was the scientific director and now is the president of the Burnham Institute in La Jolla, an independent nonprofit organization doing biomedical research.

John Reed is recognized as a world leader in apoptosis, or programmed cell death, having authored more than 450 papers on the subject. Apoptosis is intrinsically related to "telomeres," which are simple, repetitive DNA sequences that sheathe the ends of our chromosomes. Every time one of our cells divides, the telomeres shorten slightly. The process provides a scientific definition of aging, because as more and more of each telomere is shortened, it eventually reaches a point where it becomes too short to protect the chromosomes. When that happens, the chromosomes die. And so do we.

Cancer, however, encourages an enzyme called "telomerase," which stops this shortening in malignant cells, resulting in their immortality. If you could block the telomerase, you might be able to kill cancer cells. Dr. Reed is also studying a family of related genes, "Bcl-2," which stands for B-cell leukemia (or lymphoma). These genes are involved in cell survival and death control, begetting proteins that regulate various steps in apoptosis.

Among the questions I asked him through Robin was "If you could effectively spend ten times the money you now invest in research, how would you spend it?" As usual, I was trying to get a handle on what leading researchers thought could be done to cure these cancers.

Reed answered in one word: "Genomics," which is the study of the genome, all the genetic information present in a cell. Then he elaborated, "After cells accumulate the genetic mistakes that cause cancer, the Bcl-2 genes often fail to control a known 'pathway' for cell death." Scientists use the term *pathway* to represent the intricate, often unknown maze that signaling molecules travel from the genes to the proteins they create. "We're looking into a wide variety of genes to see how cell death is achieved by normal cells and avoided by cancer cells."

The staff at John Reed's Burnham Institute numbers five hundred, including almost three hundred with doctoral degrees. Reed said he easily could add staff to quadruple the rate at which they were finding new genes and tracing their pathways. I thought it was important for the lymphoma foundation to know these things. If we could focus our research funding, we might find, if not a cure, at least a way to achieve longer-term remissions in a benign way.

As I look back on it, my naïveté paralleled the optimism earlier in my life when the Bahamian government refused to approve my Island for Science—not because our technology was flawed but because the government was flawed. Again I was misinterpreting an organization's purpose, misled this time by the foundation's middle name and Ellen's enthusiasm. In reality, the directors knew little about current cancer research, declined my offers and those of others to inform them, and refused to sponsor scientific projects other than the beginning investigations of young postdoctoral fellows. But I didn't know that then.

• • •

At the end of April I flew Papa Whiskey to Los Angeles for the foundation's annual black-tie event, astutely named the "Celebration of Life Ball" and held at the Hilton. Again I took the southern route, this time with no alternator problems. As always, I felt the familiar liberation of flying above the muted colors of man, beyond his illnesses and worries, filling my lungs with the pure air of the breathing forests. After refueling at Albuquerque, I watched the white sands of the far West widen and finally yield to the low clouds that break over the coastal mountains, seeming to pour light into the

Pacific. I flew directly over downtown Los Angeles, landed at Santa Monica, and drove a rented car east to the city of angels.

The lymphoma celebration was a party—Argentine dancers tangoed over a glittering floor, and water from two giant fountains melded with the music. Yet it was more than a party; it was a recognition dinner. Ellen Cohen, elegant in her evening gown, spoke before a group of several hundred celebrants, honoring scientists and fund-raisers. The scientists could be identified easily because they stood at the centers of conversation pockets. Their eyes were controlled, and their disciples had a way of tilting themselves forward that made me think of bowsprits carved on old sailing ships. After her talk Ellen made it a point to introduce me to every scientist in that vast room.

One of them was Jonathan Said, a research pathologist originally from South Africa. A slight, serious man with a high forehead, he looked a little lost in his tuxedo. But he grew in stature as he spoke, for nowhere is a man's character so clearly revealed as when he talks about his life's work. As a professor and the chief of anatomic pathology at UCLA, Dr. Said is known throughout the world for his insights into pathology, which to him is a constantly unfolding and beguiling series of detective stories. I told him why I thought my cancer was indolent.

"How can you say you have MCL while not expressing cyclin D1?" he asked.

"Pure speculation," I admitted, "offered by Jeff Medeiros at M. D. Anderson. Yasushi Yatabe was leaning that way too in his paper. You know them?"

"Sure, I know Jeff, and he's one of the really good pathologists, and I know about Yatabe's ideas, too. But recently we've acquired more-sophisticated tests. We use microarrays, glass chips with embedded fragments of DNA that can analyze the expression of thousands of genes at one time. It's *possible* you are not expressing cyclin D1—everything seems possible in cancer—but I'd really be surprised. You see, overexpressing cyclin D1 is practically a *definition* of MCL."

Although his explanation was undermining the rationale for my hope that I could be like those MCL patients Dan Longo had been tracking—whose disease remained indolent year after year—I felt strangely remote from the discussion. Under the cathedral-like dome filled with the sounds of tango and water leaping from fountains, I felt as if locked in a dream, as though I were an academician discussing some impersonal abstract concept. I froze, half-smiling like the other partygoers, drinking Jonathan's words. Suddenly I forgot to smile.

Jonathan Said noticed, his expression changing to sympathy. "As I'm sure you know, Neil, in science when you don't *find* something you're looking for, it doesn't mean it isn't there."

"Right," I said, trying to regain some semblance of our former academe. "It only means you haven't found it." In my mind, illusion and reality were locked in battle.

"Why don't you send me your tissue blocks and slides when you get back? We'll be glad to check the RNA in your cells." It's remarkable for a pathologist to offer something like that directly to a patient, but Jonathan Said, like Jeff Medeiros at M. D. Anderson, was a remarkable man. I was hearing a bittersweet melody: a helpful scientist, but one who was pointing to danger.

I reentered the noise of the room, stopping before a mirrored pilaster for a moment, studying my image. For the past year or so I had been looking far better than I felt. Tall, reasonably good posture, heavier than David but not fat. I'd been swimming a half-mile four or five times a week since age forty, and my physical ability was intact. I looked all right, with hazel, determined eyes, and over the years my hair had increased in quantity both on my head and body. But inside, pain was my usual companion. Nothing so bad as when the lymphoma first brought me down, but there was a constant, systemic ache in my bones—arthritis possibly inherited from my mother. As Dan Longo had told me, both lymphoma and arthritis follow the same arachidonic pathway. For a while I thought my own pathway through life would resume its former course, that the lymphoma would remain indolent. But after talking to Jonathan Said, that prospect seemed remote.

Garrulous groups at the party formed between the pilasters and the dance floor. The composition of the groups changed slowly as people moved out of one and into another. These human clusters *seemed* healthy, honeycombs in a vast hive dripping with life and laughter, changing their composition in rhythm with the orchestra. *Were you ever frightened?* I wanted to ask them. But why ruin what for many—no, for most—in this seemingly plenary party of cancer doctors and victims must be a respite from grave illness? Maybe one of their patients', or a family member's. Or their own.

· · ·

While I was on the West Coast, I flew to Seattle and met Carol, who had come by airliner since she dislikes the confinement of a small plane on long trips. Seattle has become something of a mecca for biotech companies with its accessibility to the Orient and California, natural beauty, abundant fresh lake water, and mild climate. Our target there was the University of Washington's Fred Hutchinson Cancer Research Center, where we had made an appointment weeks before.

Like M. D. Anderson in Houston and Sloan-Kettering in New York, the "Hutch" is one of the thirty-seven NCI-designated research centers, employing more than two thousand people. It is home ground for one of the world's best-known professors of oncology; many times had Carol and I seen the name Oliver Press at the top of scientific papers describing bone-marrow or stem-cell transplants and high-dose chemo. Most oncologists have about as much to do with developing cures for cancer as meteorologists have in influencing the weather. But Ollie Press was not only an oncologist. He was a scientist, an applied researcher of the ilk of Mark Kaminski and Michael Blend, both of whom he knew well. Press was an expert in bone-marrow transplantation—a rather drastic attempt at saving the lives of lymphoma and leukemia patients. But he had also authored papers on radioactive Mabs and other new therapies, and he proved knowledgeable about the entire field. He holds both M.D. and Ph.D. degrees, the latter in biological structure, which he teaches as an associate director of Washington's medical-scientist training program at the University of Washington.

Oliver Press's office was small and modest, like the man. For someone with such renown, he was surprisingly young, not yet fifty. Beneath his sandy receding hair, he wore huge glasses and a ready smile, exuding openness. We talked mostly in the cafeteria, where a fresh ocean breeze wafted through open windows. Ollie began a rapid series of questions about the state of my cancer. Afterward he sat quietly for a moment, considering my answers.

"Neil, the *last* thing you ought to consider is a transplant. You haven't had chemo. You haven't had a radioactive antibody. You haven't even had Rituxan!"

"I'm at the learning stage," I said. "And not only for myself, for others in the MCL Group, too. So many of us, including me, have been told to have transplants. I suppose you know that Ellen Cohen is considering it, too."

"Yes, we talked about it."

Transplants, Ollie Press explained, allow your cancer to be bombarded with intensive chemo, radiation, or both in such extreme doses they destroy most of your blood cells, good and bad. Afterward your own stem cells, which have been removed—or someone else's, usually a sibling's whose blood is a close match—generate new cells.

That's the theory, anyway.

I had visited the Duke University transplanters working in the children's wards, who were marvelously upbeat about the process, making it sound effective and quite routine—as indeed it is for childhood leukemia. Because children do much better than adults when undergoing donor, or "allogenic," transplants, researchers came to realize that transferring cells from newborns' discarded umbilical cords or from unwanted embryos in fertility clinics would work better than using adult stem cells. Because embryonic cells are immature and not yet differentiated into specialized cells, it rarely causes graft-versus-host disease in donor transplants and eliminates the danger of reinfusing cancer cells in autologous transplants.

You could look at the lives of most cells in the body the way you do the lives of many people, I suppose. They grow up, do the same job, reproduce a couple of times, deteriorate, and die. But stem cells are almost immortal, at least compared to most other body cells. They reproduce time and again, which is why they are so useful in research for so many diseases, from cancer to Alzheimer's. There are gradations of immortality within stem cells. Those derived from embryos are especially valuable, Ollie explained, because unlike adult stem cells, they are "pluripotent"—that, is they *stem*, or develop, into a wide variety of specialized blood, muscle, gland, and even nerve cells. Adult stem cells are not nearly as self-renewing.

The controversy over using embryonic stem cells for research comes about because, on the one hand, they make excellent cell lines. These are cells that behave in repeatable ways and can be grown time after time in Petri dishes. They can be made from excess in-vitro fertilized embryos that otherwise would be thrown away. On the other hand, stem cells also are harvested from aborted human embryos and fetuses and so may promote abortion; in addition, even those that come from fertilization clinics may be viewed as involving abortion, since the embryos, which could develop if implanted in a human uterus, must be destroyed to get the cells. Some people thus see this as tantamount to killing. It is not much of a moral argument, as I see it (although I respect the opinions of those who disagree), because a tiny group of cells that has never been in a uterus is not a human being, even if theoretically it *could* become one. (Likewise, therapeutic cloning does not create a human being, but it does promise help for those who suffer from cancer and other extreme afflictions.)

The real problem with stem cells is technical: the desirable cells are awash in a sea of other cells, difficult to isolate and even harder to integrate into various organs. Stem cells from different umbilical cords can't be combined, and the volume of cells from a single cord is too small to treat an adult. Scientists have made some progress in proliferating them by using fat cells taken from liposuction. More recently researchers at the University of Minnesota have doubled populations of stem cells from rodent bone marrow more than eighty times. But such research has not yet resulted in practical use. Meanwhile, for blood-cancer patients it is far easier to use mature stem cells from their own bodies or from donors.

"Stem-cell transplants often can give you a new life. The problem is," Ollie Press admitted, "too many patients—even when we use cord blood—die of opportunistic infections in the stage between shutting down their immune system and rescuing them with the new blood cells. You can only go a couple of weeks without a functioning immune system. Transplants are a last resort."

He paused a long moment, then spoke an octave lower, as though in someone else's voice, one that had lost its timbre of enthusiasm. "I had a transplant patient die this morning."

"Sorry, Ollie," Carol and I said at the same time. Losing a patient like that must be a tragedy for the physician as well as the family.

Dr. Press updated us on progress with a new Mab called "alemtuzumab" (tradename Campath), for lymphomas and especially chronic lymphocytic leukemia. This monoclonal antibody, developed by Ilex Oncology, in San Antonio, attacks and kills leukemia cells, finding and binding to their CD52 markers. (The FDA approved Campath in May 2001.) Unlike the fludarabine chemotherapy it was designed to replace, Campath showed less toxicity to the immune system, leaving it relatively unharmed and resulting in fewer fatal bacterial, viral, fungal, or protozoan infections. Press presented these promising prospects for blood diseases but clearly had no holy grail, no absolute answer to the questions that plagued him daily.

"Look," he said to both of us, "I like what you're doing: traveling around, visiting labs and hospitals, reading scientific papers. I wish more patients did that. One of these days, sooner than you think, you'll be cross-fertilizing this field with what you know from other sciences." He peered over his glasses to look me directly in the eye. "I understand from Ellen Cohen you're going to join her board."

"I already have," I said, surprised, although I quickly realized that Ellen knew everybody in the lymphoma community and probably talked to most of them at least weekly. That afternoon Ollie told us of the broad range of his investigations into virtually every therapy that could be used against lymphoma. He also mentioned the Ceprate system developed by CellPro, whose chief executive officer, Rick Murdock, had become his patient, one of his fortunate successes. Ollie said there now were other cell-separation systems under development to remove as many cancer cells as possible before reinfusion of the patient's own blood during an autologous transplant.

• • •

Upon our return home, Carol asked Rade Pejic to order a blood sample to be drawn from me. Afterward I sent the tube of blood to Larry Rose at UC San Francisco to determine whether I was expressing HLA-DR10, in which case I could become a candidate for Oncolym. Two weeks later Dr. Rose called me to say that the test results proved positive. One more option was available, should I need it.

For the first time, I felt my "research of research" was accomplishing something. Like Ellen Cohen with her foundation, I was putting one foot in front of the other and treading, however tenuously, on the tortured pathway to a cure.

14

False Alarm

I IMAGINE MY LYMPH SYSTEM INDOLENT AS A GOLDEN LION, SATED AF-
ter his meal of red blood cells, lazing on the savanna and yawning at the sun,
his great eyes half-closed, only an occasional tail twitch attesting to his continuing life. I have seen such lions up close in Africa, and I have seen their
great muscles where the fur is thin, quiescent but quivering a little in some
dream of action, then rippling, and finally propelling the beast to his nocturnal hunt. Lymphoma, like the lion, is no pussycat. Would my cancer, indolent for the moment, awaken to attack its prey?

Our primary tool for checking whether the lion was awakening had become, wryly, my periodic "CAT" scans. As long as these scans showed the
lymph nodes either stable or shrinking, all would be well. To a certain extent I could sense the size of the lymphoid tumors by my own internal seis-
mology, for when the lymph nodes throughout my torso were large, I felt
pain and fatigue. Lately, except for occasional apprehension, I had been feeling well. The pain of surgery had long since subsided, I had regained the
weight I'd lost, and I no longer felt tired.

One day at the end of May 1999, while waiting for fuel at an airport, I
called home to find that Jonathan Said had left a message. I was eager to hear
what he had found in my tissue blocks. I stared for a long moment at the
telephone in the pilots' lounge. Finally I picked it up and called him.

"Neil," said Jonathan from his pathology lab at UCLA, "sorry to report this to you, but yes, you *are* expressing cyclin D1. In fact, you are over-expressing it, like everyone else who has mantle-cell lymphoma."

Long seconds passed as I remembered Dan Longo's insight and sought other explanations for the benign nature of my MCL. Or was I kidding myself? Maybe I was in the presaged waning phase, with my lymph nodes soon to wax.

"Neil? Are you there?"

"Yes, Jonathan. Have you mentioned it to Jeff Medeiros at M. D. Anderson?"

"I called him. I think the reason we were successful in finding your cyclin D1 was twofold. Better antibodies have become available since he did your test, and we used special retrieval techniques to unmask the antigens after fixation."

"Well, if I am overexpressing cyclin D1, then why do you think my lymphoma is indolent?" I had long passed the three-month deadline, having gone seven months since my splenectomy and initial diagnosis.

"I don't know."

"Jonathan, as a research pathologist, wouldn't you like to find out?"

"I certainly would."

"There are a lot of indolent MCL patients. Why don't we start a project?"

"I think we should," said Dr. Said. "How will we fund it?"

"Tell you what. You put the project together, and I'll make sure it's funded. If I can get the Lymphoma Research Foundation to help, I will. If not, I'll do it myself."

I didn't know at the time, but my suggested project provided the impetus needed for these scientists to focus years of their research into the phenomenon of apoptosis, or programmed cell death; why DNA is destroyed by suicidal enzymes; and why there should be such things as oncogenes. Why on earth, I thought, would we evolve genes that give us cancer?

For most of my life I had thought of myself as an agent of change, maybe a catalyst—which is what an enzyme is—a substance that speeds up a reaction without itself being used up. Like a catalyst, my input accelerated these various researchers into a specific investigation: how to keep lymphomas, if not all cancers, from progressing. Like a catalyst, I was in no danger of being consumed, happy as an enzyme to contribute to changing the poison therapies of the twentieth century into the molecular therapies of the twenty-first.

In record time—less than a week—Jonathan recruited Jon Braun, his colleague at UCLA's Jonsson Cancer Center, to be the project leader, and Phil Koeffler, a professor of medicine at UCLA, to be the principal investigator. Koeffler also is the chief of hematology and oncology at Cedars-Sinai. In turn, both scientists enlisted their postdocs and graduate students. That was how Project Indolence began in the last year of the old millennium.

• • •

It would be a long time before Project Indolence would solidify into results, let alone restore the ravages of cancer, but research has to start somewhere. As my CAT scan frequency declined from every six weeks, to two months, and then to longer intervals, time dilated with hope. Spring turned into summer. Jonathan Said's finding that I was overexpressing cyclin D1 was, so far, irrelevant. My overabundance of this cell-cycle regulator had not yet prodded my cancer to leap like that golden lion into aggression.

Other than trips to Los Angeles for the Lymphoma Research Foundation's board meetings, life returned to something approaching normalcy. Some months earlier the last of our five cats had died of old age, and in June Carol and I visited the animal shelter, where we were chosen by two enthusiastic kittens who climbed up the chicken wire of the kindergarten ward to examine us eye to eye. They agreed to accompany us home, where they have been living happily ever after as Cleo and Petra.

In past summers we took David and his family to the island in August, and I was determined not to let my cancer interfere this time. Carol flew with me on the forty-five-minute flight to Champaign, where we stopped to see a local production of *The Wizard of Oz*, whose cast included David and his wife, Marilyn. The next day I flew David and my grandsons to the island, leaving wives and friends to come by commercial airplane, since Papa Whiskey holds only four people.

On the island Ryan, Brandon, Carol, and I put on a parody we had written in secret, *The Wizard of Schnoz,* and presented it one night to the Oz players and friends. The four performers wore foot-long noses. Brandon in a makeshift cat costume played the Lion. With the help of a cut-off old shoe, Ryan became Baretoe (since we didn't have straw for Scarecrow). Wrapped in aluminum foil, I was the Tin Man, and Carol played Dorothy in pigtails. She blew with the wind not to Kansas but to the Bahamian island of Little Stirrup Cay, where we followed not the yellow-brick road but the yellow lymph node, represented by a large and yellowish tropical leaf pulled by hidden string. We had come a long way as a family to be capable of poking fun at one of the deadliest cancers known.

· · ·

After we came back home, David Liebowitz and his wife visited for Sunday dinner; they were in the Chicago area because they had returned briefly to finish moving their possessions to Pennsylvania. Mike Blend and his wife, along with David and the Pejics, joined us. Seagulls wheeled over the lake, which was churning and foaming in its early autumn cycle, raccoons led their cubs looking for handouts, squirrels were busy squirreling away acorns, and on our side of the glass wall, Cleo and Petra tumbled in their perpetual play. With so much new life around us, it seemed strange to be talking of cancer, but the conversation moved inexorably into Dave Liebowitz's T-cell co-stimulation research—and how it was too early for my participation as a patient. I mentioned that I thought it was time for another routine CAT scan. A few heads nodded in agreement.

For one who before cancer had lived his life with almost no thought of illness, I wondered more than once whether I wasn't overreacting by requesting too many CAT scans. Still, this would be the first in five months, the longest I had gone scanless since diagnosis. I reminded myself that MCL wasn't likely to go away by itself and once again paraphrased Henry Kissinger's slogan, *Even paranoids have enemies,* thinking that *even hypochondriacs get cancer.* My metamorphosis from a patient dependent on doctors to a patient dependent on science was a natural transition to me, although it seemed to alarm my friends. One of them told me, "The person who is his own doctor has a fool for a patient," neatly skewing the lawyer adage.

But what do you do when your disease is incurable? When the medical community recommends some outmoded alchemy? When the doctors don't know what's going on in clinical trials, much less in research? Besides, I wasn't really doctorless. I had Dr. John Ultmann, a science-based oncologist; Rade Pejic; the scientists at dinner that night; and the many others I had gotten to know. They were my doctors, and they gave unstintingly of their time and knowledge.

• • •

A few days later I endured the usual routine: lying on my back looking up at a backlit ceiling showing cherry blossoms perpetually budding, feeling the hot glow of iodine in my veins, and being told when to breathe. Afterwards, as had become our custom, Rade accompanied Carol and me to view the films. The radiologist on duty that day was an older, more-experienced doctor who had come out of retirement for a couple of weeks to pinch-hit for a vacationing colleague. He stabbed the big films onto the light boxes that lined the walls, comparing the new X rays with those taken in April.

"Your lymph nodes seem to be the same size or smaller," the radiologist said. We had been hearing good news like this with every CAT scan. "*Except, of course, for this one,*" he added.

The radiologist pointed out a circular shadow the size of a small grapefruit in my lower abdomen, on the right side of the mesentery, the fold surrounding the small intestine. Measuring with a pair of calipers, he compared it to a smaller but still predominant lymph node on the previous films made in April. Somehow neither the regular radiologist, whose job it was to detect such things nor any of the rest of us had noticed this single errant tumor. In April the tumor had been almost twice the size of the largest of the others. Now, in the space of five months, its size had more than doubled again. Could my intuition about the indolence of my MCL have been dead wrong? Was my recently gained peace of mind so ephemeral?

CAT scans, like magnetic-resonance imaging, tell you that something is there but not what that something is doing, in effect photographing the anatomy but not the physiology. Rade thus ordered a PET scan, which reveals biochemical activity. In PET—positron emission tomography—radionuclides are injected into the veins, and as these radioactive atoms decay, their electrons are annihilated by positrons. The action produces gamma rays (like X rays but stronger), which are detected on opposite sides of the body and integrated by computer. If there is any metabolic activity in an organ or tissue—for instance, if a mass is actively growing—it will show jet black on the film.

The tumor in my belly lit up, in negative, like a beacon. And it was the *only* spot that was completely black. No other lymph node was growing. Rade then ordered an ultrasound, which indicated the tumor to be a solid mass. What could it be other than a diseased lymph node?

A full year had passed since my splenectomy. Now I was better off emotionally, knew a host of scientists who would advise me, and had gained a fundamental understanding of mantle-cell lymphoma: enough to recognize the weirdness of this new tumor. It was truly an enigma. How could a single lymph node grow so fast while the others in the abdomen remained stable? Wasn't lymphoma supposed to be systemic? Its existence seemed like that bright leaf from our play on the island, the yellow lymph node forming a highway that led not to the wonderland of Oz but to oblivion. What should I do about it?

I asked the scientists.

John Ultmann, M.D., renowned University of Chicago oncologist with fifty years of lymphoma experience: "Watch it for two months. Do not do surgery. If it continues to grow and you need the tissue for Levy to make a vaccine, access it by needle aspiration or laparoscopy. Then shrink the tumor by radiation."

Ronald Levy, M.D., vaccine pioneer at Stanford University Hospital: "Remove the tumor surgically at Stanford so we can make a vaccine from it. Do not irradiate the tumor, because that would preclude getting into our vaccine trial."

Dan Denney, who holds Ph.D.'s in immunology and microbiology and is the president of Genitope, Inc.: "Enter my new protocol, in which we will access a small sample of tissue that the Levy lab can use to make a vaccine. While the vaccine is growing, take CHOP or CVA [another mix of chemos: Cytoxan, vincristine, and Adriamycin] for four or five months to reduce the size of the tumor."

Mike Blend, D.O. and Ph.D., professor at the University of Illinois at Chicago, radiation and radio-MAb expert, and good friend: "Don't assume a linear progression. Confirm the growth of the tumor with another CAT scan a month after the last one. If it's still growing, avoid chemo and irradiate the tumor."

Parkash Gill, M.D. and Ph.D., a geneticist who developed a method of achieving anti-angiogenesis using already approved drugs, and his boss, Alexandra Levine, M.D., a distinguished professor of medicine and chief of hematology, both at the University of Southern California: "Make a vaccine from samples taken by needle aspiration, then remove or shrink the tumor by radiation. If needed later, consider a Mab or Parkash's anti-angiogenic drugs."

Larry Kwak, M.D. and Ph.D., and his NCI colleague Wyndham Wilson, M.D., who have been working with a vaccine like Levy's but with a different adjuvant designed to stimulate T cells: "First irradiate the tumor, then enter a protocol using REPOCH [Rituxan with the chemotherapeutic drugs of ectoposide, prednisone, Oncovin, and hydroxorubicin]."

David Liebowitz, M.D. and Ph.D., investigator of the co-stimulation of T cells at the University of Pennsylvania: "Wait two months as Ultmann [his mentor] recommends because more options are coming up, such as our T-cell protocol. Whatever you do, don't get treated 'off-protocol.'"

Phil Koeffler, M.D., the UCLA professor who is one of the principals on Project Indolence and a good friend: "Send tissue to us so we can test it in mice. You can get a sample by needle aspiration, or else have the tumor excised and send it here."

Dan Longo, M.D., scientific director of the National Institute on Aging (NIH): "Don't fear chemotherapy if you need it. Get into a protocol where your first therapy is your last therapy. Be aggressive."

Ann Mohrbacher, the M.D. at the University of Southern California who is working with Alan Epstein on Mabs: "Be conservative. Irradiate the tumor and take Rituxan, which is the least invasive of the Mabs."

Missag Parseghian, Ph.D., the molecular biologist at Peregrine Pharmaceuticals who was helping develop Oncolym and other Mabs: "Since your test for Oncolym was positive, you may want to try this radio-Mab if you can get it. I'll ask our vice president to see if Oncolym can be furnished in some type of protocol or through a compassionate exemption."

Mark Kaminski, M.D., lymphoma and leukemia director at the University of Michigan: "Bexxar would be the best choice, using it to kill the tumor by radiation."

Finally, my close and decisive friend Rade Pejic, M.D., in Michigan City: "This is a discrete tumor near the inferior vena cava and duodenum. Let me get rid of the damn thing before it does some real harm. By surgery. Now."

Not surprisingly, the vaccinators had suggested making a vaccine, the radiation experts said to irradiate, the surgeon said to cut, and so on. Had I asked a clergyman, he would have said to pray. As with any incurable disease, the final decision was tough, and it was mine alone. Everyone, including Rade, told me that surgery was risky. But the greater risk was not taking one, I thought. I decided not to wait and chose immediate surgery—here—not at Stanford. I wanted the tissue for Ron Levy to make a personalized vaccine, yes, but I had an unshakable faith in the ability of Rade Pejic, who is among the planet's most accomplished vascular surgeons.

I called Dr. Levy and asked whether he would accept my frozen tumor and hold it until he had a protocol that did not first require chemotherapy—or until I became so desperate that I would accept chemo in order to get the vaccine. The Chemo Culture was becoming for me a future nightmare. Or my epitaph.

• • •

Ron Levy acceded to my rather unusual request and sent me instructions for preparing the excised tumor for shipment. Jonathan Said and Phil Koeffler, of the UCLA Project Indolence team, offered to investigate the tissue, too. Jonathan would determine what it was, and Phil would try to grow the tumor "permanently" in immunodeficient mice so he could test them repeatedly for sensitivity to various therapies. In addition, Phil and his associate Wolf-Karsten Hofmann, an M.D. and Ph.D. in hematology and oncology, would extract some of the tumor RNA and incorporate it in a chip that would let them use computer analysis to determine which of some fifty-six hundred pertinent genes were under- or overexpressed. These genes, considered to be the most likely of those involved in the regulation of cell cycles, growth, and signaling, would fit on one genechip—an optical chip made with a glass or quartz slide.

"When you find out what that tumor is," Phil said, "let me know. Don't assume I'm in daily contact with Jonathan Said."

Carol visited the local Federal Express office to find out what kind of containers could be used, and I talked to one of our local pathologists, Phil McGuire, who in the absence of my friend Tom Roberts became stuck with the mission. A bizarre and (on hindsight) humorous proceeding followed. It began with my delineating the directions I had received from the various scientists.

"On Monday, October 18, 1999, after removal of the large mesenteric tumor and one of the other lymph nodes," I wrote to those concerned, "Dr. McGuire will come to the sterile operating room and divide the large tumor into six portions—three quarters, one eighth, and two sixteenths—and will cut the lymph node into thirds. Keeping all tissue sterile, Dr. McGuire will prepare them and send by priority overnight Federal Express, with 10 A.M. promised delivery, to three locations. . . ."

Subsequent instructions discussed how to treat the various segments: some were to be flash frozen in liquid nitrogen and packed in dry ice; some to be sent in wet ice; some bottled in dimethyl sulfoxide, fetal-calf serum, or formalin, as appropriate for the use intended; . . . and on and on and on.

• • •

Surgery (by a surgeon you trust) is something like skiing: someone else, or some force like gravity, does the hard work, and all you have to do is ride it out. When I awoke in the recovery room, Rade assured me that the samples had been sent as instructed. Since we seemed to be doing this every year, I suggested he install a zipper on my belly for easier access.

"Oh, we won't let it become a habit," he said. "I cut out the old scar from your splenectomy and extended the incision downward past your navel. The tumor was *big*."

"How big?"

"Ten by twelve centimeters, pear-shaped."

"Jesus, that thing grew fast—triple the size in six months!"

"That was no lymph-node tumor," he said. "It was tan colored and hard as a rock. Literally a rock. Hard as limestone."

"What else could it be?"

"If it hadn't grown so fast, I would say it was a desmoid tumor, in other words, a fibroid—a mass of fibers. Probably has nothing to do with your lymphoma. Actually I had a hard time even *finding* an enlarged lymph node for the comparison tests—I had to reach way around behind your pancreas. Fortunately, almost all of your nodes have shrunk."

"Was the tumor malignant? Or for that matter, the lymph node you removed?" I asked.

"I don't know yet. I excised your appendix, too, because it looked a little suspect."

Removing it along with the big tumor ought to allow my immune system to concentrate on fighting the cancer more effectively, I thought, but something seemed to be bothering Rade. He looked different—less cheerful, his brows heavier. The lines of his face were creased in worry, his formerly jet-black hair streaked here and there with gray. And he was wearing glasses. Maybe it was overwork, I thought for a second. No, not that. More a sign of inner turmoil.

"What else is wrong?" I asked.

"Well, the problem is that the tumor was stuck to your duodenum, actually wrapped in and around the circular folds. I had to dissect it—very, very carefully. It took four hours and was really difficult. Eventually I separated it and got it *all*. But there could be complications."

I turned my neck as far as I could, a few centimeters, and beheld a dozen tubes from a dozen machines running into or out of my veins, nose, bladder, stomach, abdominal drain, and just about every orifice except my ears.

"One of these machines is a stomach pump," Rade explained, "to get rid of the gastric secretions before they continue through the system. Then there are your IV fluids, oxygen, and the usual monitors of blood pressure, cardiac function, and so on," he added, waving his hand to indicate the plethora of equipment.

• • •

Carol, David, Ryan, and Brandon visited, and I talked to them between my morphine dreams. At least I think I did. One late afternoon I awoke to what seemed like even more tubes, more pain, and a tremendous nausea, and I mentioned it to Carol, who was sitting next to the bed. She looked around, discovering in angry astonishment that the stomach pump had been turned off.

"Neil, you're not connected!" she said, and ran out to find a nurse.

The day nurse, hurrying to leave at the end of her shift, had forgotten to reattach the tube to the pump, and gore and bodily fluids were building up in my stomach. Rade arrived immediately, reconnected the tube, and was so angry that he found the nurse responsible and admonished her on the spot. "This man could have *died!*" I heard him yell from the hallway.

That night I awoke covered with blood and rang the nurse's station. Blythe Topa, the supervising nurse of the floor, whom I remembered from my stay there a year ago, arrived promptly. She is short, blond, and an energetic hard worker. According to Rade, things always go smoothly when she is on duty. Blythe reinserted the needle that had worked loose from my wrist, and she changed the bloody bedding.

Rade solved the needle problem when he saw me the next morning. He installed a central venous access, a device that allows delivery of antibiotics and nutrients to the bloodstream so that nurses need not keep puncturing overused arm veins. Rade also sent in a urologist and other specialists. Between their rounds of questions and tests I looked out the window, through which, between buildings, I could see Lake Michigan in the distance. The water seemed farther from the shore than before, the inland sea less attainable, cold and steely. Toward evening the hospital quieted down, heavy with the echoes of past conversation. The setting autumn sun cast bleak indigo shadows across the room. I slept.

In the middle of the night an orderly entered, moving furniture ostensibly to clean the floor but murmuring half to himself and half to me that Y2K was coming soon—the end of the twentieth century and with it the end of the world. We should prepare ourselves for a long stay in the nether regions, he said, where we would join those incombustible sinners pitchforked into hell. St. Anthony's is better than most hospitals that I've heard about. The nurses and doctors, for the most part, are especially dedicated. As in other institutions, however, a few weirdoes sneak through the employment screens. I have never felt so vulnerable as after that sinner departed for dark corners unknown and nurse Blythe had left for the night.

A rage of vigilance descended on me, and I couldn't sleep despite the drip of morphine. I called my home, where David was in bed, having planned to return to Champaign in the morning, and asked him if he would come to the hospital. For the first time in my life I was afraid I would die, worried that some other tube might fall out before a nurse could discover it, troubled that the orderly would return with his dark terrors. Carol would have come, of course, but since David was in town, I thought his knowledge of instrumentation might be more useful. He came right away, and we spent the rest of the night talking about how the monitoring instruments in the room worked, about family, about the prospects of death, about what if anything might come afterwards. I would not want to die in the hospital if I had a choice. The final moments ought to come at home or out in a boat surrounded by family and the sea. Before entering the hospital, I had left notes on my computer: for David, ideas on children, ambitions, and investments; for Carol, reminiscences; for Ryan and Brandon, thoughts on living their lives well.

I thought about my life, then shook myself as if to throw off these thoughts. I wasn't very fond of introspection. The usual crap, I thought. Let's get on with living!

. . .

A slow stream of internal bleeding started in the morning, causing Rade to add blood to the mélange of liquids flowing into my body. The days passed painfully, twelve of them with twelve blood transfusions, and I contracted pneumonia. Nights passed in slow motion. Fits of dismal wakefulness alternated with agonized dreams until finally I would be dragged by the morphine into a stupor for an hour or two, only to climb out of it like a deep-sea diver gasping for air. Pneumonia patients usually are encouraged to move around, but Rade didn't want me getting up because the bleeding had not stopped. I learned later that he had told his wife there was a strong possibility that I would die. My white-cell counts were haywire, the blood from my bladder ran a steady red, I was anemic, and infections even beyond the pneumonia were likely.

Whatever his feelings, Rade never gives up on a patient or on a friend. Like me, he believes in Ockham's Razor, the maxim that the simplest explanation accounting for the facts is usually correct. After abdominal surgery Rade uses the established method of checking for untied blood vessels, filling the cavity with sterile saline water, then pumping it out to make sure it isn't pink from blood. Mine had been clear. The simplest explanation, therefore, was that the bleeding had started from a stress ulcer at my sutured duodenum, perhaps stressed further after the stomach pump was disconnected by mistake.

On my thirteenth day in the hospital, a bevy of nurses, orderlies, and technicians flocked into the room. They carried away the other bed and two dressers and replaced them with endoscopic equipment, computers, oscilloscopes, fluoroscopes, and various machines in an area already teeming with digital monitors, bags of fluids hanging from stands, tubes, and hoses. Sour with electrical odors, the room looked as if it had been conceived by an interior decorator on LSD.

The executive of these transformations entered behind Rade. He was Juan Benitez, a gastroenterologist. Dr. Benitez told me how he planned to stop the bleeding. He would snake the long tube of a gastroscope into my mouth, through the esophagus, into the stomach, and out the other end to the duodenum, the first part of the small intestine. It seemed like an easy procedure.

Until he began to push the tube down my throat.

Benitez commented all the long way down my alimentary canal, an eternity for me, although in doctor-time probably no more than ten minutes. "Nothing in the pharynx, nothing in the esophagus," he said. "The stomach looks good . . ." Four of his assistants monitored various instruments and reported data to him. The gastroscope allowed him to slide long needle-like wires down one side of the tube while he guided a fiber-optic light and camera through the other. The scope was as miniaturized as modern technology allowed, but to me it felt as thick as a garden hose.

Finally, at the end of his tube—and at the end of my rope, since I was gagging and retching—he reached the duodenum. It was an achievement in my mind on a par with Columbus reaching America. (Soon afterward, a pill-like camera—comprising an inch-long electronic eye, a light source, and a battery-powered transmitter—was developed to diagnose gastrointestinal bleeding of uncertain origin and to locate polyps or other abnormalities. Had the camera pill been available at the time, however, I still would have had to endure the endoscope to repair the tear.)

"Ah, here is the ulcer!" Benitez announced happily. "It is spurting quite vigorously!"

No sooner had he found the bleeder than he repaired it by injecting some epinephrine through one of the wires in the tube. Epinephrine, I learned afterwards, not only is a natural hormone but is used therapeutically as a vasoconstrictor—that is, to mend local blood-vessel hemorrhages.

• • •

Three days later, requiring no new blood transfusions and my pneumonia bacteria killed by antibiotics, I was wheeled out of St. Anthony's once again a free man. And twenty pounds lighter.

By then the pathology reports had arrived from Jonathan Said at UCLA. The small lymph node was positive for cyclin D1, as well as for the CD5 and CD20 cell markers. In other words, it was consistent with mantle-cell lymphoma. But the large tumor, which Jonathan had sent to a soft-tissue expert for a second opinion, turned out to be a fibromuscular tumor, something like a desmoid but consisting of smooth muscle cells, like the duodenum itself. Both pathologists confirmed what Rade had suspected, that the rogue tumor had nothing to do with my lymphoma. It was a rare fibroid of unknown origin—rare because tumors similar to desmoids normally grow slowly.

As is usual in science—or for that matter in any kind of fact finding, as I had learned so long ago in Costa Rica—asking the right question is absolutely essential in eliciting the right answer. These scientists had varying opinions *because I had asked the wrong question.* Believing that my imaging scans had shown the tumor to be an enlarged lymph node, I had asked incorrectly, What should I do about this large lymph node? Doubtless I would have received a completely different set of answers—probably more suggestions for biopsy—had I instead asked the same twelve scientists, What should I do about this large tumor, which may or may not be lymphoma?

Walking slowly, I entered my office and made a series of phone calls, a most-welcome series, first to Ron Levy, thanking him for agreeing to freeze and store the tumor but now telling not to bother, just to dispose of it. I called the other dozen scientists who had so generously offered their advice, including my friend Phil Koeffler. Phil had already grown the tumor in mice and was sending me a printout of 5,560 of my genes.

Phil and the other sympathetic scientists were happy to hear me say, somewhat sheepishly: "The tumor I sent you was unrelated to my lymphoma. It was not malignant."

Then I called my friend Andy Raymond, who works in the hospital-equipment business, found out the name of a manufacturer of film illuminators used by radiologists, and bought two of these lightboxes and a pair of calipers. It's not that hard to compare the sizes of your own lymph nodes from one CAT scan to the next. Or to find other strange shapes that shouldn't be there. More do-it-yourself oncology.

15

Does Prayer Work?

PRAYER THERAPY FOR CANCER HAS BEEN STUDIED, RECOMMENDED, sneered at, applauded, and accepted by believers in God and by nonbelievers alike.

There are cancer patients aware and patients naïve who retain physicians scientific and physicians parochial, all thrusting upon the Almighty the same mantras: let me live; let my patient recover. Considering the eternal statistics of cancer, few of their prayers will be granted. Yet there is scientific evidence that prayer works. Why?

After my brush with death, thoughts of God and prayer returned with an urgency unfelt since my days at Loyola and Northwestern, where we students would churn the subject so thoroughly I knew I had either to withdraw or devote my life to the proof or disproof of the hereafter. Now, a half-century later, I looked up scientific studies attempting to prove the efficacy of prayer as disease therapy. The California Pacific Medical Center had done a double-blind study that indicated prayed-for AIDS patients survived in greater numbers than did a non-prayed-for control group. San Francisco General Hospital claimed patients receiving prayer did better clinically than others. And a study at Duke University had a team of believers praying over thirty cardiac patients, who enjoyed results twice as good as those for a control group. All three stated they were double-blind studies, meaning that neither the subjects nor the researchers knew who was receiving prayer and who was not "in order to reduce the placebo effect"—the power of positive thinking or willing yourself to succeed. But how can you control the control group? How can you ensure that no relative prays for someone in that group?

Other studies were even harder to believe. For instance, in order to eliminate any placebo effects and to isolate prayer as the independent variable, one study had people praying for bacteria to grow, seeds to germinate, and wounded mice to heal faster than did control groups for which prayer was withheld. I couldn't help but wonder whether they had tried it out on horses at the racetrack. At this point it began to get a little ridiculous. I mean, how can you control such experiments without ruling out the effects of billions of prayers flying around the planet on behalf of all life on earth?

To ascribe healing powers to a supernatural cause is to say that the mechanism is not natural, but how would you know that? No one so far claims to understand all the natural factors in the universe. On the contrary, cosmology constantly elicits more questions than answers. God, if he exists, certainly has shown a propensity to work through physical systems such as star and planet formation, gravitation, electromagnetism, photosynthesis, biological reproduction, mutations, the evolution of species, and the rest of nature.

My son, David, and many scientists I know believe in God. But theirs is rarely the patriarchal, personal God embraced by organized religions, nor do they think that we retain our human identity while residing in heaven or hell. Shahid, one of the most humanitarian persons on the planet, considers himself an atheist. Carol believes in a personal God. I am a skeptic, an agnostic. Four close people with four widely divergent beliefs. It's a wonder that the six billion people on the planet agree on anything!

As the procedure we have established for seeking truth about the physical world, science has been enormously successful. The scientific method works to discover what is true, whereas the blind acceptance of others' beliefs, dogma, astrology, and magic have not worked. Can science, then, shed light on the existence of God? What do the scientists themselves believe?

Recent polls of scientists, such as those taken of members of the National Academy of Sciences, show about the same number of believers today as in the 1960s and 1970s, when we used to survey them in our magazines. Now as then, about 40 percent express belief in a deity, and 44 percent express disbelief. Only 7 percent believe in a personal God, and 72 percent do not. Belief in human immortality or life after death was rejected or believed by similar percentages. The fact that scientists believe in God is of importance only insofar as it results in their desire to study the question. Whether they believe or disbelieve, of course, has no bearing on proving or disproving the existence of God. After all, it wasn't so long ago on the scale of human history that science by opinion would have proclaimed belief in a flat earth and stars as jewels in a velvet sky.

"Scientists think about these things a lot," David said in a conversation with Shahid and me one day at my home in early January after my convalescence from surgical complications. The lake was wearing its steel-gray winter armor; the logs in the fireplace were burning cheerfully. Our young cats, no longer kittens, were lying on the couch, following the conversation with twitching ears. The Christmas tree was still intact, and the holiday spirit still hung in the air. It was a good time for talking about God.

"I believe in intelligent design," David continued. "In other words, that this universe was created at a finite time, the Big Bang of fifteen billion years ago. The theory holds that since organic life, especially mammals like us with free will, is so incredibly complex after the millions of years of guided evolution, it is unreasonable to assume life created itself. If life didn't create itself, something did—some unseen intellect or spiritual force embedded in the cosmos.

"After all, we have free will. It's hard to believe that quantum mechanical fluctuations in your brain, based on past experiences and new sensory inputs, randomly converge and cause you to make decisions on—say—taking chemo or having surgery. *I am responsible* for my actions, not some confluence of random events outside my control."

"How does that make prayer work?" I asked David.

"Well, if God exists in *any* form, this spiritual force can be swayed to our advantage even if it isn't a personal God who watches our every action."

Shahid, who comes from a Muslim family in Bombay, looks at it differently. "All major religions claim there is one God. But how capricious this God! Ignoring the prayers of the millions during Hitler's holocaust . . . ignoring the millions of cancer victims praying all the way to their apocalyptic deaths. Man evolved on this planet not to understand God but to survive. He invented God to explain what he couldn't understand in nature. Meteors, the weather, recoveries from disease were seen as miracles. As we progressed, we unraveled the mysteries, one at a time, until now we no longer need to explain things by invoking supernature."

Even the Jesuits taught that the existence of God is unprovable, I thought, remembering my days at Loyola, but neither can you prove he does not exist.

Carol said, "If God is just one more superstition, like leprechauns or other green people from space, why is the belief in God so pervasive?"

"Because man in his ignorance invents superstitions to impose order in the universe, thereby reassuring believers," Shahid ventured. "Emotionally held beliefs, like psychic phenomena and astrology, are virtually impossible to dislodge. With UFO abduction stories sold in supermarkets, we need no further lessons in human credulity."

"Hordes of young, educated Muslims are waiting in line clamoring to die in their jihad," Carol said. "They've been taught from childhood that by switching the detonator to the bomb and killing innocent nonbelievers, the door to heaven will open for them immediately, that they'll see God and Muhammad, that their loved ones will enter paradise with them."

"Such fanatics saw nine-eleven as God answering their prayers," Shahid said softly as he attempted to stroke both cats with one hand. "Christians felt the same way during the Crusades."

Near the ends of our lives we feel cheated and lost, so we grasp gods out of our verisimilitude. We would be less than human if we didn't feel that our lifetimes spent learning and accomplishing and accumulating and loving and improving society were meant only to continue the species. I reasoned that either there is a God, and we lack the ability to prove it, or there is no God. If I learned anything from cancer science, it is that *just because you can't find something doesn't mean it isn't there.* Others told me they had prayed for me. I had prayed for myself. Just in case.

. . .

The millennium had arrived without plunging us into hell or even a secu-
lar disruption, and my convalescence was nearly completed. As a rule of
thumb, you need a week's exercise to make up for each day spent in the
hospital, and this January, twelve weeks after surgery, I resumed swimming
fifty lengths in our palm-lined indoor pool. When the weather permitted, I
alternated swimming with riding my bicycle ten miles along forested roads.

David, Shahid, Carol, and I were sitting under a giant wooden chande-
lier I had made that shone lights downward and sprouted Swedish ivy climb-
ing up steel pipes to cedar rafters twenty feet above. An amateur architect, I
had designed this house in the open-beam style of a ski lodge so you could
see the woods on one side and Lake Michigan on the other. While I was
running a Bahamian construction team on the island, Carol had managed
most of the building of this house by hiring, coordinating, or cajoling car-
penters and plumbers and ordering lumber and other materials. We had
hoped that we could live here one day but had built it originally to sell, not
expecting at the time to be able to afford it.

Now we looked out at the lake swells rolling in, long and leisurely, before
ice and snow broke them at the shoreline, where glaciers once reigned. Close
by a curious doe and her speckled fawn looked in at us. I was happy to be
alive in a nontheocracy, a free society in a relatively free century where you
can talk openly about God or anything else, and happy especially to talk about
these things with our son. Shahid had melted into the couch with the cats,
serene as a Buddha. David's worldview was intact, and he was equally relaxed.

Despite the idyllic surroundings, I could smell again the organic odors that
reminded me of my hospital room, still stuck in that layer of being between
the conscious and subconscious where anxiety intrudes, where thoughts of
God lead inevitably to thoughts of death. The unremitting quandary of
God's existence had never left me; it had only been suppressed these many
years. My agnosticism is not an in-between belief, not halfway to God, condemned like one of Dante's souls swimming in the vacuum between heaven
and earth. It is an all-or-nothing belief: either the concept is true or it is

untrue. The problem is that at this stage of mankind's development, we don't know enough to determine which. But maybe someday we will.

Shahid was talking: "Medieval inquisitors respected the biblical passage that 'thou shalt not spill blood' by burning their witches at the stake. Less recognized, perhaps, is how managers of the world's religions kindle mysticism by appealing to the senses: the awe of mighty temples or pyramids, Bach by organ, legends and gospels, priestly robes, stained glass, statues, incense, and even, in some cults, hallucinogens."

Carol returned from making coffee in the kitchen, where she had continued to listen with her twenty-twenty hearing. "I believe in God because it makes me feel better; it gives me an inner peace," she admitted. "Maybe there really is a heaven and hell. Maybe Jesus really did multiply loaves of bread. I think the stories in the Bible and the Koran, and all the other holy books have suffered some in two thousand years of retelling, but I believe our souls continue in some way when we die. How do we know? We *can't* know! That's where faith comes in. Faith doesn't mean that you take someone else's word for something. It means that you can't figure some things out using logic, physics, and biology, at least not yet, because it's beyond us. You can get closer in touch with it by praying, and it might work. After all, look at you, Neil, and at all the people who have been praying for you—especially me."

"Amen!" added David. "You received the gift of a new life, Dad." His voice was gentle but precise. "Now after your experience, is your life more focused?"

Three faces looked at me expectantly. A storm of emotions raged inside, but all I could say was, "I think of life less . . . indifferently . . . now. Mine and others."

I thought of St. Peregrine, about whom I had read after visiting the makers of Oncolym, Peregrine Pharmaceuticals, to see why they had named their company after him. Peregrine, a thirteenth-century monk, contracted cancer in his leg. Scheduled for an amputation in the morning, he prayed all night and was miraculously cured. If anyone ever had reason to believe in God it would be Peregrine . . . and me. God saves me from a horrible disease so that I may go forth and multiply the knowledge that splenectomies and anti-angiogenics can cure some cancers and that manmade antibodies, immune stimulators, and vaccines can cure others, all the while diminishing the Chemo Culture until soon cancer, all cancer, succumbs to man's exquisite enlightenment.

It was a great scenario, but I couldn't buy my own argument, unwilling to sacrifice integrity to emotion. My intuition kept forcing the questions: What are we really saying when we pray to God to cure our cancer? Aren't we asking God to admit he was wrong the first time and to change his mind because we so humbly beseech?

• • •

Scientists ask questions, sometimes the right ones. David made a quantum leap to the next step, saying something I took to be astounding. "Could prayer be effective even if you don't believe in a personal God and don't expect him to answer your pleas?"

"How would that work?" Shahid asked.

"Just believing that there is some reason for our existence, some driving dimension to the universe, might stimulate the immune system," David said.

I wondered whether the God most scientists favored, the impersonal, nonpatriarchal, inhuman, and sometimes inhumane God, the god of cosmic force, was nothing other than endless, perpetual time. Time that speeds and slows relative to velocity, time that governs and orders the universe. Would belief in Supreme Time make any more or less sense than any other undetectable force? These thoughts had leapt into my mind, nowhere near theory status. We were concentrated now on questions flowing from David's query: How does God allow prayer to work when he answers—or does not answer—prayer? Or can prayer work without God?

It seemed to me that the mechanism used by God, or by nature without God, is communication between the brain and immune system. When the patient himself is doing the praying or is involved by being thankful that others are praying for him, those thoughts trigger the brain to boost an immune response. The brain-immune connection has been proved by observation and experiment. Mind over matter.

I remembered something Freud said: more or less, that illusions save us pain even when they collide with reality against which they are dashed to pieces. But the illusion of prayer *is* reality. There is no such thing as objectivity—only objective thinking by a subjective brain. What's the difference between my brother's imagining that he can't eat without applying numbers to a regimen and his really not being able to eat? The distinction is meaningless to him. He can't eat! As long as the brain and the immune system are in two-way communication, "inner" thoughts and "outer" thoughts are equal in prompting an immune-system reaction.

The immune molecules called cytokines consist of more than a hundred distinct proteins produced by white blood cells. They include the interleukins, interferons, tumor-necrosis factors, erythropoietin, and colony stimulating factors—the same body substances that immunologists replicate to treat cancer. These cytokines help the body recuperate by sending messages to the brain that set off a series of responses. One of these is fever, which creates temperatures that help kill foreign invaders. Another is sleep, which has restorative and renewal properties. Yet another is the immune response against diseases like cancer. All these are triggered by the brain when we laugh, hope, will, remember our former wellness, declare our resolve . . . or pray. The converse is true, too. Negative emotions—worry, stress, panic, and fear shut down the body's immune reactions and result in the self-fulfilling defeat of illness and death.

Shahid was saying, "Many Indians believe in heavy meditation, which is like prayer without God."

"Scientists have confirmed the power of positive thinking," David added, his blue eyes vibrant. "To a person in touch with this kind of 'spiritual' awareness—in other words, a believer—prayer can be extremely positive thinking. Prayer sets your mind in a certain frame. Call it fervent meditation, free will, being in control of our lives, whatever. The familiar ritual of a repeated prayer, such as saying an 'Our Father' or a 'Hail Mary,' exerts calm. Whether a prayer is answered doesn't matter."

Carol smiled agreement with matching eyes.

Shahid said, "What you seem to be saying is that, whether you believe in

God or not, your prayers—not someone else's—can bolster your immune reactions."

"Seems possible," said Carol, "since God works his other wonders by natural means."

It was food for positive thought. Experiments over the years have shown that the cells of the immune system are profoundly sensitive to messages from the brain, and vice versa. Amazingly, among all the physiological systems in the body, only the immune and brain communicate both ways. When immune-system cells are isolated outside the body and exposed to chemical signals, extreme modifications in their responses have been observed. Both the immune system and the brain possess specific receptors that allow them to talk to each other, so much so that the immune system becomes a neurochemical extension of the brain swimming around in the bloodstream. Thus, our immune response to cancer can be enhanced or suppressed by our thoughts—which goes a long way in explaining the mechanism of prayer.

Prayer, whether God exists or not, I thought, stimulates the T cells, revs up the helper T cells and the natural killer cells, kick starts the antibodies, and the rest of it. I found myself kneading Cleo's muscles, digging rhythmically through the fur, knowing automatically how hard to massage by the strength of her purr. I suppose prayer is like massaging a cat. It lowers *your* blood pressure, not the *cat's*.

"You can look at prayer that way, as some kind of ritual to spark the immune system," David said.

"Or you can see it as proof that God can be flattered, like everybody else," Shahid pointed out.

"What!"

"Well . . ." He lengthened the syllable into a long liquid sound. "Prayer praises God, telling him he's great so he can grant you favors—love, money, health."

If God does exist, I thought, we know he operates through the laws of physics and biology he created, through the evolution of atoms into stars spinning off planets, through organic progression ending, at least so far, in mankind. If God answers your prayers to cure you of disease, he does it by stimulating your T cells.

"I can accept the usefulness of prayer regardless of God answering the request," Shahid continued. "What I can't accept is the idea of God, who by definition is good, wanting so many billions of people to suffer, because if he didn't want them to suffer, then the all-powerful God would prevent their suffering. And if there is a good, infinitely powerful God, there would be no need for prayer—at least not prayer to God—in the first place."

"Christ promised an *afterlife* without suffering—not heaven in this life," David said. "Even Christ had doubts and prayed when he was dying on the cross. Prayer in traumatic situations works."

"Not only is prayer known to be therapeutic," I said, "but so is laughter."

"And writing!" said Carol.

Laughing—and expressive writing—both are known to relax blood vessels and ease muscle tension. Laughing increases an antibody called immunoglobulin-A, as well as T cells and natural killer cells, all of which fight infection. I had just read several studies purporting to show that people who laugh more have fewer heart attacks, lower heart rates, and lower levels of a stress hormone called "cortisol" in their blood. In addition, Carol had given me an article from Stanford showing that "ventilation of negative emotions" through writing is similarly therapeutic.

Over dinner that night, we didn't start writing or praying, but therapeutic laughter reigned over stories told.

• • •

In the following weeks I often directed my neurochemical brain to consider God and prayer, watching through the glass wall the chunks of ice crunching along the shore and the great lake churning from blue to choppy gray as it responded to the planet's cycle of atmospheric temperature change. I saw only nature there, nothing supernatural. I felt intuitively that man created God, not the other way around, but that doesn't stop me from hoping. For God and for an afterlife. Who in his right mind does not hope that life continues after death?

Whether God is out there answering prayers selectively or not, whether the placebo effect or faith healing is at work, and whether the mechanism ever will be precisely understood, the fact remains that prayer kick starts the immune system. I keep coming back to that. The finding sheds no light on the proof or disproof of God but becomes one more example of how nature—whether started by God or not—functions through physical instead of supernatural systems.

However it works, the millions of cancer victims dead and struggling show that prayer is efficacious sometimes to some people, but used alone it rarely cures malignancies. It seems to be a good idea to learn about the new biotherapies instead of waiting around for the intervention of a deity. The evidence is overwhelming for the observation—sometimes made ironically, sometimes in faith, sometimes tritely said, and yet incontrovertible—that God helps those who help themselves.

16

Project Indolence

MISTAKES HAPPEN IN NATURE, ALLOWED BY GOD OR OTHERWISE—
chief among them our faith that nature rarely makes blunders. One-eyed sheep
and human babies with deformed brains usually die in the womb. Our immune system, which reinvents itself every day by producing new white blood
cells, is somewhat tolerant of blunders, such that a few malfunctioning cells
don't lead to devastation. The malfunctioning of more than a few cells, however, or of just one gene pair at a precise location, can lead to catastrophe. Our
approximately thirty thousand genes replicate billions of proteins—all the
while being bombarded with cosmic rays, sunshine, pollutants, and pathogens
that mutate our cells. The process is so complex, it makes you wonder not that
there is cancer in the world but that everyone doesn't have it.

In my pursuit of a cure, I began slowly developing a plan of action should
my lymphoma become aggressive. I started reading about Judah Folkman,
the surgeon turned scientist at Harvard who almost single-handedly invented the now-thriving field of anti-angiogenesis. One of his findings suggested that cancer grows in spurts—alternately resting and growing—growing especially between sessions of chemo and eventually becoming resistant
to the toxins. Folkman and his colleagues spent decades isolating natural
biochemicals in the body that prevent cancer in most people by depriving
tumor cells of blood nutrients. His early trials of these substances, which he
named "angiostatin" and "endostatin," had not proved efficacious—so far—

although they certainly might later. Meanwhile, I knew that trials were soon to commence on hundreds of other angiogenic inhibitors, including Celebrex. I began to view anti-angiogenesis as a good mechanical method to stop my own cancer for a long time.

Simultaneously, I regarded cloned antibodies and especially customized vaccines as therapies closer to a cure, because instead of merely inhibiting the growth of cancer cells, as do anti-angiogenics, these biological therapies attack cancer cells directly by replicating B and T cell fighters. In effect, they help the body cure itself. Yet even the new biotherapies were mere stopgaps along the scientific raceway to a universal cure—one that would apply in one form or another to everyone's cancer.

Finally, though, I had arrived at the frontier of molecular biology.

A molecule is the smallest quantity into which matter can be divided without losing its characteristics. The idea that you can examine the molecular structure of cells, determine the interplay of their electrical charges and chemistry, see how they interact and communicate, and understand how they live, die, fail to die, and form pathways—not long ago all this was the stuff of science fiction. Now it's routine laboratory research.

When Project Indolence began in May 1999, three laboratories became involved: the large Phil Koeffler lab at Cedars-Sinai, Jonathan Said's small lab, and another run by Said's boss, Jon Braun, who became the project leader and coordinator. Starting together, they used different approaches to determine what triggers lymphoma into taking that final leap off the brink of normalcy into uncontrolled cell immortality.

Phil Koeffler is both a professor of medicine at UCLA and the director of hematology and oncology at Cedars-Sinai. This medical center, the largest nonprofit hospital in the western United States, is separated from the university by some six miles of busy palm-lined streets that were made even busier by the constant travel between the Koeffler, Braun, and Said laboratories. For his end of the project, Koeffler recruited several young scientists with M.D. and Ph.D. degrees in molecular biology, including a new assistant professor, Mike Teitell, and the then-postdoctoral fellows Sven de Vos and Wolf Hofmann, both from Germany.

Although these investigators were looking for specific genes, their task was sped by the international effort to map the entire human genome to precise locations on various chromosomes. The Human Genome Project, supervised in the United States by the NIH and the Department of Energy, would not produce the final sequencing of human genes until 2003. Long before that, by January 2000, less than a year after Project Indolence began, the Cedars-Sinai–UCLA collaboration found *four hundred genes responsible for triggering indolent into aggressive lymphomas.* With this beginning, their inquiries would require no less than a fundamental explanation of cellular mechanisms that have evaded researchers for a hundred years.

Finding a gene is not the same as identifying its function. A map can bring you to a certain address, but it doesn't let you inside the house to see what's going on. Even by 2003, fewer than half the human genes have been identified for function, and their pathways to aggressive cancer are only partly understood.

All cancers are "genetic," although only about 5 percent are hereditary. In other words, 95 percent of cancer results from the accumulation of genetic changes—mutations caused by environmental factors. Sometimes the process occurs fast and younger people and children get cancer. Usually, though, the chain of mutations requires decades, which is why older people are more prone to develop malignancies. Mutating cells trigger hundreds of safeguards or checkpoints, striking a balance in healthy human cells between the high and low manifestation, or "expression," of genes. By changing their own "expression profiles," normal cells constantly adapt to adversities such as an invasion of viruses or bacteria. In the ensuing battle, the normal cell overexpresses genes important to stopping the infection.

Less often the cells accumulate mistakes in the genes that cause them to grow uncontrollably. These cells retain their aberrant gene expression, permanently stopping the apoptosis pathway—in other words, stopping their normally built-in cell death. The ultimate aim of tracing the pathways from these genes to the proteins that they beget is to keep those complex pathways permanently turned off or on, whichever will prevent the final march toward cell immortality. A related approach is to restore normal cellular control by forcing cancerous cells into the apoptotic pathway, where they can be destroyed. Armed with a truly fundamental understanding of the process, just about any pharmaceutical company would give its corporate teeth to take it from there and spend the billion or more dollars required to develop and test drugs that will short-circuit those pathways or otherwise achieve apoptosis of wayward cells.

It would be tantamount to a cure for lymphoma. From there it would not be far to curing other cancers as well.

• • •

The Project Indolence investigators at Cedars-Sinai had already begun writing papers on their results, and I wanted to see how we could speed their progress. When I asked for a meeting in late January 1999, the research team gathered to talk to me and three other directors of the lymphoma foundation: Bill Hawley, a quiet, unassuming, highly skilled thoracic surgeon from Oklahoma City; Michael Becker, a young venture capitalist from New York; and John Kornet, a six-foot-five businessman from Boston. Vested in our interest, the four of us were lymphoma victims, and as bad as that sounds, it is not the most horrific of tragedies. Recently Bill and John had suffered worse: Bill's wife had been diagnosed as having nonsmoker's lung cancer, and John's daughter, a mountain climber, had fallen to her death at the age of twenty-nine. Conversation during our drive to the meeting on the UCLA campus was understandably restrained.

When we arrived in Westwood Village, five miles from the Pacific, we had a close look at the University of California's blend of architectural styles, a mix of Italianate basilicas and stacked five-story pigeonholes sprawling over more than four hundred acres. The buildings are separated by meadows, and although spring was still distant, meadowlarks were singing in the sunny Mediterranean-type climate.

I had been there before in my magazine-publishing days, meeting the Nobel-laureate chemists Willard Libby and Glenn Seaborg, members of my editorial board. Today we met with a younger generation of scientists. Some (perhaps swimming at the top of the gene pool) were of future Nobel status, and twelve of them crowded into a small conference room. All were participating in Project Indolence, although only one, Sven de Vos, worked on it full time. By shifting salary allocations and borrowing resources from the university, the lab directors Jon Braun and Phil Koeffler had persisted long beyond the first contribution made by me and the MCL Group.

Phil dimmed the lights and showed us the slides, charts, tables, and graphs describing those four hundred "aggression genes." The lymphoma genes had been identified using the same "genechip" technology that had enabled the Human Genome Project to sequence some three billion pairs of chemical bases—the molecular building blocks of DNA and the source of the genetic code. There were two genechip inventions, both utilizing glass or quartz slides to analyze DNA activity in tumor samples. One had been made only months earlier by Patrick O. Brown, a Stanford University M.D. and Ph.D. molecular biologist. The other, developed about the same time by Steven Fodor, Ph.D., the founder and president of Affymetrix, was the one used by the Project Indolence team.

"Genechips signify a tremendous advance over traditional assays," Phil Koeffler explained. "That's because the nucleic acids—the information-bearing molecules of a cell's nucleus—are made part of the chip, allowing rapid data analysis. It is a complex process that proceeds first with a chemical separation of an RNA sample of interest, such as diseased tissue, which then is bound to an array something like a computer chip."

Unlike computer chips, however, genechips contain no silicon to conduct current. Instead they use either a photographic mask or a half-million tiny aluminum mirrors that shine light in specific patterns to construct segments of DNA. DNA comprises four nucleic acid components—adenine, thymine, cytosine, and guanine, the A, T, C, and G alphabet of life. These four then are arranged into different combinations, or sequences, at tens of thousands of locales on the chip. The result is a fast, computerized way of determining the functions of various genes—in this case, genes that trigger indolent into aggressive lymphomas.

• • •

When the lights came on, everyone was smiling. The scientists, not given to premature celebration, were quietly excited. The dilated pupils of the rest of us wobbled in wonder. "My God!" Bill Hawley said, "Four hundred aggression genes . . . How long will it take to get to the stage where a pharmaceutical company can begin drug development?"

Among the three other foundation directors present, Bill was the most in a hurry, having given up his practice to visit laboratories throughout the country, racing to a cure not for himself or other lymphoma patients but for his wife, whose aggressive cancer could not wait. As a surgeon who had been studying cancer, he knew that genetic-based biotherapies designed for a systemic disease like lymphoma might apply to inoperable lung and other organ cancers as well.

"At this rate, five or more years," Koeffler said.

"Can you speed it up?" I asked. "Only Sven is full time, right?"

"Yes to both questions," he said. "All we need is money to hire more people."

"How many scientists could you use and be realistically effective?"

"We could put to work, with no duplication of effort, ten full-time Ph.D.s or M.D. scientists and another ten or twelve technicians. That would cut completion time to eighteen, maybe twenty-four months. It would cost $1.8 million a year for no more than two years. Or . . . we could hire five professionals and supporting staff for half that, and it would take three to four years." Their various projections and detailed budgets lay before us.

"Could you actually find ten researchers?" Bill Hawley asked. "Experienced scientists who would be willing to drop what they're doing and work full time on the project?"

Phil Koeffler was nodding his head up and down even before the end of the sentence. I could feel the electric concentration of this scientist so completely immersed in his work, his optimism illimitable. "We already know who they are. We've talked to them. You get us the money and we'll get the staff. But we're going to need it all at once—or at least half of it and a firm pledge for the rest. We can't start hiring M.D.s and Ph.D.s and then face the prospect of letting them go after a few months."

John Kornet and Michael Becker, the two money men in the room, thought that financing the project at either of these increased rates of activity was manageable for the Lymphoma Research Foundation, possibly with matching funds from other charitable groups.

That night at the board meeting the three of us gave a brief, enthusiastic summary and made the request. The ensuing silence hit me as though it were an electric current. I looked around at the dozen other directors assembled around a large conference table, drinking coffee, shuffling papers, obviously anxious to return to their printed agenda. I was stunned by their blank stares, temperamentally unable to comprehend the workings of minds more concerned with raising money than fulfilling the foundation's purpose. With Ellen in the hospital, we could muster absolutely no enthusiasm for Project Indolence. At the time the foundation retained $2.5 million of contributed funds in the bank—held, the executive director said, "for a rainy day."

I pointed out that it was raining pretty hard right then, with the lymphoma epidemic raging nationwide, 61,000 new cases annually, 26,000 deaths a year, and the numbers growing by 4 percent annually.

The board members voted to consider funding such a project . . . after they had the time to form a scientific-review committee to look into other university research that might be equally worthy of the donated money in their stewardship. Just then, however, they were "uncomfortable" in sponsoring any research project.

There is a fine line between funding a "research project" and sponsoring an individual postdoctoral fellow who does research. The lymphoma foundation makes annual career-development grants to postdocs—notably to Mike Teitell, whose work at UCLA proved significant—but not for wholly formed senior-level projects as such. By limiting support in such an artificial way, I felt we were missing an enormous opportunity to further the understanding of phenomena that could control or even cure lymphoma.

Six months passed before the answer came from the foundation's scientific director, and it was "no . . . for now." More months slipped by, months that for me and for Bill Hawley were filled with increasing adrenaline and decreasing hope. I ended up funding the second, third, and fourth year's Project Indolence effort myself, with small but important contributions from dozens of members of the MCL Group. Gifts from the group were difficult to make because most of these patients were financially stressed, most of them too young to qualify for Medicare.

• • •

Given minimal funding, the Koeffler lab, although armed with forty postdocs, graduate students, and technicians, could advance Project Indolence at only a slow pace because of the demands of several other cancer programs underway. At the top of the laboratory hierarchy, Phil Koeffler himself split his time directing the research, teaching, and seeing a limited number of patients. At the junior level, the team was buttressed by graduate students, who do the drudgery of research in any field of science. In between, postdocs designed new experiments, prepared specimens, made cultures, analyzed genechips, and amassed data—only to start the entire cycle over again when first tries failed. Like those in a hundred other laboratories at UCLA and thousands more throughout the world, their discoveries are made gradually, progressively, written in dispassionate scholarly papers that reveal little of the underlying passion, the long hours in the laboratory, at the computer, and at the blackboard exchanging ideas with peers.

One of the techniques the Project Indolence team used was "polymerase chain reaction," or PCR. This elegant process had been dreamed up in the 1970s by Kary Mullis, a Ph.D. biochemist turned writer, while he was driving down the road in Newport Beach, California, where he lives; it later won him the 1993 Nobel Prize in chemistry. PCR uses one of those strange heat-stable bacteria, *Thermus aquatics* (so-named because it lives in hot springs), to prime nature's method of copying DNA. When a cell divides, an enzyme called polymerase copies the DNA in each chromosome. Mullis replicated the event in the laboratory, and every scientist in the field now uses his technique routinely. A scientist heats DNA to separate the two chains of the double helix. As the material cools, primers anneal to the ends of the DNA strands. When heated again, the polymerase adds nucleotides to the primer and makes a complementary copy. That's the general idea, although the process is more complex than that.

PCR also makes possible "DNA fingerprinting," employed most famously in the O. J. Simpson murder trial. It is one of those developments so ingenious that it revolutionizes the way science works. It allows DNA fragments to proliferate exponentially, reminding me of a constantly accelerating rocketship eventually achieving fantastic speeds on the way to a distant planet. The DNA doubles, then doubles again—2, 4, 8, 16, 32, 64, 128—reaching a million clones on the twenty-fourth doubling, arriving at *a billion* on the thirty-first. Using this propagation of living fragments, today's scientists analyze the cloned DNA exhaustively, down to its sequence, down to the positioning of those four "letters," A, T, C, and G, which run the long length of a gene. The message deciphered reveals the proteins our cells can make, such as enzymes, or workers, or signalers.

Using both PCR and genechip technology, by the spring of 2000 the Koeffler lab had determined the functions of 203 genes commonly "upregulated"—that is, genes that increase a cell's responsiveness. The upregulated genes included ribosomal proteins (the site of messenger RNA attachment and amino-acid assembly), various translation factors, and genes important for DNA replication. The lab also analyzed 91 genes commonly "downregulated"—genes that decrease responsiveness, for instance, by producing immune-system molecules.

Today's technologically advanced hospitals use gene-expression profiling to predict which patients who have undergone cancer surgery will develop secondary tumors, or metastases. Having the ability to profile genes in this way is like being able to spot bomb-toting passengers in a crowded airport. Of course, profiling gene expression is infinitely more precise than profiling the proclivities of terrorists. (With such predictive ability, incidentally, breast-cancer patients so profiled these days are being advised *not* to undergo chemotherapy, which until recently had been considered standard procedure after surgery or radiation.)

The Koeffler team working on Project Indolence was more interested in finding the chain of events that causes cancer than in predicting which people might get it. They compared gene profiles of patients who had various lymphomas with a control group whose lymph nodes, although non-malignant, were swollen. (Bacteria from simple infections often drain into and enlarge lymph nodes.) To make the comparison, they extracted RNA from about ten million tumor cells and from another ten million cells from the nonmalignant lymph nodes of the control group. After running a series of biochemical reactions, the researchers were able to insert some six thousand genes into a single computer chip. At that point they measured the intensity of the genes with a laser scanner, which yielded an expression profile as a single number for each gene.

Both PCR and genechip technology are prime examples of the way scientific research creates better techniques, which in turn generate greater knowledge, an unending cycle of progress.

• • •

On one of my trips to Los Angeles during 2000, Phil Koeffler handed me a ream of paper listing almost four thousand genes in my mantle-cell lymphoma, neatly organized by computer under the headings: *Identification, Expression, Common Name,* and *Gene Description.*

"I didn't print out some three thousand other genes that had no expression," Phil said.

I picked out one at random that seemed to have a high expression—listing number 85 called "D12763"—and learned that it was expressing precisely 29.99 times the normal quantity, that its "common" name was "IL1RL1," and that its description was "interleukin-1, receptor 2."

"Is that good?" I asked.

"Well it means your interleukin-1 level is high, as you would expect in lymphoma. IL-1 originates in macrophages during the early, nonspecific phase of an immune response. It's one of the fever-inducing molecules."

• • •

Just as rocketry depends on computer technology to get us to the moon, so now does analyzing what is probably the most complex system in nature:

the molecular makeup of the human body. To extend the limits of knowledge faster, the largest chip maker, Intel, is in the midst of linking some four thousand computers across the world into a "Teragrid" capable of 14 trillion calculations per second. When completed in late 2003, the Teragrid will become the most super of supercomputers, able to store and access 450 trillion bytes of information. With all that computer power, scientists may still be unable to make perfect simulations of the incredibly complex behavior of human cells; yet even imperfect models will prove valuable. Headquartered at the University of Illinois in Urbana, the grid also will be used for drug discovery, weather forecasting, and other complex projects.

In science, however, you can't wait for the latest supertool. Wolf Hofmann, said, "We used whatever software we had at the time. The results were what was important, no matter how long it took. We selected single genes and gene clusters that were expressed differently in tumor and normal cells. Now we're comparing them to discover which genes are changed the most and which pathways to the tumor cells had been altered."

"Sounds like a meticulous job," I said. Wolf and I had gotten to know each other; later he served as the science editor for this book.

"It was . . . but it was worth it. We confirmed that the signals important for normal programmed cell death are reduced or absent in cells from MCL patients. That seems awfully obvious and intuitive, but what if it was wrong? What if there were some other mechanism instead of apoptosis? The absence of normal cell death in mantle-cell lymphoma had never been precisely established before. Now it is no longer a mere assumption." Cell suicide. Confirmed.

Project Indolence and similar inquiries are leading inexorably to a new paradigm. It may come sooner than you think—provided we can get the cancer-research direction of this country turned around and pointed toward molecular biology. In the near future, if you request it, your family physician will have your own personal genome profiled on a chip, filed neatly along with those of his other patients. After consulting an international database, he will treat you with specific drugs to alter any errant genes that have started to produce cancer or other chronic disease, doing so long before you experience symptoms.

The exact mechanisms that make lymphomas and leukemias progress into their aggressive, disastrous stages remain elusive, but the UCLA–Cedars-Sinai investigators are hot on the trail. By employing human tissue on a chip, the molecular scientists are doing nothing less than seizing temporary custody of cellular life and ordering it to reveal its secrets. "You could call it a scientific art form," Wolf said to me in a philosophical moment.

The Project Indolence discovery—that genes in a distinct set known to be critical in cell transformation are altered during the transition from indolent to aggressive blood cancers—is a vital first step in keeping those genes indolent. Permanently.

17

Cure Cancer in Ten Years

EVERYONE AGREES THAT CONDUCTING AND FUNDING RESEARCH TO cure cancer is the primary reason for the National Cancer Institute. Not everyone agrees on how to spend the money the NCI requests each year from Congress. Building and maintaining cancer centers, training, educating the public in prevention, developing new technologies, studying cancer trends, and especially running clinical trials are essential to the process, but they leave less for research. For what's left, there is fierce competition

Each year the House subcommittee in charge of health funding decides how much the NCI will spend on preventing and curing cancer as opposed to other diseases, and it was my honor to represent the Lymphoma Research Foundation in Washington, D.C. Chaired by Congressman John Porter, who represented Chicago's North Shore, the first subcommittee hearings of 2000 met (on the Ides of March) to hear testimony from . . . *supplicants.* There is no more precise way of putting it. These petitioners, representing foundations and societies, attempt to channel the finite pot of federal money into research to help stop *their* disease.

I flew into Reagan National, my first time there in Papa Whiskey, with some trepidation. The airport is lined with high-rise buildings that are virtually surrounded by another hazard, the winding Potomac River. Worse, if you get too close to the White House, defenders of the president may shoot you down with shoulder-fired missiles. The early spring morning that I arrived, however, was sunny and clear, and it turned out to be an easy landing, in part because the controllers keep a runway available for private aircraft. Already finished with his meetings at NASA headquarters, Shahid was waiting for me, having flown his plane in earlier. A young woman who worked for the firm that lobbied on behalf of the Lymphoma Research Foundation met us at the airport as planned and drove us to the Rayburn House Office Building.

The cherry blossoms were in full bloom. Gray squirrels were running up and down the trees, happy to be warm again in the March thaw. The huge Rayburn Building, with its white marble façade and pink granite base, named for the speaker from Texas who died in 1961, stood serenely at the end of a spacious field of grass southwest of the Capitol. Inside, it was a warren of wide corridors and tall doors opening to offices and conference rooms. Pillars, ornate plaster, solid balustrades. Rock solid like a castle. The third-floor hearing room was packed with cancer-foundation representatives. Most of these supplicants suffered from the cancer whose research they were trying to get extra-funded: cancers of the lung, breast, colon, prostate, or skin. A few others had debilitating maladies such as diabetes and Alzheimer's; some were semiconscious in wheelchairs, on display as articulate spokespersons made half-hour presentations.

When my turn came, following other funding pleas concerning specific organ cancers, I seated myself before a microphone at a small table. Above me on a raised platform sat the subcommittee chairman—a precise man with sandy hair wearing a well-tailored suit—his two aides, and a court reporter with a stenotype machine. No one else. The other ten members of the committee were absent, which surprised and angered me. Surprised because years ago I had been in this same building testifying at well-attended hearings about NASA funding for space exploration. Angered because these testimonies were on behalf of people who were suffering and dying.

"Chairman Porter," I began, adding somewhat uselessly (unless the absent members read the testimony later), "and members of the subcommittee. I have lymphoma—cancer of the lymph system. So do a half-million other Americans. Our country is suffering a lymphoma epidemic, which has spiked 82 percent in the U.S. since 1973. Lymphoma is increasing faster than any other cancer except melanoma. Unlike melanoma, which can be prevented by staying out of the sun, and unlike lung cancer and smoking, the causes of lymphoma are complex and largely unknown. Each year another sixty-one thousand Americans are contracting lymphoma, which has become the fourth leading cause of death by cancer.

"Studying lymphoma is central to curing other cancers. The white blood cells that fight infection move freely between the lymph and blood systems," I explained. "So a comprehensive cure for lymphoma must begin with a basic understanding of the interplay between these systems and how the immune system works, how the chromosomes and genes function, how the actual molecules of the cells fit together. Because leukemia and lymphoma are systemic—they pervade the whole body—most new discoveries are applicable to organ cancers as well."

I stole a glance at the Lymphoma Research Foundation's lobbyist sitting next to Shahid. She seemed pleased at the emphasis on lymphoma. My duty to the foundation done, I then proceeded to commit heresy. I urged that spending for *all* cancer research should be increased, pointing out that some 12.7 million Americans were being administered mostly ineffective toxic chemotherapies and that these poisons were still being used despite the revolution in molecular therapies now underway.

"We need *less competition* among the cancer advocates—the people in this room," I said, indicating them all with a wave of the hand. "We need cooperation. We have to end this wrangling for funds that achieves nothing but institutional sclerosis. We have to elevate the whole mission to cure cancer. Discoveries in *any* life-science field will help all others."

The shuffling of papers and whispering to colleagues among the other health delegates subsided when some of them heard me advocate cooperation. They were here to compete! Others saw them looking and turned their heads to the front, making me feel as though I were on the table in an operating room and they were medical observers. The court reporter peered up a moment from her steno machine. Chairman Porter looked down at me intently.

"Every year, one and a quarter million people are being diagnosed with cancer, adding to the six hundred thousand Americans who already have it. The almost thirteen million of them that are taking chemotherapy in any one year are weakening their immune systems, which makes them less responsive to new biotherapies. It's hard enough for a new biotherapy to fight cancer without expecting it to work on poisoned patients."

I told a little of the tremendous progress in the understanding and manipulation of genes that was being made, adding that the answer lay in more basic biological research. "Yet federal cancer spending for basic research is not appreciably larger today [2000] than when President Nixon declared his war on cancer—"

"Wait a minute," Congressman Porter said, glancing at an aide and then at me. "I thought we had something like a tenfold increase since Nixon started all this in—what—1971?"

"We did. Funding for the National Cancer Institute, adjusted for inflation," I said, "went up from $2 billion in 1971 to $3 billion." (That was in 2001. By 2003 the NCI budget had roughly doubled again. Federal and private spending on conventional cancer research has totaled $40 billion since the war on cancer was declared in 1971. In addition, the pharmaceutical industry spends almost $30 billion annually on applied research and product development.)

Departing from hard numbers, I explained that about half the budget was lumped under research, and the remainder went for promoting prevention, conducting clinical trials, or improving the infrastructure of the sixty-four cancer institutions supported by the government, such as M. D. Anderson and Sloan-Kettering, but also including nonresearch centers providing care or conducting trials.

"Sounds like the scientists ought to be happy with that," Porter said.

"The problem is the half that is lumped into research includes a lot of other things, such as administrative costs, testing, and trials of chemotherapeutic drugs. With chemotherapy soaking up so much of the research budget, funding for basic research is far less than reported."

"Well," Porter asked, gamely continuing the game, "if most of the research money doesn't find its way into actual basic research, how much does?"

"God only knows. I certainly don't."

Porter chuckled.

"My guess is that probably a third of the money actually gets to the scientists doing the work, for their salaries and equipment."

"What kinds of basic research need more funding?"

"Molecular biology. Immunology. With the new genomic profiling, we have an unprecedented opportunity to discover the precise biochemical interactions that progress to cancer."

"All the cancers? I've heard a million times that cancer is not just one disease; it's a hundred or so."

"Cancer could be considered a single disease in the sense that, no matter which organ or blood or bone is affected, the malignancy begins by a failure of programmed cell death. Cancer is one disease because basic research into human biology knows no borders of inquiry and because most of the new biological therapies are applicable to more than one type of cancer. On the other hand, you could think of cancer as being millions of separate diseases—one for each patient—because we are all unique, all different."

"Okay," Porter said. "How can we do better? God only knows we're throwing money at it. Billions."

"Yes, but we're throwing the money at proving or disproving preconceived ideas. Trial-and-error experiments that someone thinks up with more sophistry than science, like new combinations of chemotherapy toxins—without first doing the difficult basic biology to find out *how* the cells work."

"Are you saying that chemo doesn't work?"

I was silent for a long moment, thinking of the MCL Group's e-mails filled with tragedy, thinking of respected scientists still using chemo when more-benign treatments fail or when a patient has already had so much chemo that nothing else will work. "Not exactly," I began, hoping that Porter or anyone else reading the testimony later would have the patience to wade through a thoughtful answer. "I'm saying that chemotherapy has become part of the doctor-patient culture, that it is too widely accepted and relied upon as the first instead of the last choice. After all, if chemo worked for most cancers, there wouldn't be so many millions of people dying. We have spent a trillion dollars on chemotherapy during the thirty-year war against cancer. What is the result? We have more cancer in the country today than when we started."

Porter didn't appear to be offended by my audacity. But why should he be? The antichemo argument was probably news to him.

• • •

"What should we do to stop cancer?" The question came from a new voice, a deep voice from a second member of the congressional subcommittee who had just walked in and heard the gist of the discussion. Still standing and looking to me to answer was Congressman Jesse Jackson, the son of the widely known Reverend Jesse Jackson, both of Chicago.

"If Congress wanted to make the investment to expand basic research substantially," I ventured, *"we could cure cancer in a decade."* It was a premeditated statement loaded with emotional vitamins.

Porter and Jackson looked at me quizzically, as though not comprehending the pageant of pure power vested in the 535 members of Congress when it comes to wining the cancer war. They could understand shooting wars. Understanding science is not a long suit in our nonscientific Congress.

"Look," I said. "I realize that massive spending wouldn't have worked even a few years ago. These days it's different. Molecular biologists and other scientists can put dramatically larger funds to good use. The NCI funds less than 28 percent of cancer-research projects—well-thought-out, peer-reviewed projects. The other three-quarters of research projects go begging for funds elsewhere, or they don't get started at all. What we need is a creative, ambitious undertaking that will focus the tremendous energy of America: inaugurate a national goal to cure cancer in ten years."

As I was talking, Congressman Jackson whispered something to one of the aides, received a whispered answer, and left the room. He was a member of this subcommittee but had dropped in only to check something else. I was encountering a glimpse of our government at work—or nonwork.

Porter, on the other hand, seemed to compensate for his colleagues' lack of interest. I have met senators and representatives over the years through various strivings—advocating returning to the moon or limiting the National Park Service in taking over our town—and for the most part have found them locked in a bored attitude of censure. Not this one. Chairman Porter kept asking questions and seemed willing to alter the status quo, despite having announced the month before that he would be retiring from the House at the end of his term. Fortunately, subcommittee hearings are made public through the *Congressional Record*. I hoped someone would read them.

"Ten years," he repeated. Not a question. He was back on track, and you could tell he wanted to purse the idea.

"If research labs working on understanding these basic phenomena could be tripled or quadrupled," I said, "new areas could be explored as they come up—those 72 percent of projects that are going unfunded by the NCI. And not only for bench science. For software, too. The government could help establish a creative and prolific industry devoted to three-dimensional mapping of antigen expressions. Of all cancers. Then scientists could do pattern-matching by computer. There are all kinds of initiatives like that which ought to be encouraged."

"Do you think a national commitment to curing cancer in ten years would work?"

"Yes, I do. Let's say for a moment that the president announced a ten-year goal and Congress appropriated the money—and then we mobilized for it with the same dedication brought to bear in World War II. The challenge before us isn't only the amount of money allocated but what it goes for. The only way we could accomplish a ten-year goal would be to spend massively for basic research—to find out exactly what's going on in our bodies."

"We've always hoped big programs would work, but as you said, the more we spend, the further we are from curing cancer."

"It's different now."

"What makes it different?"

"Genomics. For the first time in history, scientists have the tools to understand how, why, when, and where the genes mutate to produce cancer in the first place. Never before have we understood the fundamentals, knowing what's happening at the cellular level, at the molecular level. Never before have we had the ability to study the interaction of actual molecules! Scientists do that now using computer chips containing DNA. They make mathematical simulations of how cancer cells behave in the body. The way it used to be . . . we were just guessing."

Porter leaned over the long narrow table set on the dais, a barren barrier behind which sat no other representatives, only aides. "Let's get back to curing cancer in ten years." He glanced at his notes to find my name. "Mr. Ruzic, how would you suggest we wage an *effective* war on cancer? Specifically?"

It was the question I'd been hoping for.

• • •

I took an index card from my pocket and glanced at the five words I'd listed: mobilize, ask, simplify, compete, coordinate. I looked around. Shahid and the lobbyist were attentive. The court reporter seemed poised for a flurry of typing.

"First, *mobilize for a blitz of science,*" I said, "to recruit the soldiers to fight this war. Proselytize college seniors into following scientific careers in medicine, computer simulation, immunology, genetics, biophysics, biochemistry, and molecular biology—*from everywhere in the world.* Do that at both the professional and technical-support level. Sure, this takes time, but the sooner we build our army of scientists and link them to computer wizards, the sooner they can join the battle. Offer full scholarships and economic assistance for students earning combined M.D. and Ph.D. degrees. That would relieve professors from having to pay their graduate students out of their research grants and make them a lot more productive. We're good at advertising in this country. Publicize the hell out of the new war on cancer to recruit the most brilliant people.

"Second, *ask the researchers* themselves. Fighting a cancer war isn't only about money. Ask the principal investigators in cancer research what they would do differently if they had *ten times the funding requested.* If the answers make theoretical sense, peer-review their project proposals *fast* and get them started. That may not sound like the most efficient way to spend money in the short run, but even theories ultimately shown to be wrong often have positive consequences. Lives are at stake here. And the investment will return manyfold. With people dying, time is the enemy. Any money wasted on the way to faster results will pale in comparison to the overwhelming financial benefit of a cancer-free economy. We can't afford the zero-sum game we're playing, where spending on breast cancer, for instance, detracts from, say, lymph cancer.

"Third, *get rid of convoluted FDA regulations.* Laboratory heads have to satisfy too many committees: radiation safety, biosafety, animal use, human subjects, ethnic diversity of patients—countless reviews, internal and external. Scientists spend more time writing proposals and filling out forms than they spend on doing science."

I glanced around at the room. Porter and his aides seemed to be soaking up my words like thirsty travelers at a fire hydrant. Even the delegates from the other health organizations were listening.

"Fourth," I continued, "*Encourage competition among researchers.* Competition works whether you are selling computers or researching cancer. Give prizes. Endow more chairs in medical research laboratories. The ten thousand universities in this country are America's greatest asset. Use them to the hilt. All graduate students in science perform basic research. It's this constant probing into fundamental molecular biology—and into seemingly unrelated research in bioengineering and three-dimensional simulation and the development of artificial intelligence to maximize computer searching—that will cure cancer. The research freedom at the universities and peer reviews to decide on worthy ideas are good practices that shouldn't be changed. Instead, the government should seek opportunities to expand the existing system and infrastructure.

"Finally, *coordinate*—really coordinate—the research results of both private drug companies and the National Cancer Institute with their own laboratories and those in universities. Only 1 percent of pharmaceutical-company research contracts with universities now require that researchers have access to the clinical data at other sites conducting the same trials! Coordination of both research and trials also must take place globally. Lives are lost and millions of dollars wasted on redundant clinical trials because each country has to repeat trials testing the same drugs. One day you read a scientific paper from a lab in the U.S. and a few months later you hear about the same trial conducted in Italy or England."

To his credit, Congressman Porter heard me out without interruption. Now he looked at his watch but asked one more question, "How would we implement all that? More bureaucracy? A cancer czar?"

"A *research* cancer czar. One person with a hundred staff members. A leader who is both a basic-research scientist and a competitive business leader, somebody like Craig Venter, the head of Celera, who sped up the human-genome project. . . . Whoever that someone is, charge him with coordinating a global central database and ultrafast communications system. So that scientists in cancer-related subfields wouldn't have to request pertinent information on a hit-or-miss basis. They'd be informed instantly of discoveries elsewhere that relate to their work."

Chairman Porter thought about that for a moment and smiled. He seemed to go for the activism. Aggression against an aggressive adversary. "If it worked, it could change the world. Cancer. Human misery. All those suffering people would be healthy and productive."

The chairman thanked me, which meant I had to stop, realizing he'd allowed me to run overtime. It would be a long day for him. The spokeswoman for diabetes was next to testify.

Porter's interest in my ideas vibrated within me like a sympathetic cord. It was ironic that the one member of this subcommittee charged with recommending appropriations for cancer and other health legislation, the one who was truly interested, who asked all the right questions, would retire at the end of that year. What I hadn't realized was that John Porter would continue his health campaign in a different role.

• • •

Since then I have talked again to John Porter about speeding up basic research for cancer. The ex-congressman, now Mister Porter, is now an attorney with Hogan and Hartson, in Washington, advising Congress on health issues. He is an effective spearhead, selling ideas to a Congress he understands firsthand. He and patient lobby groups, such as Research America, are leading the drive toward changing the way government spends our health dollars—107 billion every year—on therapy, which for cancer means chemotherapy. It is a tremendous sum, more than enough to find cures for chronic diseases if more of it were directed to basic research. The return on those dollars if, say 10 or 20 percent of them were spent for basic research, would be astronomical.

In 2001 Kevin Murphy and Robert Topel, economists at the University of Chicago, estimated cancer's total costs to society by calculating the years of productivity lost from patients dead and dying. Murphy and Topel concluded that if all forms of cancer were eliminated in the United States, the economic value to the nation would be $46.5 trillion!

Their calculation had been buried on the inside pages of newspapers. When I read it, I was incredulous. I called Prof. Topel in Chicago. "Forty-six *trillion?* Did you say *trillion?* That's more than all assets in the United States!"

"It is," he said. "It includes the gigantic health-care expenses that drain Medicare, the wasting of so many otherwise productive years of relatives tending helpless patients, and the *trillions* of dollars unearned by the sick and dead victims themselves."

"How did you calculate the cost of a life?"

"We estimated the value of lives saved—now and in the future until actuarial death—and discounted them back to the present at a 3.5 percent rate of interest. We figured the value of one working lifetime at about $5 million."

A pregnant pause. I had never thought of the value of lives in economic terms.

"Exporting cures for cancer and other diseases would make great foreign policy," I said.

"Yes," he said, thoughtfully.

• • •

I am aware of the other side of this argument, that curing disease allows people to live longer, further crowding the planet and diminishing resources. Being an optimist, I see it the other way around. Healthy people have time for education, for democracy, for resisting dictators. As once before I had urged that we "wage peace," in a widely read article I wrote by that name, now I found myself advocating that we *wage heath*. Exporting health would empower people to develop other resources, such as wind, solar, and nuclear energy; to slow population growth; and to lead themselves out of poverty and into education and democracy. The benefits are incalculable. Democracies, for instance, do not go to war against one another (at least not so far), an astounding conclusion based on analyses that have been documented but not publicized.

Global prosperity through curing cancer and other diseases is feasible for the first time in history. The dramatic funding increases in the United States for fiscal 2003 have set health science on an uphill road, driving slowly but steadily toward new research to cure cancer.

Whether that cure arrives in ten years, or in thirty years, is primarily a matter of money—redirecting tax dollars already allocated.

18

Think Tanks

AN EASY WAY OF TALKING TO SCIENTISTS ABOUT THEIR RESEARCH IS
to attend their conferences, and while my helpers or I attended quite a few,
three stand out for their marked differences. The first was a small think tank
sponsored by the Lymphoma Research Foundation and held at Stone Mountain, Georgia, to which I flew Papa Whiskey directly from Washington after
giving my congressional testimony. Arriving northeast of Atlanta, I circled
the stony mountain and its evergreen-lined valley, landed at the Peachtree
airport, and took a limo to the lodge, arriving early and eagerly for the four-
day meeting.

The think tank consisted of some twenty heads of university laboratories, mostly from the United States but also from Britain, Italy, and Germany,
and foundation staffers, who like me were observers. It was one of the
foundation's more-important undertakings because it encouraged participants to bond with one another in a smaller, less-formal setting than the big
conferences. After giving a slide presentation of his lab's latest work, each
principal joined in discussions around tables set in a square. Meeting their
colleagues from across the ocean at tables of six at breakfast, lunch, and dinner was the main point of the think tank, however, not the prepared papers
or the subsequent question-and-answer sessions where the introverts
watched the extroverts convey their views.

Subjects ranged over the gamut of blood-cancer research. Ronald Levy discussed the allure of the CD20 marker for monoclonal antibodies, since it appears on the surfaces of 93 percent of B-cell lymphomas (like mine). Yet CD20 is absent on plasma cells, normal tissues, and unfortunately on precursors to B-cell lymphomas. The anti-CD20 Mab Rituxan was proving highly successful for many lymphomas, Levy acknowledged, as were manufactured antibodies specific for some organ cancers. Others immersed in this think tank suggested that the lab directors keep in mind the goal for developing therapies that would be more universal, treating all lymphomas or all cancers.

In answer, one participant mentioned how many biotech companies were hot on the trail of novel approaches. This fact has not gone unnoticed by the giant pharmaceutical companies—all of which were either acquiring promising biotechs or infusing cash into them in trade for partnerships on semiproved research that would lead to new drugs. Whereas monoclonal antibodies and vaccines use the immune system to fight cancer, one promising method called "antisense" seeks to block production of proteins necessary for cell immortality. The group discussed several compounds capable of that feat that were emerging from clinical trials conducted by Genta, Inc., together with Avertis Pharmaceuticals and by Isis Pharmaceuticals with its partner Eli Lilly. Both Avertis and Lilly are among the world's largest pharmaceutical companies.

To understand antisense you have to look at DNA, which comprises two interwoven strands bound by unique molecules called nucleotides. These DNA strands—one termed "sense" and the other "antisense"—create the proteins that help maintain normal cell growth. Antisense drugs are short strands of modified DNA designed to oppose the sense message carried to cancer cells by proteins. Animals, plants, all living things perform the dance between sense and antisense in maintaining cell growth. Antisense cleaves, or knocks out, the sense protein that carries the message to make cancer cells, literally changing the design of that protein so it no longer can shield cancer cells from normal death. And it does so without altering any other protein. This potent-but-safe biological therapy has been shown to inhibit the expression of Bcl-2 (B-cell lymphoma number 2), which is found also in other cancers. Genta's antisense therapy would become of intense interest to me in late 2002. By then it had entered clinical trials for lung cancer, acute myeloid leukemia, prostate cancer . . . and mantle-cell lymphoma.

Other research that came to light at the think tank included "kinesins." These are enzyme proteins that run along microtubules, tiny tracks within a cell that transport bits of DNA, and they were being disrupted selectively in experiments at Cytokinetics and its giant partner, GlaxoSmithKline. I had known about kinesins from my days publishing *Oceanology* magazine, for they were discovered a quarter-century ago in the nerve cells of a squids. A human cell contains about forty-five kinesins, which power motion within cells like tiny motors. They are efficient little critters, converting chemical energy into work at about 50 percent efficiency (mechanical engines usually convert less than 15 percent of energy into work).

To inhibit kinesins, Cytokinetics investigators interrupt cell division selectively, inducing cell death in tumors. Trial-and-error screening of 200,000 compounds finally resulted in one that reduced tumor growth by more than 75 percent in a mouse that had been given human pancreatic cancer, a particularly difficult disease to treat. Unlike antisense, the as-yet-unnamed drug for stopping kinesins was a long way from human clinical trials.

Although only an observer at the think tank, I was regarded by the scientists not exactly as an equal but more as a representative from some other world of science, perhaps an early Mars when it held oceans. Between sessions I talked to two lab directors from Britain who became genuinely interested in the indolence of my lymphoma and more engrossed as they drew me out about my aquaculture research. They were Andrew Lister, an M.D. at St. Bartholomew's Hospital, and David Mason, an M.D. at Oxford's Radcliffe Hospital, both world-renowned institutions in or near London. David Mason looks and talks somewhat like the actor James Mason. I gave him a copy of my novel about the Island for Science. At dinner that night at a table with Lister and three others—an American, a German, and an Italian—Mason made me a gift of a beguiling book, *The Faber Book of Science,* containing passages by the world's great scientists—Galileo, Newton, Darwin, Einstein, Feynman, and many others.

"My favorite," Mason said, "is Priestley's honest description of how pure chance was responsible for most of his discoveries. It is the kind of chance, however, that comes only to those who position themselves in the path of serendipity."

He opened the book to the Priestley chapter, and while he watched, I speed-read the four-page chapter entitled "Two Mice Discover Oxygen," which is how Joseph Priestley put it in 1775 when he separated the mixture we breathe into "two types of air." He had managed to separate oxygen from nitrogen without knowing what he had done. He put a mouse inside a glass jar containing "the other kind of air" and was surprised that it was active for a full half-hour, twice as long as another mouse that had been placed in a closed jar of ordinary air.

"I'm glad to see he kept hold of their tails," I said, smiling at Priestly's antique words and concern for his animals, "that they may be withdrawn as soon as they begin to show signs of uneasiness." Although the mouse immersed in what became known as oxygen came out unconscious and seemingly chilled, "it presently revived on being held near a fire and appeared not to have received any harm from the experiment."

The conversation, soon joined by the other scientists at our table, turned into a full-scale discussion of the treatment of lab animals, a topic that concerned them. I knew that mice constitute the overwhelming majority of mammals used for experiments in the United States and Europe. What I didn't realize until the German scientist mentioned it was that chimpanzees, monkeys, dogs, cats, rats, and rabbits are used, too, especially in Europe and Asia. The scientists at our table expressed a certain reverence for animal life, as have other men and women of science I have met.

"Do any of you go hunting?" I wanted to know.

"Shooting animals for *sport?*" said the Italian, spitting the last word. "This is sport?" The others laughed in agreement.

"Every time I experiment on animals, I have to remind myself that it's for the greater good of humans," Mason said, adding, "and for the good of the animal population as well."

I told him my son's dog recently had contracted lymphoma, and the vets gave him chemotherapy, which helped for a few months before he died.

"In a sense, we share the problem inherent in veterinary," Mason said, "working with several species. I can't help but notice how even tiny mammals such as mice and hamsters possess four-chambered hearts, spleens, and other organs and possess essentially the same genes as ours for the same bodily functions. The problem in extrapolating data from mice to humans is not because we are that much different—all mammals are closely related—but because our cancers occur by environmental mutations, whereas mouse cancers ordinarily have been transferred to them full-blown in the laboratory."

The German mentioned that he had been mulling over the ethics of laboratory animals, a problem these days with animal-rights activists on the march. "What really is the difference between us and the other mammals? They have feelings, yes? The difference is only the quantum of intelligence."

"Self-awareness seems implicit in elephants, whales, and nonhuman primates," offered the Italian.

"Not only mammals," I said, telling them that while diving off the Island for Science, I once made eye contact with and then befriended a two-foot octopus who lived under a coral head.

The other American at our table described how experimenters in the United States proceed according to stringent humane rules: fruit flies are used when feasible; otherwise, a lab animal must be anesthetized sufficiently to be insensible to pain; if injured during an operation to the point of suffering, it must be destroyed while still insensible; an animal who has undergone one operation cannot be subjected to another; authorizations must be sought, records kept, and so on. The Europeans said they worked under similar regulations.

I thought laboratories surely treated mice better than do most households, where a mouse receives slow death in a dark basement after a steel spring breaks its backs and leaves it to suffer. Between ten and twenty million unwanted dogs and cats are euthanized in the United States every year, and several million more starve to death, are shot, or are killed on highways. By contrast, there are twenty-five million laboratory animals in U.S. laboratories today, the overwhelming majority of them rodents. Putting these numbers into perspective, only a fraction of lab animals are destroyed in any one year, and these animals die humanely and with purpose. I am an animal lover, but I know we need animals for experimentation, for there is no better way to conduct tests in advance of human clinical trials. We must—and do—use them humanely.

· · ·

A few months later, in May, a super think tank was held in New Orleans. It was the annual meeting of the American Society of Clinical Oncology, attended by 25,000 cancer doctors. Rade and Leslie Pejic were at O'Hare, waiting for a flight to New Orleans, where their son, Rade Jr., was graduating from medical school. A friendly, outgoing woman, Leslie started talking to a bevy of oncologists waiting for the same flight.

"There were dozens there," she said, "from all over the States and Europe. The first thing I asked was how effective they thought the monoclonal antibodies were, especially the radioactive Mabs. The silence was stunning. They didn't know what I was talking about. I repeated the question to others. Same results."

"How about on the way back?" I suggested.

"Same thing. After the graduation and the parties were over, our return flight coincided with the end of the oncology meeting. We saw some of the same people. They still didn't know anything about Mabs, vaccines, stimulation of T cells, or anything of what you and I have been studying."

Intrigued, I accessed the conference's Web site to see what on earth the five days of meetings had been about. "Comparative Cost-Effectiveness of Paclitaxel-Cisplatin vs. Cyclophosphamide-Cisplatin in Ovarian Cancer," "Non-Small-Cell Lung Cancer Treated with Concurrent Thoracic Radiotherapy and Chemotherapy," "Combined Radiation and Chemotherapy Improves Survival in Adenocarcinoma of the Stomach," "Thalidomide for Multiple Myeloma after Stem-Cell Transplant," and so on. There were a few preliminary papers on using celecoxib, or Celebrex, to starve tumors by killing their blood vessels, but nothing on low-dose thalidomide as an antiangiogenic.

A year later I retrieved a list of papers given at the next oncologist's meeting, this one held in San Francisco. Chemotherapy still dominated the sessions, but some papers addressed Celebrex, the breast-cancer Mab Herceptin (approved three years earlier, in 1998), and genomics. To its credit, the society awarded $2.2 million to promising research projects leading to biological therapies. Chemotherapists *do* learn about scientific treatments beyond chemo at these conferences. Then they return home and continue administering chemotherapy and radiation.

. . .

A third conference was the annual ASH meeting—the American Society of Hematology. In December 2001 I flew my plane to Orlando and drove to the nearby convention center, a sprawling building set amid a mass of parking lots, like a big-city airport. As does the clinical oncology meeting, this conference draws 25,000 attendees. These, however, are mostly scientists humbled before the immense alter of complexity that is the human body.

For six days and nights they select from an incredible menu of 3,500 lectures and poster sessions (informal discussions in the exhibit hall between the presenter and passers-by). The subjects include every aspect of blood— bone marrow, immunology, transplantation, diagnostic tests, new therapies. Blood being central to human function, its study contributes to the understanding of all cancers. Virtually all research hematologists are oncologists; that is, they treat patients. In contrast, as I realized from the oncology society's meeting, few oncologists are hematologists—or for that matter, scientists of any stripe.

When they were not listening to papers being presented, conferees ambled through a room the size of a football field half-filled with booths displaying the science behind new drugs under development by pharmaceutical houses and biotechs. The other half of the vast hall contained research posters, some colorful, arranged in rows like vials of blood in a lab rack.

Standing a little apart from a small group that had assembled at one poster session, I recognized Dr. D, the man I had tried to ask about a chemo-free vaccine trial. It had been, I calculated roughly, fifteen months since I'd talked to him on the phone. During that time he appeared often at lymphoma meetings, and I had read several interview articles in our foundation newsletter that included his photo. I sidled up to him and read his name tag, confirming that it was indeed the same Dr. D. It's no fun to approach someone impenetrable, but I gritted my teeth, hoping by now that he had changed his mind. It was important.

Introducing myself as a director of the Lymphoma Research Foundation, I asked him about Mark Kaminski's plan to start a clinical vaccine trial using Bexxar instead of chemo to reduce the tumor burden.

He glanced at my name tag, trying to be intensely elsewhere. "Chemo works to lower the tumor burden," he said with exaggerated patience. "Why try it with something else that may or may not be as effective?"

One more instance of short-term solutions steamrolling long-term survival, I wanted to say, but instead I spelled it out for him: "Because if a Mab would work as well, we could get vaccines without the dangers inherent in poisoning the system with toxins."

"You don't know the technical problems involved, and I don't have time for such . . . ," letting the word *nonsense* hang in the air between us. "I wish you'd stop bothering me about this . . . idea."

It had been more than a year since I'd talked to him for thirty seconds, not exactly bestowing nuisance status on me. Dr. D looked haggard, unwell, which could have accounted for his intransigence. I wondered where his arrogance came from—maybe from years of deciding treatments for incurable cancer patients too sick or too weak in spirit to think for themselves. At least he cited "technical" problems instead of hiding behind the FDA. He knew that I knew trials such as those using a radio-Mab plus vaccine could be approved when the request came from a scientist as entrenched with the FDA as himself.

Dr. D was obviously anxious to end this conversation. I changed the subject, hoping to get into anti-angiogenesis. "You may remember a year ago I mentioned my MCL was indolent, that my lymph nodes were shrinking. Well, since then they have continued to shrink—"

"Don't count on it," he said. His nose twisted as if smelling the words he heard, words that were giving off an offensive odor. "Lymphomas are notorious for waxing and waning," he added.

"But mine have only waned."

"So far."

"I wonder whether Celebrex could be killing the capillaries feeding my tumor cells," I asked.

"Not likely," he said. He took his cell phone out of his pocket and started dialing, moving away in a dazzling display of pedantry.

• • •

Dr. C from Chicago—Dr. CHOP—was at this conference, too, although by then he had become "Dr. CHOP + R." That is, he had added Rituxan to his mix of chemotherapy, and I attended a paper he gave on that combination therapy. I was puzzled in this way: obviously Dr. C was knowledgeable about the molecular sciences and radioactive Mabs. They were under discussion at hundreds of sessions at this very conference, if nowhere else. Why, then, did he persist in treating his mantle-cell lymphoma patients with outmoded recipes for disaster instead of enrolling them in clinical trials where there was some hope, actually excellent hope, for their long-term remissions? I really wanted to hear his answer. I waited until after the session, after the last questioner had left him at the podium. As he strode out of the conference room and along the broad hallway, I kept pace with him and asked why he continued to use CHOP for mantle-cell lymphoma patients, albeit with Rituxan, as first therapy.

He stopped, glancing around to make sure no one was listening, and said, "Because these new treatments are not approved. *I don't have time for lawsuits.*" His unsocial veracity amazed me, as in having "thank you" answered by "you are not welcome."

"Lawsuits for getting patients into clinical trials?" I asked.

"No, of course not, but patients don't stop at trials. You get one patient into a trial, then a dozen more want the same therapy after the trial is closed. You bend for one, you bend for all. One guy dies and you're charged with malpractice." He kept turning his head as though hoping to find something—escape, maybe.

Today, as I write these words, I have learned that Dr. C became a garrulous spokesman for the radioactive antibody Zevalin after the FDA approved it in 2001 (surprisingly ahead of Bexxar, which was developed much earlier). Like most cancer therapists, he simply waits for final approval. As he said, if you bend for one, you bend for all. With an attitude like that, I realized why 85 percent of cancer patients are unaware of clinical trials that could save their lives, instead led by their noses into the Chemo Culture.

As I went my way at the Orlando conference, I had to ask myself whether this apparent truth about Dr. C and other chemotherapists was real or only a manifestation of their own phenotypes, a convenient cop-out designed to hide their indolence regarding patients. There was no way I would ever know, but it made me thankful for Phil Koeffler, Mark Kaminski, Mike Blend, Ollie Press, Dan Longo, and the rest of the dauntless researchers who double as practitioners and persevere in helping their patients to restored health. They were tearing down the wall between medicine and science.

• • •

The next day I had lunch at a convention-center restaurant with my friends Phil Koeffler, Sven de Vos, and Wolf Hofmann. Wolf recently had left the Koeffler lab and moved back home to Germany, at the University Hospital in Frankfurt.

Koeffler—early fifties, princely, tranquil, soft-spoken—is an effective leader, alert to nuances where creativity lurks in his protégés. Sven, the other German, and Wolf are both in their thirties, both unusually tall, especially Sven who is tautly drawn to six-foot-five. Wearing shirts and ties without suit coats (the scientist's uniform of the day), they were obviously happy to be among their colleagues. Not for the first time, I realized how intriguing was their science, made more so by its importance. Three other postdocs joined us: another German, a Japanese, and a young American woman in her twenties. Her appearance here surprised me, not because she was female, but because she was American, a vanishing nationality, it seems, in this country's research laboratories. Those at the table, all M.D.s, Ph.D.s, or both, work or have worked for Phil, their mentor. They made up one of the Project Indolence teams then in its third year and well on its way to determining why lymphomas change from lazy to hostile. Phil Koeffler told me about a related study they were beginning, one specifically for mantle-cell lymphoma.

"We've already identified candidate genes," Phil said. "Now we want to find how these genes cooperate with cyclin D1 in the development of MCL to try to reverse the aberrant pathways."

"How are you going about it?"

"Initially by replacing genes that are either poorly expressed or reversing the expression of genes that are too highly expressed. If this works, we'll team up with a pharmaceutical company to identify molecules that can reverse the abnormal pathways."

"Who's funding it?" I asked.

"Nobody yet," Phil said.

I volunteered and wrote him a check I would cover later by selling stock. By year's end I induced several MCL Group members to join me. Few projects could be as specific for mantle-cell lymphoma as this one, but few in the group had money they could spare. My own funds were dwindling, too. I am not one who sees the answers to society's problems in bigger government and bigger bureaucracies. Clearly, however, this kind of fundamental research requires action by government, whose first responsibility is the defense of its citizens.

• • •

There is a maxim that you can reach any one of the earth's six billion inhabitants, no matter where he lives, by asking someone you know, who knows someone, who knows someone else—going through a succession of no more than a handful of steps. Before the election of 2000, I needed only two intermediaries to contact the man soon to be president. My first step was to call a friend who, the year before, had bought most of my island lodge. He was a prominent businessman in Houston and knew George W. Staake, a former Texas secretary of state, who knew the then-candidate George W. Bush. Staake promised that if I wrote a letter to Bush, he would ensure that Bush would read it.

My letter, sent May 2, 2000, suggested that the future president make a campaign promise of curing cancer in ten years and detailed how the promise could be implemented. Some months later Staake wrote, "It looks to me that much of your plan was adopted by Bush when he came up with his $91 billion over *ten years* to renew the war on cancer."

It was more than a campaign promise. President George Bush's request of $27.3 billion for the National Institutes of Health was adopted by Congress, an impressive first step and double the 1998 level of $13.6 billion. Of that amount, $5.5 billion was directed specifically for the National Cancer Institute. Maybe letters to candidates running for high office truly are read. (I am sure mine was not the only such letter.) Maybe ordinary citizens do get attention in our democracy.

No one can fault the government's new commitment to the war on disease in terms of money thrown at the problem. The new challenge is to change the government's agonizingly slow status quo, to alter the spending mix in favor of basic research so that laboratories like Koeffler's can recruit more scientists, and to streamline FDA regulations. In this country, in our time, lives matter. As much as we need to fight terrorists, we also need to recognize that the daily war waged against cancer in our bodies is far more devastating, for it is killing not three thousand Americans in New York and Washington but six hundred thousand throughout the nation. Every year.

· · ·

In December 2002, well after the NIH budget for cancer had been doubled, I went to another annual ASH conference, this one in Philadelphia. By then there was a preponderance of papers presented on targeted, biological therapies. And yet—even at this most scientific of large medical meetings on cancer, attended by hematologists and oncologists from throughout the world—the doctors who see patients revealed themselves unready to practice what they were learning. At one session, called "Challenging Cases in Lymphoma," attended by about two hundred oncologists, the discussion leader asked this question: "What would you use today as first therapy to treat a fifty-seven-year-old man diagnosed with mantle-cell lymphoma?"

Approximately half the practitioners answered "CHOP with Rituxan," some 30 percent said "hyper-CVAD with Rituxan," and 20 percent chose hyper-CVAD alone. None in the room ventured to recommend monoclonal antibodies, vaccines, anti-angiogenics, or other targeted bioagents as first therapy for this most aggressive of blood diseases.

Despite conferences, think tanks, and other scientific meetings, practicing physicians are slow to adopt fundamentally new cancer therapies. The problem resides not only in lengthy FDA approvals. The scientists themselves, those who make the discoveries, are reluctant to promote their new therapies as cures, having been thwarted so often in the past. Even those so inclined are severely limited by time. Scientists are arguably the busiest worker bees on the planet. Many of them, especially the principal investigators and heads of labs, spend most of their time seeking funds; publishing in order not to perish (the adage is true); managing research, budgets, and graduate students; devising and repeating experiments in their own laboratories; attempting to replicate results discovered elsewhere; reviewing the papers of their peers as kindly or as critically as expected by the golden rule; serving on boards of foundations; and occasionally testifying before congressional subcommittees. Some M.D. researchers, such as Phil Koeffler and Dan Longo, also make time to treat a limited number of patients. And often, as does Koeffler, they teach. Making discoveries under such severe time limitations is difficult enough, let alone convincing the world to use them.

For the work they do, the incremental discoveries they make, the lives they ultimately save, they earn a bureaucrat's wages while working an entrepreneur's hours. On average, the 25,000 clinical oncologists, who are mostly chemotherapists, earn about twice as much as the 25,000 hematologists, who are mostly scientists. I endorse free markets and the freedom to work where you please. All the same, I am thankful that there are those who forsake the more-lucrative branches of medicine and choose scientific research instead, finding the pursuit of truth to be its own reward.

19

Transplants: Risk vs. Cure

PICTURE YOURSELF LOST AT SEA IN A WOODEN LIFEBOAT. A SMALL airplane like Papa Whiskey flies by at dusk. You have two choices. You can pour the gallon of gasoline saved for this purpose over the boat and set it afire to attract the plane, hoping while you flounder in the water that the pilot and his technology are capable of rescuing you. Or you can remain in the boat and continue to drift for an unknown time, hoping for ultimate salvation. In both cases the key word is *hope*. The benefits of immediate deliverance are partly real and partly emotional, for when you are a cancer victim, you are adrift in a vast and empty ocean, in agony bordering on panic. Isolated from health and therefore from life, you imagine your malignancy widening, engulfing your entire body. You need to do something for yourself, for your family. Now.

After years of chemotherapy, when a cancer patient becomes refractory, a bone-marrow or stem-cell transplant, like setting fire to your lifeboat, can be seen as a necessity. Statistics vary tremendously, and while not an especially good guide to helping a patient decide, they can be seductive. My friend Ellen Cohen, president of the Lymphoma Research Foundation of America, had chronic lymphocytic leukemia and was intrigued by a study at M. D. Anderson. It reported that CLL patients have a 40 percent chance of long-term survival after transplants but only a 26 percent probability when treated with chemotherapy. Ovarian-cancer patients have less chance—25 percent disease-free survival at eight years, according to some studies—but that's because for many, their immune systems already have been damaged by the cancer itself by the time they are diagnosed.

Ellen was as youthful and energetic at fifty as when she founded the foundation fifteen years before. We had been talking for a year about potential cures for blood cancers—on the phone every few days and in person every third month before the foundation board meetings. She was as convinced as I that the university emphasis on molecular biology would lead to real cures, and she urged me to find out about them and recommend significant projects for funding to the rest of the board of directors.

"I don't want us to focus on CLL, my own disease," she emphasized. Most of Ellen's work involved fund-raising for the foundation, and she was worried that contributors might think she was using their money to cure her own cancer.

"Ellen," I reminded her, "CLL is the most prevalent form of adult blood cancer in the Western Hemisphere. It affects sixty thousand in the U.S. and an equal number in Europe."

"Still, if we sponsored a CLL study, it would give the appearance of impropriety."

"That may be a moot point," I said. "If we're going to back research leading to biotherapies, it doesn't matter what form of lymphoma or leukemia scientists start with. Whatever they discover will apply to them all."

The funding of research projects soon became irrelevant for Ellen. By the spring of 2000 her CLL erupted again, forcing her to divert her attention from the foundation to her own survival. She'd had chemotherapy off and on over the years—primarily the toxin cyclophosphamide and the more-specific fludarabine, which interferes with DNA formation so new leukemia cells cannot grow. She had also taken a drug called "filgrastim" (or Neupogen), which stimulates the production of white blood cells. Her white-blood-cell counts had fallen dramatically despite these medications. She had arrived at the point where she was refractory to chemotherapy—unless toxins were administered in lethal doses. The only way to do that without killing the patient was to administer the assault to the cancer cells in conjunction with a bone-marrow or stem-cell transplant.

• • •

Ellen certainly knew of biological alternatives to transplants. She had been looking over my shoulder into laboratory science for the past year and was intrigued by a new biotherapy drug for a disease that might be similar to hers. In February, at Ellen's suggestion, I called Brian Druker (pronounced *DREW-ker*), the now-famous professor of medicine at Oregon Health and Science University. Druker was working in collaboration with the Swiss pharmaceutical giant Novartis on what soon would be known as Gleevec in the United States (and Glivec elsewhere) to combat chronic myelogenous leukemia—CML, not Ellen's CLL. One of the rare, often-fatal forms of leukemia, CML originates in the bone marrow and causes uncontrolled growth of white blood cells that can clog blood vessels, leading to strokes or heart attacks. Chronic myelogenous leukemia affects only about five thousand people in the United States and a similar number in Europe. What was exciting about this drug wasn't that Gleevec itself would help thousands of people but that it targets the genetic defects underlying the cancer. It shuts down the abnormality produced by the translocation of chromosomes 9 and 22—a genetic jumble known as the "Philadelphia mutation," named for the city where it first was identified.

"Dr. Druker," I said after introducing myself on the phone, "isn't CML pretty close, genetically, to CLL?"

To a nonspecialist like me, the cancers seemed awfully similar: both are chronic, both are leukemic, but one is myelogenous (in the bone marrow) whereas the other is lymphocytic (in the lymph system). While I was still trying to formulate a plan against my own lymphoma, I also was helping Ellen with hers.

Druker, whose portrait stared out at me from his Web site, had penetrating eyes under heavy brows and a high forehead. Although in his late forties, he looked too young to have been working on the genomic pathways to CML for almost two decades. I could picture him as a young resident in a lab coat marching off with his stethoscope to fight cancer—and then being surprised two decades later to have done just that.

"Yes and no," he said. "Some cancers that *seem* close—like CML and CLL—have a way of moving further apart the more you study them. Our drug is unlikely to work against lymphomas, including CLL," he said, "because these cancers are not caused by the same mutation that is blocked by Gleevec."

"Now that you've had such great success with C*M*L," I asked, emphasizing the middle letter, "would you consider turning your attention to the mutations that trigger CLL?"

"A lot of researchers are trying to adapt this model to treat other cancers," Druker said. "For the forseeable future my focus will remain on diseases that are genetically closer to MCL."

Neither Ellen nor I—and probably not even Brian Druker—could have imagined the rapid progress of Gleevec during the next year or two. Gleevec was approved in May 2001, and the event made headlines as the fastest FDA drug approval in history. Gleevec's manufacturer, the big Swiss drug company Novartis, produced it immediately and gave it free to cure formerly hopeless CML patients. Phase-three and -four trials came afterwards. The entire medical-science community hailed Gleevec as the first in a new class of agents known as growth-factor inhibitors. If Gleevec could recognize and alter the unique molecular defects that caused certain cancers, could other biological drugs be far behind?

Even while their researchers continue to penetrate the genomic mechanism of a successful drug, pharmaceutical companies don't wait to try it out on related diseases. Novartis was no exception. Like IDEC and Genentech with Rituxan, like Pharmacia with Celebrex, Novartis saw Gleevec as a potential cure in search of other cancers. They started trying Gleevec against tumors in the brain, lungs, breast, and prostate, often in combination with other drugs—with little success. Surprisingly, however, a seemingly unrelated cancer called gastrointestinal stromal tumors, or GIST, takes a similar gene-to-protein pathway that *can* be disrupted by Gleevec. Stromal tissues are those that support an organ, and this type of cancer is among the most

• deadly of intestinal malignancies, its only other effective treatment being early surgical removal. In February 2002 Gleevec was approved for GIST.

. . .

Before the Gleevec success, at the time of Ellen Cohen's need in 2000, biotherapies were largely unapproved except for a few monoclonal antibodies, and she asked me what I would do if my lymphoma should turn aggressive. The quickness of my answer surprised even myself, since I had not been dwelling in those terms for a while.

"Okay, I would take Rituxan first, then high-dose Rituxan, then—even if Rituxan worked—I'd try hard to get an idiotype vaccine without taking chemo first."

"Without the FDA's pet gold standard? Good luck. What next?"

"Another anti-angiogenic to work in synergy with the Celebrex I'm taking."

"Which one?"

"It would depend on the state of the art at the time. Right now, probably vinblastine or thalidomide—with the Celebrex."

"And if all that didn't work?"

"If co-stimulation of T cells or some gene-modification therapy wasn't available by then, I'd want a radioactive antibody. . . . How about your plan, Ellen?"

"Well, you know about the Berlex monoclonal antibody alemtuzumab, or Campath?"

"Right. It's now in clinical trails. Why don't you get into a trial?"

"I've been talking to my oncologist about it. He seems reluctant."

Just as Rituxan attaches to the cell surface marker CD20, Campath homes in on the CD52 marker, which is prolific on CLL and other leukemic cells. Patients in Swedish trials at the time—actual CLL patients given Campath, not mere human cells in a laboratory dish—showed an overall response rate of 87 percent. Campath wasn't yet approved, but Rituxan was. High-dose Rituxan either alone or in combination with fludarabine or another drug commonly given for leukemia (pentostatin) had been found in randomized human trials in the United States to be statistically effective against CLL. They sounded like a low-risk option for Ellen.

"I don't know what to do," Ellen said. "My doctors are so wary of anything experimental, it's hard for me to insist on something. I mean, what do *I* know?"

And, I thought, what do I know? I'm not an oncologist. How could I advise someone like Ellen, who as the head of the foundation could have a good part of the lymphoma medical community at her disposal? I could only make sure she knew about various options and encourage her to talk to the scientists who were developing these drugs. For years Ellen had been spending the larger part of each day talking on the phone, raising money, and directing the business of her foundation. Nevertheless, she was reluctant to talk to scientists. She said she had trouble understanding them and comparing their suggestions.

Possibly because Campath was still in clinical trials and would not be approved until the following year (in May 2001), her doctors recommended a transplant. As in my analogy of the shipwrecked sailor, Ellen decided to "burn the boat" in an attempt for a true cure. There is enormous pressure to make a decision when you are a cancer patient holding out for something new. I know. I have been there. The pressure comes from your doctors, from your family, from yourself. Such life-and-death decisions often segue insidiously and automatically into your consciousness. Instead of asking yourself whether you should have the transplant, your thinking shifts to a more-limited framework: *If I am going to undergo a transplant, what kind of transplant?*

Ellen considered a "mini-transplant," so called because it is preceded by minimal quantities of chemotherapy or radiation. Usually employed on elderly patients unable to tolerate full doses, minimal transplants, as the name implies, require less therapy and therefore are less dangerous than full transplants, but they are also less successful. The patient's bone marrow is not completely wiped out with total body irradiation (or a radio-Mab), and minimal chemotherapy is administered—just enough to allow a donor's stem cells to engraft in the recipient's system. The hope in jumping into this sea of therapy is that the donor's T cells will recognize the recipient's cancer cells as being foreign and mount a response against them.

This is called the graft-versus-tumor effect. The risk of going too far and fighting the host instead—chronic graft-versus-host disease—however, is still significant in either a mini- or a full transplant. Oncologists who perform transplants try to deplete only those types of T cells that cause graft-versus-host disease without removing other cells that confer the beneficial graft-versus-tumor effect.

• • •

As Ellen Cohen was deciding which kind of transplant she would undergo (she was young enough to qualify for a full transplant), dozens in the MCL Group where making similar choices, discussing options with one another by e-mail and phone. "It's no fun to have your bone marrow sucked out of your pelvis day after day," wrote one member of the group. Most opted for less-invasive stem-cell transplants. Unfortunately, graft-versus-host disease occurs more often in transplanting stem cells from the blood than during bone-marrow transplants. As in heart or other organ transplants, if even tiny bits of a cancer recipient's own immune cells survive, they can generate an unwanted immune response that kills the transplanted cells.

In these transplants, the patients' immune systems are exterminated temporarily, so a failed graft leaves them extremely vulnerable to infection. Given that problem, coupled with the difficulty of finding a donor with perfectly matched blood in anyone other than an identical twin, transplant scientists have thought of using umbilical-cord blood. The three ounces of blood typically contained in placenta, or afterbirth, and the umbilical cord itself are rich sources of stem cells, the precursors of everything in the blood.

Cord blood can be stored. It avoids graft-versus-host complications because its stem cells are immature and therefore far more tolerant than adult stem cells or those in bone marrow. Its benefits extend beyond leukemia and lymphoma, to restoring normal red blood cells in sickle-cell anemia and in several fatal inherited deficiencies that result in progressive neurological degeneration and death. Cord blood is being stored at centers throughout the country, including Duke University, UCLA, the New York Blood Center, and a company called the Cord Blood Registry. Those who oppose using cord blood (such as Jehovah's Witnesses) on the "moral" basis that it is somehow wrong seem to me to have their ethical concerns backwards. The real ethical travesty would be to let cord blood go unused, thrown away after the birth of babies, when it could save lives.

. . .

In the end, like so many other shipwrecked blood-cancer sufferers, Ellen fired the boat in a courageous attempt at full rescue. She decided on a full stem-cell transplant instead of a mini and instead of first entering a clinical trial for Campath or another biotherapy. Plagued for years by recurrences, worried about her son and daughter nearing their teenage years, wanting a normal life with her husband, and desperate to get rid of the dogged enemy, she developed an inchoate yet fervent hope. If it worked, her chances of being cured, ending her fifteen-year struggle in the rough seas of cancer, would be excellent. Given her history of chemotherapy, started many years before anything else was available, and given the advice of her oncologists understandably distrustful of new experimental drugs after decades of failed science, most cancer victims would have made the same decision.

Time slid around my emotions. There was never enough of it to examine all options in detail. There was never enough time for Ellen, for me, for any of those in the MCL Group, never enough time for cancer patients or for their doctors. Ellen was influenced in her decision by the fact that her donor, her brother, was an exact match for the six major genes comprising the human leukocyte antigens, or HLA proteins, that transplanters look for in the blood of donor and recipient. These HLAs, which vary widely from person to person, are responsible for antigens presenting themselves to T cells, thus permitting the immune system to distinguish its own cells from those of foreign invaders. Matching blood, like anything else in cancer research, turns out to be more complex than previously thought, more involved than matching those six genes. Fortunately DNA testing had become fairly sophisticated in time for Ellen's transplant and could detect differences that don't show up in conventional antigen testing.

Ellen's transplant at the City of Hope Hospital in Los Angeles was successful . . . as such. That is, she did not reject the transplanted tissue. With her brother's blood type soon to be her own, she was on her way to being cured.

Before rescuing a patient with new stem cells, however, transplant protocols elevate the ordeal of chemotherapy to lethal intensity, destroying much of the bone marrow along with the cancer cells and temporarily turning off the immune system. Ellen responded well to the transplant and was rescued as planned with her brother's stem cells. But while her immune system was shut down—despite sterile precautions including positive air pressure in the tented-off portion of her hospital room, despite accessing her via a glove box through the tent, despite every human precaution against invading bacteria and fungi—she developed two types of infections. The bacterial infection was controlled by antibiotics. It was the fungal infection in her brain that killed her. Ellen Glesby Cohen died on August 23, 2000, at the age of fifty-one.

• • •

Many of the MCL Group transplant patients, too, were dying or undergoing complications from "opportunistic" infections—that is, pathogens that attack when the immune defenses are shut down. One member of the group who had an autologous, or "self," transplant left the hospital with his lymphoma cured but his immune system not fully restored. He contracted a virus that resulted in the loss of 75 percent of both temporal lobes of the brain, affecting his short-term memory. Now, four years later, he asks his sister every day what happened to him the day before.

The horror stories are legion, but so are success stories, including some transplants Oliver Press conducted on mantle-cell lymphoma patients at the Hutch in Seattle. The theory behind transplants is sound, if perilous: shut down the immune system, poison all the cancer cells, and then restore immunity with stem cells or bone marrow. The renowned transplant scientist Jerome Groopman, chief of experimental medicine at Beth Israel and a Harvard professor who performed the procedure many times, said that when transplants work, the results "appear almost miraculous." Cancer victims on the edge of survival have become whole again after transplants. They need no more treatment. They are cured.

But Groopman wrote of transplants, "I cannot regard it without a measure of horror. Even when all goes well, it represents an experience beyond our ordinary imaginings—the ordeal of chemotherapy taken to a near-lethal extreme. . . . It is a treatment of last resort. . . . For all the effort and resources devoted to mastering the technique, we can only hope that it will become obsolete because something more effective and less punishing will take its place."

Three years later I asked Dr. Groopman by e-mail whether he now felt that "something more effective" had arrived.

"The most promising are the monoclonal antibodies that may ultimately obviate the need for transplants," he wrote back.

"Not now, though? Shouldn't Mabs be tried *before* resorting to transplants?"

"Well, first," Groopman replied, "since I wrote that, considerable progress has been made in reducing the side effects of transplantation. And second, the reason I use words like 'may obviate' or 'ultimately' is there are not sufficient data over a long enough time period to speak definitively."

"How about the other targeted agents like co-stimulation of T cells? How about vaccines? How about anti-angiogenic drugs?"

"In time," he answered, "they will find their place . . . when they are proved."

• • •

Today, in 2003, transplants continue to be conducted, often without first trying the approved monoclonal antibodies or the vaccines with excellent twenty-year records, let alone the experimental therapies in clinical trials. The year before Ellen's death, Jordan's King Hussein—the longest-ruling head of state in the world (and a private pilot!)—died from graft-versus-host disease following a stem-cell transplant at the Mayo Clinic. Afterwards, Ellen had been able to get Queen Noor to serve as an "honorary chair," a figurehead for the foundation's fund-raising effort.

Being privy to the story of the king's death made me wonder, yet again, how complacently we enter the Chemo Culture. It is not only the man in the street, without resources to determine options, who makes the wrong choice. Wealthy and famous people do so as well: lymphoma victims include Jackie Kennedy Onassis, Senator Paul Tsongas, the CIA director William Casey, baseball's Roger Maris, and many others.

I wondered why some of these wealthy celebrities, especially the powerful king of Jordan, who possessed virtually unlimited resources, hadn't used their resources to do something exceptional. The king could have hired and equipped a hundred (or a thousand) lymphoma scientists to investigate his particular subset of disease and recommend short-term stabilizing biotherapies while searching for long-term solutions. He could have established an international team in Jordan, first to keep him alive and then to continue as an active institution collecting data from cancer research projects throughout the world, collaborating and catalyzing other efforts worldwide. I wondered whether the idea ever occurred to him.

• • •

Back here in the land of reality, chemotherapy and radiation—because they are used both with and without transplants—are typically the last therapies you receive before your life is claimed by lymphoma or leukemia. The annual twenty to thirty deaths within the MCL Group are almost all due to complications of today's standard therapies.

As if these people were insufficient grist for the cancer fiend who presides over that exclusive hell of incurable malignancies, my own oncologist succumbed. The internationally renowned and beloved John Ultmann, who made friends of his patients, inviting them to call him at home at any hour of the night, was one of our time's leading figures in lymphoma research. John helped create both the University of Chicago's Cancer Research Center and the *Journal of Clinical Oncology.* His research direction started the team that later joined T-cell co-stimulator Carl June at the University of Pennsylvania. Dr. John Ultmann died of "complications" (his physician refused to tell me what they were) in October 2000 at the age of seventy-five, two months after Ellen.

• • •

I know how to live with death and grief, fear and pain, but I can't live with ✕
helplessness. I have to try something, as long as it is rooted in sound science.
It is not possible for me to accept a chemotherapist's standard treatment, not
when I've seen the results, not when it violates the cardinal principle of medicine: first, do no harm. I wanted to say these things to the board of directors
of the Lymphoma Research Foundation of America after Ellen died, but I did
not. You don't speak passionately to people who have entirely different out-
looks on life, not even to friends, not in this culture, not in this time.

Instead, I advocated—because we were directors of a *research* foundation—that we sponsor actual research projects beyond those of postdoctoral
fellows, who usually can be funded by the National Cancer Institute. The
other directors agreed with me in principle but said they weren't sufficiently
oriented in science to select among the myriad projects devised by the universities. They did promise, eventually, to gather a committee of scientists
to look at research proposals. (Following the merger in 2002 the Lymphoma
Research Foundation did create an advisory board of erudite scientists as
the first step in funding research projects.)

At the time of my last board meeting in October 2000, however, some
of the directors felt that my personal funding of projects constituted a
"conflict of interest." I resigned in amazement, feeling I could do more on
my own to catalyze cancer research and urging those who remained on the
board to look carefully at projects in the middle of the research spectrum.

I put it like this. At one end of the spectrum are the *untargeted long-term
basic research projects* at universities, which usually find adequate support
from the government. At the other end are *applied research projects* conducted by the pharmaceutical companies to develop drugs based on university or their own fundamental research.

It was in between, in the middle of the project spectrum, where the foundation could make a real difference. These are basic research studies, yes. But
they are *projects targeted to specific goals,* with time frames of perhaps eighteen to thirty-six months. Let others fund long-term groundbreaking experiments, for instance, in gene therapy. Small foundations ought to sponsor
research based on important ideas that slip through the cracks of the big

funders. They could contribute to research that would render transplants obsolete, such as Project Indolence. Here was a body of research that sought not to solve the elusive grail of gene therapy but more simply to alter the metabolic pathways that trigger cancers into becoming aggressive, answering the elusive question: *Why is one man's lymphoma indolent, while another's is aggressive?*

20

Pathways to Success

THE YEAR 2001 OPENED WITH MORE SUCCESSES BY THE UCLA PROJECT Indolence teams despite a lack of real funding. These were not dramatic breakthroughs, as had been Gleevec. Rather, like most science, the project proceeded slowly, tracing step by step the pathways from the four hundred "aggression genes" the team had found to the proteins they produced. Progress by the centimeter.

The term *pathway*, so graphic and omnipresent in biology, conjures images of a foot trail through a dense and extensive forest, forking here and there in the darkness at unexpected places, splitting off at the slightest provocation into new lanes that themselves rift, break off, form again, and finally arrive at some welcomed—or dreaded—destination. Picture, instead, an infinitely more complex forest containing millions of paths, a multiplex running from our thirty thousand genes and through to the *billions* of proteins they beget. These proteins act like switches, activating or deactivating the genes that made them; they also decide which pathways will be formed and followed by other proteins, which forking roads will be taken.

Just as different trails through the woods can lead you this way or that, the convoluted protein pathway chosen by the genes can determine the outcome of a signal in diverse ways. For instance, one pathway may lead to the death of a cell when DNA is destroyed by suicidal enzymes. Or signals along a different pathway may reprogram a cell for dramatic changes, such as morphing a fertilized egg into structures that become a newborn baby. Or, when obstacles change the paths and "unprogram" cells that should die and instead make them relatively immortal, these alternative paths allow the cells to explode into cancer.

Determining tens of thousands of gene expressions is an enormous step forward. But that does not mean we understand—or even that we are close to understanding—how networks of genes regulate one another's expressions or the pathways they take in order to progress into cancer.

Having marveled at the intricacies of spaceflight, it was hard for me to acknowledge that the simplest cell—a unit of life so tiny it is to the human body as the body is to all the water in the Great Lakes—is so utterly complex that determining its every function makes sending a spacecraft to other worlds seem like child's play.

Although I often visited Phil Koeffler, Jon Braun, and the other scientists working on Project Indolence, usually for a hurried lunch, the two smaller laboratories (as opposed to the large Koeffler lab at Cedars-Sinai) were on the UCLA campus, and I came to see them in November 2001. I found my way through the maze of the university buildings by asking directions, then stopped to watch a student ride by on a bicycle with a dog on his horizontal bar, pausing again to smell the cut grass mingling with the California warmth rising from the pavement even in winter. I feel about universities the same way some people feel about New York or Chicago, finding them invigorating, full of energy, in a way I've never experienced in a city.

The Braun lab measured less than a thousand square feet, into which were crammed a dozen workers: postdocs, grad students, undergraduate assistants, and technicians working while studying to become scientists. Rows of black chemical-resistant benches lined the room with cherry cabinets below and black shelves above, each cluttered with scores of hundred-milliliter glass bottles containing colorful chemicals, serially numbered lab notebooks, reference books, bags of translucent test tubes, Petri dishes, and equipment of diverse design. Adjacent desks sprouted laptop computers, notes and reminders, photos of DNA gels, and printouts of instrument measurements.

I arrived at night because the student workers were not in class, and anyway, scientists seem to be a nocturnal species. Fluorescent lights lent an extraterrestrial hue to the frenzy that usually lasts past midnight. Jon Braun moved through this confined place not like a prisoner examining his crowded cell but like a space traveler on the verge of arriving on an exotic new planet. Braun and I had kept up with each other on a weekly basis after meeting in 1999. Reed thin and humble voiced, he shows the world a warm smile that spreads from his short black beard, flecked with gray, to eyes set deep under prominent eyebrows. Intensely analytical, he combines a humor and determination that seem to make him appear larger than his physical build. Braun received his M.D. and Ph.D. at Harvard. He is an award-winning national leader in both pathology and immunology with a string of patents for the diagnosis and treatment of immune disorders of colitis.

As befitting a man as unique as Jon Braun, he is an identical twin (born, incidentally, on my birthday), and his brother is also a physician. The Braun lab is staffed with mostly young investigators, an eclectic mix of men and women from China, India, Europe, and occasionally America. Many have lost loved ones to cancer, and they acted as though they were lieutenants not in the war on cancer but in a shooting war, conducting experiments as if probing clusters of the enemy. They were defined by the usual hard work of science but something more as well . . . I could think of no better word than *patriotism*—our side of normal cells against an enemy that outnumbers us by the billions. It was that characteristic, I believe, that led them to rise again and again after experiments fail, knowing as they started anew that in cancer research 90 percent of experiments must be repeated or scrapped.

Next to the lab was Jon's office, where I sat beside him in front of his computer. The opposite wall was lined with cages of white mice. Leaning back in his chair, his fingers laced behind his head, he brought me down to fundamentals.

"We knew that an impaired immune function results in a high frequency of cancer, particularly lymphoma," he explained, as though holding back adrenaline. "Various antitumor vaccines are successful in mounting an immune response against established cancers. Here's the question we needed to answer: why are these tumors insensitive to the natural immune response?"

Glancing at the mice running around in their cages, he continued. "We used a mouse lymphoma which was available in two variants, one sensitive and one resistant to immune recognition. When we compared the two, we found some two hundred genes were either over- or underexpressed in the immune-resistant tumor."

The Braun lab painstakingly analyzed these genes. The investigators first ranked them in terms of biochemical properties that might be related to immune recognition. Then they studied suspected genes for the effects of their over- or undermanifestation on tumor formation and immune recognition. For overexpression, they isolated the full length of the gene and transferred it into a form that would be constantly produced at high levels in the recipient cells. For underexpression, they used a "ribozyme" (a catalyst that recognizes RNA in a sequence-specific manner) encoded for an enzyme designed to cleave and destroy the gene's messenger RNA in the recipient cell.

One gene stood out: EMP2, named for the epithelium, the layer of cells forming the epidermis, or linings, of the skin, lungs, and intestines. This second in a series of three genes that produce "epithelial membrane proteins" is a newly discovered member of the "tetraspan" family comprising fifty or more genes involved in cell-to-cell communication.

If you think of a cell as a vast sea—in this case, a sea not of water but of liquid fat—the tetraspans may be visualized as long spaghetti strands coiling in and out from the depths of this ocean four (*tetra*) times and forming four loops. The ocean is dotted with floating pockets of these tetraspans, each of them anchoring a specialized collection of proteins spanning the floating pockets and thereby connecting them in order to recognize, communicate, and signal each other. When the researchers manipulated these tetraspan molecules, they found the EMP2 gene everywhere in the epithelium *except* in cancer cells of the same epithelium! What was it that prevented this gene from forming in epithelial cancer cells?

The Braun lab experiments went on to prove that tumors with high EMP2 were being killed efficiently by T cells, whereas tumors with low EMP2 were resistant. "In fact," Jon said, "pockets of the EMP2 gene actually harbor the tumor molecules recognized by killer T cells. In the absence of EMP2, the pockets and their target molecules are not displayed, rendering the tumor cell invisible to the immune system."

"What we hope to do," Jon went on, gazing at the cages, perhaps seeing in them not mere rodents but vectors of the secrets of cancer, "is to manipulate EMP2 or the molecules it controls in order to restore immune susceptibility of tumor cells, thereby improving antitumor vaccines."

$$\cdot \ \cdot \ \cdot$$

Jon Braun coordinates Project Indolence not only in his own laboratory and across town at Cedars-Sinai but also in Jonathan Said's nearby lab. Jonathan Said had not come new to this inquiry. For more than a decade, he had been comparing highly aggressive HIV-initiated lymphomas to lymphomas arising in the general population. The question was related to the aggressive genes found by the Koeffler lab at Cedars-Sinai. Afterwards, aided by Jonathan Said's staining of tissues, another UCLA investigator, Mike Teitell, began large-scale analysis using genechip technology on donated mantle-cell tissue blocks (including mine).

Jonathan Said and Mike Teitell are physical opposites. Mike is young, tall, curly haired. Jonathan is in his late fifties and balding, a slight man who seems hidden behind huge glasses when he peers up at you from his desk—or more likely, from his nearby microscope. They share much in common. Both men earned dual doctorates in medicine and molecular biology. Both are robust, rushing from laboratory to conferences to animal cages. Both have imagination and pay extreme attention to details, an unusual combination in any one person.

Far more than most investigators, who tend to be lone wolves, Said has built scores of individual relationships with colleagues throughout the United States, his native South Africa, Europe, and Japan. Communication among laboratory investigators usually is limited because scientists like to make sure their information is validated and adequately conceptualized. But Said, Braun, Koeffler, Teitell, and the scientists in their labs were exceptional in collaborating on Project Indolence. You could say that they inspected those protein pathways together, following them step by step until they revealed molecules that decided to take one route instead of another.

Mike Teitell's contribution came after months of poring over internet databases. He found scores of genes that were either elevated or decreased in the two types of aggressive lymphomas, eventually focusing on a gene called "TCL1," for T-cell leukemia number 1. At one of our meetings Mike Teitell explained that the TCL1 gene seemed to be protecting abnormal cells from normal programmed death—"at least in AIDS-related lymphoma," he said. "So we devised experiments to confirm whether T-cell leukemia-1 was indeed an oncogene."

The concept of an oncogene—that is, a gene in our bodies that contributes not to our welfare but to the generation of malignant tumors—is terribly counterintuitive, pushing against every nuance of evolutionary theory. And yet, more than a hundred oncogenes have been discovered within us, along with our immune fighters helpless to conquer them. To carry out his experiments, Teitell used an antibody he produced by immunizing rabbits with a TCL1 gene to beget a protein.

We think we understand the word *protein* because we eat proteins in beans and meat. Proteins, though, are incredibly complex compounds, acting sometimes as catalysts (enzymes), sometimes as signalers, and sometimes as transporters of molecules into and out of a cell. The simplest cells in our bodies contain more than two thousand diverse proteins made of a long chain of molecules. They are built from only twenty amino acids, the nitrogen-carbon-water precursors of life that appeared soon after the formation of the earth. Proteins virtually *are* us. They construct the cells, turning sugar and fat into energy. In the process, they enable us to compose music, visit the moon, and discover how we are made.

Mike Teitell treated ultrathin wafers of tissue, one-hundredth the thickness of a single hair, with an antibody that attaches to rabbit cells in the tissue expressing the protein. The approach yielded the discovery that TCL1 is expressed by normal B cells at a single stage of development: the mantle-zone stage. Mantle-cell lymphoma—which emerges from this stage—exhibits high levels of TCL1, whereas *the gene is almost absent in follicular lymphoma*. You could think of lymphomas stretching out in a long continuum, with follicular on the left as the most benign and mantle-cell on the right as the most aggressive, because they arise from different life cycles of developing B cells.

Building on their discovery of how TCL1 develops, Mike transferred his T-cell leukemia-1 gene into mice. As soon as the mice were injected, an overgrowth of B lymphocytes promptly appeared! The experiment revealed that the cells' abnormal behavior was caused by some disturbance in apoptosis—the programmed cell death investigated endlessly in cancer research because it truly defines cancer. Since then, Mike and his colleagues have been studying these mice to understand how this gene promotes lymphoma formation so that—ultimately—they can block its pathway and cure the cancer.

Working separately, yet still pooling resources and ideas with the Koeffler team, the scientists from the different laboratories converged into a single biological insight. They discovered not only that two extremely different but aggressive cancers—mantle-cell lymphoma and HIV lymphoma—express the TCL1 and related genes but also that these genes disrupt the normal pathway toward apoptosis. Thus one more step had been taken in finding the way through that dark and winding trail toward the opposite of cancer: the normal death of cells.

"The correlation they discovered between this gene and aggressive behavior in lymphoma was unknown before," explained Jon Braun. "It was an electrifying connection," Jon said with his subtle humor, alluding to the cellular flow of electrons in the process. "First, Mike's TCL1 gene has been proved to be absolutely critical—kind of a rheostat for controlling cell growth. And second, the disordered TCL1 and its gene cousins are regulated in an exotic way by an enzyme—previously known to exist only in plants and fungi—that marks genes either for expression or silence."

. . .

The investigations described are multiplied in a hundred other UCLA laboratories, typical of twenty-first-century genomic research stretching across thousands of laboratories throughout the world, between which collaboration unfortunately is not the rule. One of the most prevalent targets of research is the often-duplicated research on the role of the rather famous family of "p53 genes," which are known as "the most frequently mutated genes in human cancer."

The p53 family consists mostly of control genes that tell a cell when its DNA has been damaged. The cell either fixes the damage or, if too severe, kick starts commands that cause the errant cell to commit suicide. If p53 is inactive—as it is in at least half of all cancers—the cell has no way to respond to DNA damage. The result is a cell mutated into cancer. Several biotech companies are developing drugs that would turn p53 back on. Introgen Therapeutics, in Houston, is in phase-three trials with a drug called Advexin, which uses a deactivated virus to deliver a working p53 gene to breast, lung, ovarian, and other cancers.

Designated by different letter prefixes, certain members of the p53 family encode tumor *suppressors*—the opposite of oncogenes—and many cancer cells evade programmed death by inactivating p53 itself. For instance, mice with high levels of one form of p53 (called "trp53") are resistant to cancer, as you might expect. Recent research, however, has shown that mice with abnormally high trp53 activity *age prematurely*—making it hard to win the p53 game and suggesting that targeting these genes may not be a good idea. In fact, there is a theory that aging might be a side effect of the natural safeguards that protect most of us from cancer.

On the other hand, researchers at the University of Illinois's Chicago campus have isolated the p53 protein secreted by bacteria that kills cancer cells in mice but appears to have no aging or other harmful side effects. The protein is the well-studied molecule *azurin*, which is involved in the everyday process that cells use to generate energy. Normally, the p53 protein is short-lived, surviving only a few minutes in the cell before degrading. But azurin winds its way into the nucleus of the tumor cell where it binds to the p53 protein and protects the protein from degradation, thus raising its level within the cell.

In addition to universities, some five hundred to a thousand U.S. biotech companies, working separately, are systematically identifying the functions of genes and proteins that are expressed differently in diseased and normal tissue, seeking to alter interactions that lead to cancer. In one example, Myriad Genetics, in Salt Lake City, added a drug to lab dishes containing human cancer cells that had been unresponsive to chemotherapy. The drug dutifully *forced* virtually all prostate and lymphoma cancer cells into apoptosis.

The idea of repairing our bodies from the molecules on up has been a dream of scientists since the concept of the molecule was formulated in the eighteenth century. Only in the last few years, however, have immunologists discarded the naïve idea that you can restore apoptosis by inhibiting only one gene or one protein. A physicist would look at the conglomeration of immune-cell molecules, disintegrating by mutation and trying for immortality of the parts at the expense of the whole, like a broken engine still pumping its piston, and he would see entropy at work. In the end, entropy—the universal drive toward chaos as energy subsides—claims everything. Stars burn out, planets spin into their suns, and plants and animals turn to dust and then, as equilibrium is achieved, become hydrogen and other elements to be recycled somewhere, someday.

But while we are alive, we fix the house, repair the car, bring the cat to the vet, and generally restrain entropy. We postpone final chaos by doing what we can to keep our immune systems healthy. With its long-term memory of everyday battles against billions of living things trying to convert us into bacteria or other organisms, it is our immune system that protects and *defines* us, separating each person from other living things, assigning us our inimitable identities, our unique phenotypes. Trying to understand this distinctive immunology, one small step at a time, investigators like Jon Braun and his allies are among the formidable builders of the new edifice of biology. The edifice grows taller each year and its rate of growth faster, reaching to conquer cancer, mental illness, and other maladies once considered incurable.

21

From India with Results

AMONG MY FRIENDS WHOSE LYMPHOMAS WERE HIGHLY AGGRESSIVE
was Ron Edwards, whom I had "met" through the MCL Group. Though I
had never seen him face to face, I communicated with Ron regularly by
phone and e-mail. A peripatetic MCL documenter and retired children's
book author in England, Ron Edwards goes down in my history book as a
unique humanitarian. Why award fame only to politicians, basketball stars,
and a few scientists? Even historians possess too few memory cells to record
all those deserving recognition.

Yet I feel someone should tell the story of Ron Edwards, known to those
in the group by his e-mail name, "Papyronnie." He worked harder than any
of us to document every case history of the six-hundred-member MCL
Group, to accumulate facts about experimental treatments, to explain different diagnoses, to describe hospitals in the United States and elsewhere,
to advise newcomers to our exclusive club, to help them find their ways, and
finally to console the widows and widowers. Many in the group came to rely
on Papyronnie's Web site for information to funnel to their oncologists.

Mantle-cell lymphoma, considered among the most aggressive, includes
a multitude of subsets, and Ron's was one of the worst, the kind that grows
polyps in your gut and renders it a nightmare simply to eat. In the summer
of 2001 it was his turn to be helped. He was dying.

Ron's e-mails were saying that his National Health Service oncologist had come to the end of his rope (as though it were *his* rope) and suggested no further treatment. Ron had long since become refractory to CHOP, fludarabine, and other chemos, and this chemotherapist "did not believe in" rituximab (Rituxan in the United States; Mabthera in England).

In August 2001 he wrote, "Although I have not told the whole Group yet, yesterday I learned that my onc has declared himself defeated. He wants to install a colostomy to make me more comfortable. Here in the U.K., even as a private patient, one cannot just change oncologists, and Dr. S seems to have taken against Rituxan."

I had been reading about the beneficial results of high-dose Rituxan—administered in quantities up to six times the dosages first approved by the FDA. This monoclonal antibody is the most successful lymphoma drug yet created. By the beginning of 2003, it has been used to treat more than a hundred thousand lymphoma patients, racking up sales of over $1 billion a year. While its action is known insofar as it attaches primarily to CD20 cell markers, clinical trials are continuing to extend its limits. Indeed, Rituxan is now being tried against rheumatoid arthritis because a B-cell mechanism similar to the one that produces lymphoma can provoke the immune system to attack the joints.

In doses much higher than normally given, Rituxan may kill cancer cells only partially expressing CD20 and perhaps other malignant cells as well. Clinical studies at M. D. Anderson and elsewhere show "clear evidence of a dose-response relationship" in chronic lymphocytic leukemia. The study showed that higher doses result in higher responses with no unusual toxicity. The Anderson scientists tried doses of Rituxan up to 2,250 mg per square meter—well beyond the usual 375 mg—repeating the high dose for six or more weekly infusions. (It is sometimes better to link dosage to area, as in square meters, because using weight may mean that children and other low-weight patients, like the starving Ron Edwards, receive an insufficient amount. Thus pharmacologists calculate dosage based on body surface. When a dosage of 375 mg per square meter is recommended, a person with two square meters of body surface would receive 750 mg.)

Admittedly, giving thirty-six times the standard quantity of Rituxan (six times the typical dose times six treatments) was experimental, especially for MCL, but why not try it on a dying patient who has nothing else? Ron regarded the high dosage of this antibody as benign. I saw it—or hoped to see it—radiating from the M. D. Anderson paper across the Atlantic and into Ron's bloodstream, where it would pervade his system like bursts of light from a double sun.

Ron wrote, "I am doing my best to change Dr. S's mind about Rituxan, even in normal doses, but it is rather rigid."

I sent the Anderson paper to Ron so he could show it to his Dr. S, but the physician refused to give him standard doses, let alone high-dose Rituxan, or radioactive Mabs, or Celebrex—all of which were approved drugs in England. Celebrex itself had been shown to reduce precancerous colorectal polyps, and I had been taking it in larger doses since February 1999. Any or all of these drugs seemed worth a try. What malevolence was this man of medicine trying to preempt by his inaction? What was his emergency plan? Was Dr. S simply unconvinced that Rituxan would help Ron because his cancer was so advanced? Rituxan treatments are expensive, about $7,000 in the United States (including preliminary medications) for each infusion of 700 milligrams, or $42,000 for a course of six infusions. I couldn't help but wonder whether we were seeing British socialized medicine at work, the cost-cutting scheme that makes Brits wait three years to get a hernia fixed.

I am aware of the fear of change and the certainty of those in charge that they alone grasp the problem, that "if I haven't heard of it, it's probably wrong." But this was too much. Ron was more knowledgeable about various treatments for cancer, especially mantle-cell lymphoma, than most people on the planet, far more so than his doctors.

Ron Edwards and I had a mutual friend, Martin Strauss, who suffers from the same type of polyp-generating mantle-cell lymphoma. Another member of the MCL Group, Martin lives in Tel Aviv. Two years earlier, when he had come to Chicago to visit his sister, Carol and I met them over dinner. Martin was in remission at the time, but now his symptoms, though not nearly so devastating as Ron's, had started again. He and I discussed a wide range of new experimental therapies that both he and Ron could bring to their doctors. These included the following:

—Hyperthermia (raising tumors to high fever temperatures) and hypoxia (starving tumors of oxygen) together have produced remarkable survival statistics in trials at the University of Munich.

—Another option was the monoclonal antibody called epratuzumab, developed by Immunomedics and Amgen.

—A drug from Sweden, so far tested only in mice, might repair the mutated p53 gene responsible for at least half of all cancers.

—ImClone Systems had developed a drug that jams various cancer-growth pathways (while it has produced no cures, it seemed pertinent to Ron's disease because it significantly shrank tumors in a quarter of patients with terminal colon cancer at Memorial Sloan-Kettering; shrinking tumors is not always as beneficial as rendering tumors stable, in terms of an ultimate cure, but doing so can prolong life until something better comes along).

—Molecular "nanogenerators," also developed at Sloan-Kettering, release a cascade of alpha particles on the inside of cancer cells. (Alpha particles are essentially helium nuclei ejected by unstable atoms. They are much weaker than the beta and gamma rays emitted by Zevalin and Bexxar—too weak to penetrate a sheet of paper or skin—but at the ultramicroscopic distances involved, they are sufficiently toxic to kill cancer cells. The method, tried so far only in mice and in human cancer cells cultured outside the body, uses a single radioactive atom of actinium-225 carried by an antibody to cells of cancers including lymphoma, leukemia, neuroblastoma, and breast and ovarian cancer.)

I included information about alpha-ray Mabs in my messages to Ron and Martin, thinking that there could be clinical trials going on in England or in Israel of which I was unaware and feeling that in an emergency any rational therapy ought to be considered.

"We have none of the freedom you folk in the U.S. have," Ron wrote back. "If I could get *any one* of these therapies, or change my oncologist, I would, but it is not possible. As for a radioactive Mab," Ron wrote, "it is out of the question here, and that goes too for any of these new therapies." His Dr. S finally agreed to give him a standard course of Rituxan—not high-dose—along with fludarabine, cyclophosphamide, and other toxins. Ron continued to lose weight while the polyps grew uncontrollably in his intestines.

"If I had the money," Ron wrote, "I would hire an air ambulance and fly to the States forthwith, although in my present state no scheduled flight would take me!"

Much earlier I had offered to send him a ticket here, and Shahid proposed putting him up at his house in Virginia and flying him back and forth to Bethesda for a vaccine at the National Cancer Institute.

"Your kind offers nigh made me weep, my friends," wrote Ron, "but my pride is such that I could not dream of accepting it, even if I weren't too ill to travel."

I am not a physician, but like many other lymphoma patients, I had learned something about my disease—ironically much of it from Ron Edwards himself. Finally, I sent him a paper on a hit-or-miss, trial-and-error therapy he could show to his doctors in a last-ditch effort to save his life. The treatment was almost incredibly simple, consisting of taking a rather common organic chemical called methylglyoxal, which recently had achieved some fame in India. In case Ron's doctors were reluctant to try it, and since Ron couldn't make the journey either here or to India, Shahid and I started working on a plan to bring a physician on the methylglyoxal team from Calcutta to Ron's town in England.

• • •

It was Shahid who first came across the idea of using methylglyoxal against cancer when he read about it in the May 28, 2001, issue of the *Hindustan Times*. In fact, the article compared it to Gleevec: "While Americans are going ga-ga with their new anti-cancer drug 'Glivec'—that was featured on the cover of [today's] *Time* magazine—the low-profile, cash-strapped Kolkata researchers have been working quietly for over a decade shunning publicity until they obtained proof from human trials nine weeks ago."

Shahid then procured a paper authored by the biochemist Manju Ray at the Indian Association of the Cultivation of Science, who lauded the drug as a "magic bullet against cancer." Methylglyoxal—also called pyruvic aldehyde or simply pyruvaldehyde—is a common organic chemical produced by Sigma Chemical, in St. Louis. It costs $319 per liter. Glyoxol gets its name from the word for sugar, as do glucose and the sweet-tasting glycerin used as a hand lotion. Produced naturally when various strains of bacteria break down glucose in the intestinal tract, it's found in various foods, coffee, and even tobacco smoke.

After experimenting for decades with human cancer cells in vitro and with mice, Dr. Ray and her group treated twenty-four volunteers who were in extremely advanced stages of lymphoma, acute myeloid leukemia, and cancers of the lung, breast, ovaries, colon, pancreas, liver, gall bladder, bone, and mouth. Most of these patients had received surgery, radiotherapy, or chemotherapy. From January to June 2000 these people were administered ten to twelve milliliters of methylglyoxal diluted in water, along with vitamin C, four times a day—equivalent to twenty to twenty-five milligrams of methylglyoxal per kilogram of body weight per day (about fifty cents' worth daily).

In the summer of 2001, when Ron Edwards was desperately sick, Dr. Ray reported that of these twenty-four, nineteen continued the treatment. Three of the nineteen died during the course of the study, five were in stable condition, and most remarkably, eleven improved quickly to "excellent physical condition."

What's going on here?

"Methylglyoxal inactivates the enzyme needed for ATP production in cancer cells and thereby starves them to death," Ray said in an e-mail. "Normal cells remain unaffected."

ATP is "adenosine triphosphate." Present in all cells, it predominates in muscle cells. When it is split by enzyme action, energy is produced; therefore, the energy of our muscles is stored in this compound.

Shahid and I talked by phone to Manju Ray several times. She seemed the epitome of the quiet and humble scientist. I looked her up on the internet and found a picture showing a studious woman in her midfifties with glasses and short light-brown hair bent over her desk against a background of laboratory glassware. The winner of several biology prizes, she was first in her class at the University of Calcutta, where she received her master's degree in physiology and in 1975 earned a Ph.D. in biochemistry, later becoming a professor. Since then she has authored scores of impressive papers on glucose, mitochondrial respiration, and methylglyoxal. Her latest scientific paper, the one that brought her to our attention, was coauthored by an M.D.-equivalent (an M.B.B.S. in India) and three other Ph.D.s: a biochemist, a biologist, and a biophysicist.

Though glad to see an interdisciplinary team at work, I wondered what role the biophysicist played. It turns out that methylglyoxal inhibits the electron flow of mitochondria—the tiny threads of the cell that contain the enzymes necessary for cell respiration and production of ATP.

In other words, methylglyoxal blocks the electrical energy of living cells!

• • •

But was I, in my attempt to search out a possible cure, becoming nothing more than an adversary of chemotherapy? Like those extremists who say all chemicals are harmful? Isn't methylglyoxal a chemical and its use therefore a chemotherapy?

Yes, it is a chemical. But then, we ourselves and everything on our world, including the planet itself, are made of chemicals; the distinction is that methylglyoxal is not a toxin, as are chemo drugs. I made a call to UCLA and asked Dr. Jon Braun whether this isolated body of research and the remarkably successful clinical trial in India was in the mainstream of science, whether it was truly significant.

"Absolutely," answered Jon. "The effect of methylglyoxal has been a famous and interesting story. For half a century there has been a recurrent recognition that cancers—especially solid tumors like colon, lung, and breast cancers—often derive their metabolic energy from biochemical pathways distinct from their cell types of origin. Some of the enzymatic reactions these tumors prefer for their pathways seem to be more efficient than those taken by normal cells."

Jon explained that, because the first stage of cell respiration involves various glucose enzymes in the release of ATP energy, "there's a lot of interest in finding out exactly which enzymes distinguish between tumor and normal cells and how they might be targeted by a drug."

Methylglyoxal is such a drug. It is a small molecule originally identified for another reason, when its derivatives were found to inhibit the synthesis of arginine and polyamine, metabolites thought to be important in the growth of leukemic cells. In fact, argenase, an enzyme that breaks down arginine directly, was used for a long time in conjunction with chemotherapy for acute leukemia, until it flunked phase-one and -two clinical trials a decade ago.

"The really interesting finding that emerged from Dr. Ray's group," Jon said, "is that methylglyoxal has an effect distinct from its role in the arginine and polyamine metabolism. It blocks one of the pivotal enzymes in the glycolytic energy pathway."

This pivotal enzyme, which has the tongue-twisting name glyceraldehyde-3-phosphate dehydrogenase, is stopped cold by methylglyoxal. Because this enzyme is needed for ATP production in malignant cells, methylglyoxal literally starves cancer to death. Normal cells remain unaffected. Isn't that a goal of cancer researchers worldwide?

Jon Braun agrees. He applauded Manju Ray's effort and thought that more research ought to be devoted to these nonsexy, economical, and rather ordinary metabolites—in addition to the exotic ones that have been so much the focus of his own field of molecular biology.

I learned from Manju Ray that the great Hungarian biochemist Albert Szent-Györgyi, who won the Nobel Prize in 1937 for his work in cell oxidation, championed the idea that methylglyoxal could be used to treat cancer, and since then countless cancer-bearing animals have been cured completely, with no toxic effects. Previous research at the Ray laboratory showed that methylglyoxal strongly inhibits the electron flow through the mitochondrial respiratory chain of specifically malignant cells. Some 85 percent of ATP generated in the cell is produced by this electron flow. By deactivating the glyceraldehyde enzyme, methylglyoxal depletes cancerous cells of their ATP. And without their ATP, the tumor cells die.

• • •

Ron Edwards lived in Grantham, Lincolnshire, a village almost in the center of England, 120 miles north of London. Grantham is best known for its fifteenth-century grammar school, which was attended by Isaac Newton. (His name, carved on a window ledge by Newton himself, is still legible).

While Shahid and I were beginning to make arrangements for a medical member of the Indian laboratory to journey to the center of England, Ron's son, Vince, helped him get into the private wing of a National Health Service hospital. Ron told us he was now in good hands and asked us to abandon the effort with the Indian scientists. He told us that if you want private treatment in England, you can have it by paying both your national-health subscriptions *and* the costs of the private hospital. While public hospitals are typically dirty, understaffed, and third-worldish, he said, private wings of public hospitals and private hospitals offer television, menus, wine lists, and less-overburdened doctors.

His new physicians gave Ron another standard course (not the high dose) of Rituxan—along with the inevitable toxins of chemo. A surgeon at the private hospital excised the intestines that were the major site of Ron's mantle-cell lymphoma. Alas, it was too late. Ron died at the end of October 2001. (Vince took over his father's invaluable Web site.)

• • •

Two years later, in 2003, I wondered what had happened to Manju Ray's patients, so I asked her. The patients in the original group, who had suffered from many types of metastasized malignancies, had been close to death. Dr. Ray answered that, although two of the eleven previously described as being in "excellent physical condition" died a year after treatment, two others went their ways and lost contact with the hospital staff—not unusual in India, she said—and she had no way of knowing whether they were alive. The remaining six stayed in touch and continue to be in good condition.

Whether methylglyoxal would have saved Ron or other lymphoma victims is anybody's guess. Yet the mechanism of its action and its efficacy against many types of cancer seem to warrant widespread clinical trials. Why has this promising therapy, which has been proved to be nontoxic, been ignored in Western nations?

. . .

About the time of Ron Edwards's death, a friend of Shahid's and mine found he had a particularly devastating subset of lymphoma. Thayer Sheets, a big and vigorous NASA-Langley engineer in his early sixties, radiated a native cheer undiminished by the remembrance of his first bout with malignancy. At age fifteen he had been diagnosed with testicular cancer and underwent thirty-five cobalt treatments.

Now, a half-century later, his cancer was a form of cutaneous T-cell lymphoma, said to be the fastest-growing cancer in the United States. It is particularly insidious because it destroys the very T cells that are supposed to rush to the rescue. It first attacks the largest organ of the body, the skin, and then spreads to the bone marrow, lymph nodes, and viscera. Median survival is only three years. If the lesions are on your feet, as in Thayer's case, you can't walk. If they overrun your body, merely wearing clothes is painful. If the sores are on your hands, you can't do anything, much less work. As is unfortunately typical in detecting a rare disease, Thayer's first diagnosis was incorrect. Detecting a small red spot on the back of his thigh in late 1999, he saw a dermatologist, who thought it was a rash and treated it with steroid creams.

As his lymphoma grew worse, Thayer went to the University of Virginia, where physicians diagnosed him correctly and sent him to another cancer center that offered total-skin electron-beam radiation but for some reason wanted to exclude his hands and feet. Physicians at still another center explained to him, "We do irradiate hands and feet, but not the head."

"I found the disparities somewhat unnerving," Thayer said, "when you realize that intensive radiation for me is a once-only shot." Radiation of all kinds is cumulative in the body, and Thayer had used up most of his lifetime allotment long ago as a teenage cancer patient.

Thayer and his wife, Betty, searched the Web for cutting-edge research, finally learning about a professor of dermatology at M. D. Anderson named Madeleine Duvic. The world-renowned Dr. Duvic had devoted a good part of her life to treating this disease and had developed a mutifaceted treatment consisting of immune-system enhancers, dermatologic applications, and radiation. Over the years Madeleine Duvic's treatments resulted in a galaxy of long-term survivors, near 90 percent. (I had heard of her because she also championed taking Celebrex to prevent skin cancer. Together with scientists at five other cancer centers, she began a national study in 2002 to see whether Celebrex reduces precancerous skin conditions.)

Madeleine Duvic's results against cutaneous T-cell lymphoma were irrefutable. Thayer's immediate problem was getting an appointment with Dr. Duvic, because her laboratory research allowed her only one day a week to see patients. Thayer's T-cell lymphoma already covered 17 percent of his body. He had no time to lose.

I called my pathologist friend Jeff Medeiros at M. D. Anderson and asked whether he knew Madeleine Duvic. He did. A few hours later she called Thayer and gave him an immediate appointment. Thayer and Betty moved to Houston for four months, where he became Dr. Duvic's outpatient. He received a combination of interferons, isotretinoin (a drug that decreases oil produced by skin glands), total electron-beam therapy (including hands, feet, and head), and nitrogen mustard applied over the sores.

Today Thayer Sheets has no trace of the disease and leads a normal life.

• • •

Contrast Thayer's victory with another story. A few months after Thayer left for Houston, Rade Pejic asked me to come over to St. Anthony's Hospital. He wanted me to talk to a man named George Farley, whose physician in another Indiana city near Chicago had referred him to Rade for a biopsy. George's tissue proved to be cutaneous T-cell lymphoma—the same gruesome lymphoma from which Thayer Sheets had suffered. Rade is a surgeon, not an oncologist, and of course I was only a patient, but we wanted to do what we could.

When I arrived with Rade at George Farley's hospital room, I saw a gaunt man in his late fifties wearing only a loin cloth, like Mahatma Gandhi, his skin so knotted and gnarled it was painful for him even to lie down. Scores of ulcerated, cauliflower-like lesions made him look like he had advanced leprosy. I told him about Madeleine Duvic's successes, talking to him quietly for a long time, letting him know that despite the hideous nature of his disease and his terrible pain, that there was a good chance of a cure awaiting him in Houston. He nodded, perhaps in thanks, but said nothing, his eyes showing him inaccessible to hope. Fear of the unknown is the greatest of human fears.

I could see him rejecting what I had told him, unwilling to try, unwilling to fight, perhaps thinking that if the unknown could become known, as death is known, he would consent to it.

22

Anti-angiogenesis

I HAD YET TO COME UP WITH A FULLY SATISFYING EXPLANATION FOR the cause of my cancer or its continued indolence. Maybe I had spent too much time in the tropics earlier in life, accumulating too much radiation from the sun, taking too much heat from foreign politicians, or breathing too much diesel exhaust from bulldozers. By July of 2000 about a year and a half had passed in which my lymphoma, originally aggressive, turned and then remained indolent, a time of taking an increasing dosage of Celebrex. It was a period of escalating hope. It was also a time, though, when others were suffering, and the MCL Group's e-mails were filled with silent screams.

"I'm really glad for you, Neil, *but why are you so healthy?*" John McKenna and his sister, Michele, friends in the MCL Group, called to ask.

Their question implied another: could John avail himself of whatever I had taken? John McKenna was the six-foot-two lawyer in his late thirties whom I had met several times in New Jersey. Though he had undergone a splenectomy six months before, now he was sick in bed once again with the familiar fever, fatigue, and pain of mantle-cell lymphoma. In other respects he was atypical of MCL patients, for he'd endured no chemo, no therapy other than the removal of his four-pound spleen.

The twenty-first century brought a bombardment of information on vaccines, Mabs naked and radioactive, immune stimulators, and anti-angiogenics. The McKennas had been kept informed about biotherapies entering clinical trials—which patients would be eligible and which trials would admit patients who never had chemotherapy or, conversely, who were refractory to it. Despite daily communications within the group, most members had long since followed the authoritative advice of their physicians, who, having moved them into toxic chemo as first therapy, now felt there was little choice other than more chemo, often coupled with bone-marrow transplants. Those patients still alive were sick, most of them. They were in agony, some of them—hardly in shape to inform, cajole, or argue with their doctors. Although the size of the MCL Group remained stable due to new entrants, about four died each month—an indelible horror not unlike terrorists shooting an innocent victim every hour until their demands are met.

My experience was an anomaly. Somehow, after the first few months since diagnosis, I had remained symptom-free while the others suffered from fatigue, swollen lymph nodes, raging fevers, drenching night sweats, or wheezing respiratory infections.

"What are you doing that we are *not* doing?" A desperate question from so many near the grave.

• • •

Until this year I had maintained an uneasy silence born of both doubt and fear of raising unfounded hopes. I had known about Dr. Judah Folkman's pioneering work on anti-angiogenesis and long since suspected that Celebrex was keeping my tumor capillaries suppressed. When CAT scans continued to reveal a steady shrinkage of my lymph nodes, I called Dan Longo, the helpful scientific director of the National Institute of Aging, and asked whether he'd found out anything more about Celebrex since last we talked. Dan, who was constantly performing research while keeping up with the progress of other laboratories, immediately cited a dozen scientific papers showing celecoxib (Celebrex) to be effective against various organ cancers.

I located the papers and devoured them, learning that Celebrex is a potent inhibitor of cyclooxygenase-2—Cox-2—which performs the first step in creating prostaglandins from a common fatty acid. During my Island for Science years, we had collected the coral animals from which these naturally occurring substances were derived, and I knew that prostaglandins are not exactly hormones, yet they produce diverse hormonelike effects in mammals. Prostaglandins were discovered in 1935 by a Swedish physiologist who coined their name from *prostate glands* because he found them first in human semen. In extremely minute concentrations prostaglandins can raise or lower blood pressure, increase or decrease the clotting ability of blood, stimulate muscle contraction, and execute myriad other marvels.

Some kinds of prostaglandins not only contribute to the inflammations of arthritis but also support tumor growth by inducing angiogenesis. While both Cox-1 and -2 are responsible for creating new capillaries from tumors to the bloodstream, Cox-2 is the major culprit, promoting microvessel formation more effectively and in more tissues. Celecoxib, and possibly other anti-Cox-2 drugs, stop these tiny blood vessels from growing without incurring stomach ulcers or other gastrointestinal disorders often produced by Cox-1 inhibitors. Studies suggesting that anti-Cox-2 drugs are no safer than aspirin in reducing the inflammation of arthritis are of little or no importance for anti-angiogenesis. The fact is that Celebrex—unlike other Cox-2 inhibitors—has been shown to stop microvessel formation feeding tumors.

Investigators across the United States and Europe had been injecting mice and rats with human malignancies, inducing lung metastasis and huge breast cancers, and then drastically reducing both tumor size and incidence by adding Cox-2 inhibitors to the rodents' diets. Epidemiologists, who study the incidence and prevalence of disease in large human populations, have shown that Cox-2 levels are extremely high in virtually all kinds of cancer. Indeed, my own Cox-2 expression prior to taking Celebrex was sixteen times higher than normal, according to tests conducted by scientists at Koeffler's Cedars-Sinai lab.

Now armed with information beyond intuition, in possession of scientific papers, I answered the group, elaborating on my very different therapies. What had I done?

1. I had refused all demands for chemotherapy.

2. I had undergone excision of my oversized, diseased spleen, an often therapeutic event in itself.

3. I had taken an increasingly higher daily dose of Celebrex for almost two years.

No one else in the group had experienced anything like this combination of one negative and two positive therapies, although many had undergone splenectomies for grossly oversized spleens. In fact, it was John McKenna who found the abstract of a paper yet to be written that linked splenectomy with lymphoma remission, about which most oncologists seemed to know nothing. The abstract described a retrospective study conducted at the Mayo Clinic. Four of twenty-six MCL patients who had not been administered chemotherapy after surgery had "maintained disease stabilization" thereafter for more than a decade. "The five-year actuarial survival rate following splenectomy was 53 percent," according to the Mayo hematologist Thomas Witzig and his colleagues, who wrote the abstract and later the full scientific paper. (See next chapter.)

My investigation of splenectomy would have to wait, I reasoned, for at this point in my survival strategy it was academic. After all, my spleen was gone, the decision concerning it already having been made. What I desperately needed to verify was my impression that Celebrex had inhibited the growth of the capillaries feeding my tumor cells.

The latest of the papers to which Dan Longo had steered me was written by Jaime Masferrer and Alane Koki, developers of celecoxib at the G. D. Searle division of Pharmacia in St. Louis. In 1995, while seeking to increase arthritis in mice to observe the mechanisms of inflammation, Masferrer added a fibroblast growth factor, a known angiogenic, to produce faster growth of microvessels. He quickly found that Celebrex blocked the capacity to induce new blood vessels; in other words, it was anti-angiogenic. After widespread clinical trials, the Food and Drug Administration approved Celebrex for arthritis in 1998 and a year later for FAP, or "familial adenomatous polyposis." FAPs are glandular polyps that occur frequently among members of the same family, the poyps invariably developing into colorectal cancer.

I made an appointment with Jaime Masferrer and his colleague Alane Koki.

• • •

It was a lusty, ineffable morning in mid-July 2000. The clouds parted, spilling sunshine into Papa Whiskey. The earth below seemed greener than usual, the corn taller, the trees more photosynthetic. I descended over the dome of the university's Assembly Hall to land at the Champaign airport, picked up David, and took off again for St. Louis.

G. D. Searle/Pharmacia was only a two-minute cab ride from the Spirit of St. Louis Airport, where I landed. Masferrer's office was located in a long three-story brick building that wore, like multiple hats, a series of glass greenhouses, evidence that until recently the company had belonged to the agrochemical company Monsanto. Jon Braun had come from California at my request and was waiting for us in the lobby.

After our greetings, Jon, David, and I looked at a display that told how the name *Celebrex* had resulted from a celebratory contest among the company's employees. Alongside, graphic posters showed that although other drugs had contributed to Searle's profitability, Celebrex was the company's shining star. Easier on the stomach than aspirin, it had become the leading arthritis medication, with $3 billion in annual sales. Aspirin and other nonsteroidal anti-inflammatory drugs (NSAIDs), explained the exhibit, partly inhibit Cox-2, but their primary action is to stop Cox-1. Some 25 percent of people using NSAIDs experience some kind of side effect, we read, and about 5 percent develop serious problems, such as intestinal bleeding or kidney failure.

Jaime Masferrer found us at the display and gave a hearty welcome, singling me out and adding, "I'm glad to see you looking so healthy!" After cordial handshakes all around, he ushered us into a small microscopy room where Alane Koki joined us. Both Masferrer and Koki are Ph.D. research pharmacologists, the emphasis being on *research*.

Masferrer, the Cox-2 project leader, hails from one of most scenic parts of Chile, a land of countless waterfalls, my favorite country in South America. In his late forties, he has the penetrating eyes of a conquistador and in his own mild way is as fierce a fighter, spearheading research on Celebrex for its use against cancer. Alane Koki, a decade younger, is a reddish blond and vivacious third-generation Hawaiian whose hobby is raising pit bulls (which, she later convinced me, are lovable). Jaime and Alane are talented in so many ways that they could have embraced any career. It is a gift to the world that they chose laboratory science.

. . .

The microscopes were connected by light pipes such that when the five of us peered into five binocular lenses, we were looking at the same image. Jaime and Alane sat at the right. Jon Braun—because he is a pathologist in addition to being a molecular biologist—was invited to take the middle microscope, where his comments could be heard better. Jon smiled in anticipation above a short beard recently in the making. David, looking less like a physics professor than, perhaps, a quarterback—physically a younger version of me—sat at the far-left microscope. I took the chair next to him, both of us out of our elements bending to the microscopes, hair spilling slightly, his once yellow now brownish blond, mine once brown, now gray.

The pharmacologists shuffled boxes of slides that I had brought with me—my tissue—placing them in order. Five pair of eyes lowered to the instruments. Alane began with medium magnification, running the focus in and out until the stained cells came up razor sharp.

"These first slides are of Neil's lymph nodes from December 1998," Alane said. I glanced up from my microscope as she paused, pulling her hair back, her eyes provocative, waiting to make sure her audience was seeing what she saw. "Note the neoplasms, the cells fairly bulging—literally bulging."

With cancer, I thought. We peered at slide after slide, listening first to Alane and then to Jaime recount the morphology of mantle-cell lymphoma. After visiting so many laboratories around the country, the scene under the microscope was becoming familiar. I could see the pattern of cells arcing into an oblong plume like the incombustible hood of a gas lamp, forming a zone separate from the mass of other cells.

"Now this next set of cells," Alane said, "is from Neil's noncancer surgery a full year *after* taking Celebrex, eight months after increasing to 400 milligrams daily." That surgery for a benign tumor occurred in October 1999, and I had remembered the date, the last day of the previous February, when I had doubled the 200-mg dose to 400 mg at Dan Longo's suggestion.

The slide we were viewing showed a landscape new to me. The cells were as large as cancer cells I had seen before, but their insides were different.

The pathologist in Jon Braun could be restrained no longer. "My God! Look at those cells! They are *scarred!* . . . See the *scarring?*"

Jon changed the magnification twice, probing deeper into the nuclei. These cells, now static, once had lived within me, producing pain and fatigue, deadly enemies now smeared onto a slide of glass like dead bugs. Jon inserted other slides, again and again, some forty of them. All told the same story.

"This scarring within the cells," he said, "looks exactly like those of a lymphoma patient who has received chemotherapy or radiation. *But Neil hasn't had either one!* So he is not likely to regress!" Five faces serious with suppressed enthusiasm segued into five excited smiles, erupting suddenly in a spontaneous cheer.

Alane Koki (who is now the chief scientific officer of Ipsogen Laboratories in Marseilles, France) was elated. "We've known for a long time that Celebrex is anti-angiogenic in many animals—especially when the microcapillaries feeding the tumors haven't had a chance to grow very large. We've seen it both in mice and in patients with epithelial cancers." (Later I would learn about the human trials she referred to, in which Celebrex dispensed together with other agents proved efficacious against various cancers.) "But we've never seen *anything* like this before in human hematologic cancers—such as lymphomas and leukemias."

"Why not?" I asked.

"We've been concentrating on the most widespread cancers: lung, breast, colon, and so on."

Everyone sat back from the microscopes, talking, exclaiming, happy for cancer science, happy for me. Within minutes the discussion took a practical turn. Jaime and Alane suggested collaborating with Jon's laboratory at UCLA on this research. They would try to discover the precise mechanisms by which Celebrex achieved and sustained its remarkable starvation of capillaries. Ideas flew back and forth like paper airplanes, ideas for future tests and proofs, suggestions for higher, regular, periodic dosing, for various drugs in combination.

My mind reeled with the supposition that those two mediators from science heaven—splenectomy to destroy the majority of the diseased lymph system followed by a year of Celebrex to starve the lymph tumors to death—had cleared my body just in time. My own medical deus ex machina.

. . .

During lunch Jon summarized what the five of us had seen—or what *he* had seen—in those before-and-after-Celebrex slides during the session at the linked microscopes.

"Okay," he said, "besides the welcomed scarring within the cells, I could tell that total Cox-2 expression had decreased because the microvessel density was reduced. I detected an increased population of T cells and a vastly greater percentage of normal germinal centers." In other words, the number of capillaries was reduced. At the same time, the quantity of noncancerous "germinal centers"—the areas of lymph cells in the center of the lymph nodes—had increased.

He turned to me with a smile that quickly turned to laughter and impulsively slapped my back. It looked like my plan for further action could be postponed indefinitely.

"This really is terrific!" David said, "but I hope we're not wrong in attributing this great outcome to Celebrex instead of something else."

"It would be presumptive to conclude that Celebrex induced the apoptosis we observe in the cancerous cells," Alane said. "However, spontaneous regressions like this are rarely observed."

"Not splenectomy alone," said Jon. "The only other probable cause might be the residue of destruction of Neil's mantle cells when they subsided from their formerly high level. It's difficult to narrow the speculation."

"What should my dad do now?" David asked, taking a bite of whatever it was we were eating. I doubt that anyone quite knew or cared.

"More of the same," Alane replied.

"I could put Celebrex in Lake Michigan," I joked, recalling Dan Longo's tongue-in-cheek suggestion of adding it to the water supply, and then asked, "What's the optimum dose? Can you scale up by body weight from all those mice who responded?"

"Oh, we've got better ways to extrapolate than that," Alane said. "For instance, the dosage for precancerous polyps, the FAP, is well-tolerated at 400 milligrams twice daily."

• • •

Now that I knew 800 milligrams a day could be taken, once home I doubled the dosage. Of course my supply of pills diminished twice as fast. Try sometime to buy double the quantity of a prescribed drug after you've run out! The drugstore pharmacists treat you as though you are asking for a year's supply of arsenic or heroin. So you take your two allowable 200-mg capsules in the morning and two nonallowable capsules at night, and then, when the supply dwindles and the druggist won't sell you more, you borrow for a few days from your wife's cache, since she is taking only a small amount for arthritis. Few rheumatologists will give you a prescription for a larger dose. Your world-renowned oncologist in Chicago, John Ultmann, is sick with his own lymphoma. What do you do?

You go to your surgeon. Rade Pejic, knowing what I have learned, rides to the rescue and writes a prescription for 1,460 pills, a year's supply at four a day. Let Walgreen's argue with *him* if they want.

• • •

It was more difficult for the other MCL Group members. With nothing to lose, many of them started taking Celebrex, although only a few found a way to get 800 mg a day. Some complained of indigestion and nausea at only 400 mg, even swallowing it with food. Some couldn't stomach the drug because of allergies, especially to sulfa, for which Celebrex is specifically contraindicated. John McKenna tried but said he couldn't continue due to pain in his digestive system, which surprised me, since a major reason for developing this drug was that it would be easier on the gut than aspirin. At the stage John was in he probably couldn't have tolerated any drug by mouth. He dropped the dosage little by little, eventually to zero, leaving nothing between him and the multiple hells of mantle-cell aggression.

David Cardin, the Ph.D. biochemist with mantle-cell lymphoma, asked his chemotherapist for Celebrex only to be told that it was a barren effort. When Cardin persisted, the doctor wrote him a prescription with extreme reluctance. After only a month on 400 mg of Celebrex, David Cardin's condition worsened, and he was given CHOP plus Rituxan three times, which helped him only for a short time. Several others in the MCL Group discontinued Celebrex "due to the expense" and after their chemotherapists told them it was a waste of money. I found the expense argument specious. Celebrex costs a little more than five dollars a day for 400 milligrams—less than most health foods, far less than chemotherapy, and exponentially less than transplants, which can cost in the hundreds of thousands of dollars per patient.

• • •

Judah Folkman, the surgeon who thirty-five years ago came up with the innovative idea of starving cancers to death by cutting off their blood supply, spent half a lifetime being ridiculed by colleagues, a fate often endured by pioneers in any field. Of course, as a surgeon Folkman had been aware of the value of promoting angiogenesis. Agents such as fibroblast growth factor had been used to induce microvessel formation so that blood flow could be restored to organs, for instance, in patients with severe angina. He conceived the possibility of anti-angiogenesis during operations, when he realized that blood vessels somehow were being stimulated to grow and feed tumors that had metastasized far from their original sites. He began searching for tiny quantities of naturally occurring substances that might inhibit those unwanted capillaries from forming. After years of study at Harvard and Children's Hospital in Boston, he and his colleagues isolated two of these minute biochemicals and concentrated them into drugs he named endostatin and angiostatin. They are now in clinical trails.

Other scientists followed in Folkman's footsteps, notably a Ph.D. biologist at the University of Toronto named Robert Kerbel. Two years before my English friend Ron Edwards died, he had brought the Toronto research to my attention. Bob Kerbel was experimenting on mice with a combination of drugs that worked in synergy to prevent angiogenesis more effectively. The drugs he tried were low doses of toxins routine in chemotherapy—cyclophosphamide, vinblastine, Adriamycin, cisplantinum, and Taxol—compounds normally administered in standard aggressive doses to try to poison tumors directly.

Folkman and his hematologist protégé Tim Browder had long before confirmed that chemo drugs could be anti-angiogenic. "It's just that they had always been used incorrectly," Dr. Browder said, according to Robert Cooke in his book *Dr. Folkman's War*. Cooke explained, "Browder was boldly pointing out that many of the drugs employed in the preceding half century could have been given in a different way, and they might have saved more lives if their anti-angiogenic properties had been known."

Browder blamed "modern medicine's absolute reliance on the phenomenon called MTD—a drug's maximum tolerated dose." These same toxins might work better if they were used not to overwhelm tumors with the toxins of chemotherapy but to target the vasculature instead. You can give the conventional "maximum tolerated dose" only so long without poisoning a person, and then you have to wait a month or so to let him recover before starting again. During that wait, that customarily month-long rest from chemo, the microcapillaries from the tumors typically start growing again. The idea of anti-angiogenesis is to dispense a drug in small but frequent doses . . . drip, drip, drip . . . like a metronome marking the beats for a pianist—a slow pianist who plunks a note only once or twice a day.

• • •

Over the previous year I had been talking by phone to Bob Kerbel and his colleagues Yaacov Ben-David and Giannoula Klement, and I finally made appointments to see them to learn firsthand about their unique extensions of Folkman's thesis. Flying down the middle of Lake Erie in August 2001, viewing both north and south shorelines at the same time, gave me an odd sensation, a flicker of confidence that my extended odyssey was paying off at last.

The Kerbel labs were at the Sunnybrook and Women's College Health Science Center, a large University of Toronto teaching hospital. They are like laboratories everywhere, the same bench tops of polymers impervious to chemical spills, the same glassware, centrifuges, incubators, and microscopes—except for one notable difference. These large rooms were not walled off from one another. The laboratories opened to a long corridor the length of the building, promoting interaction among the scientists. On the other side of the hallway lay a warren of offices, and in one I found Robert Kerbel. Short, sturdy, and balding, he was fully in charge of his domain. I asked him his view of Cooke's statement that chemotherapy administered over the years could have saved more lives if given "metronomically."

Kerbel was vehement in his answer. "There is no evidence for such a statement! Indeed, versions of low-dose chemotherapy were used extensively in the seventies without any discernible benefits in terms of survival. Our work utilizes continuous low-dose chemo in combination with one of the new molecular-targeted anti-angiogenic drugs—which were not then available."

I asked him about the term *metronomic* as applied to dosages of drugs.

"Doug Hanahan, a biochemistry professor at UC San Francisco, came up with it, and it stuck. . . . You're taking Celebrex, right?"

"Yes, twice a day, every day. My new circadian rhythm."

He introduced me to his colleague, Yaacov Ben-David, a solid, self-effacing Ph.D. biologist who spoke in a thick Iranian accent with a steady cadence, as if heeding his own inner metronome. Afterwards I met an opposite personality, Giannoula Klement, then a postdoc working in the Kerbel labs. Quick, striking, late forties, wearing a diamond stud in the left side of her nose, she had come from Greece, where she had been a veterinarian. In Toronto she lost any trace of her accent and earned an M.D. at McMaster University. Giannoula and Yaacov were studying the genetic instability of tumor cells, distinguishing the tumor-associated endothelium (the lining of the blood and lymphatic vessels) from its normal mature counterpart.

Bob Kerbel explained the focus of their research. "There's never been a demonstration of an antitumor agent to which resistance didn't develop. The toxic effects of chemotherapy destroy many cancer cells, sure, but descendants of these cells soon develop a resistance to the drug. Then the tumors return. The process seemed inevitable. Why? That is, why don't the endothelial cells of the capillaries feeding the tumors develop the same acquired resistance to the drug?"

• • •

That question was far more than a casual inquiry. It was among the pivotal questions that led to the anti-angiogenesis revolution by Folkman and Browder after years of painstaking research. Giannoula Klement's experiments confirmed the answer.

"These drugs do *not* work by killing the actual cancer cells of blood vessels," Giannoula explained. "Cancer cells can mutate and evolve to avoid being killed by the toxins. Instead, the drugs kill the *normal* endothelial cells in the developing blood vessels! Normal cells have no evolutionary experience in evading toxins, no way to resist them."

She added, "There is a different sensitivity between endothelial and tumor cells to these low doses, which are not strong enough to kill the tumor directly, so it doesn't matter whether the tumor is mutating or not."

As the first to confirm this important distinction, Giannoula Klement found that, unlike the linings of normal mature veins and arteries, the endothelial cells of newly forming blood vessels are not quiescent. These tiny capillaries wither, and continuous small doses prevent them from redeveloping, thus causing the unfed tumors to die. Here was a youthful woman finding adventure not in some mindless disco of eternal youth but through a microscope, her discoveries adding to the paving blocks on the long upward steps to the goal of stopping cancer—literally by starving it to death.

Giannoula asked me, "Are your lymph nodes continuing to shrink after all your celecoxib, or are they stable?" The Searle scientists had long since sent my slides here, and she was aware of my successful outcome.

"Most of them have shrunk to between one and two centimeters and stayed that size," I said. Realizing that half a centimeter, the size of a pea, is normal, I added, "Jon Braun explained it by saying that the scarring in all those cells of the lymph nodes takes up quite a bit of room." As anyone who wears a scar on his skin knows, scars can be thick; something similar takes place at the cellular level.

"Well, stability of lymph nodes is better than shrinkage in any event," Giannoula said, doodling on a yellow pad. "When you use an agent to kill cancer, you cause necrosis. Cell death from lack of oxygen. The tumor struggles against it." A wiggly, pugnacious tumor took shape on the paper. "When you stop the blood supply, you give it a slow death—without causing necrosis." Now she filled in the dwindling circle of dying tumor, blackening it steadily with short strokes as if the process of growing a theory were itself a matter of angiogenesis. "Tumors develop mutations to withstand toxins. This genetic instability in the tumor cell derives from evolution, since cancer cells double much faster than most normal cells."

"So," I summarized, "the slow death results in what we see on a CAT scan as stability, whereas if you attempt to kill the tumors fast with the typical overdose of standard chemotherapy, some cells die but others soon take their place, having evolved to evade the poison."

"Yes," said Bob Kerbel, who had come into the lab as we were finishing. "But," he warned, "just because you seem to be cured doesn't mean that your response was related to Celebrex. No one knows. It will take rigorously controlled, randomized clinical trials involving thousands of patients over the next five years or so to really begin to determine the merit of the idea."

It is true that history teaches us to be cautious. Kerbel hadn't seen the scarring in my cells, nor had he offered alternative explanations. Nevertheless, he might well have been right that Celebrex alone may not have accounted entirely for my long remission, perhaps not even with the prior benefit of splenectomy. He certainly was right that one apparent cure cannot be extrapolated to other lymphoma victims without meticulous clinical trials. Yet the logical extension of this argument escaped me. In five years, I thought, millions of cancer patients will die, and I could be one of them. While lymphoma scientists await the results of the trials, what could be the harm in giving patients a Cox-2 inhibitor, or for that matter other low-dose synergistic anti-angiogenics?

• • •

The Toronto team is devising clinical trails for lymphoma and leukemia using combinations of vinblastine with Celebrex, cyclophosphamide with Celebrex, and other paired inhibitors of capillary formation. The synergy of such double agents has cured hundreds of mice injected with human cancers. Currently some three hundred biotech companies and hundreds of university laboratories worldwide are engaged in testing agents to kill the blood vessels feeding tumors. There are some two thousand anti-angiogenics identified or suspected, and at least sixty human trials are in progress.

These anti-angiogenics work in various ways. Some, such as interferon-alpha and the Mab bevacizumab, block the activators of angiogenesis. Some inhibit genomic signaling in forming endothelial cells. Others, like Celebrex or the polyphenols in green tea, are agents with nonspecific mechanisms. Still others interfere with the intercellular material of a blood vessel.

One of the signaling inhibitors acting against enzymes involved in anti-angiogenesis, called "SU011248" by its developer, Sugen, a company owned by Pfizer/Pharmacia, showed remarkable effectiveness against a variety of cancers in phase-one trials conducted in Germany beginning in late 2002. One in four renal-cancer patients who had secondary adrenal or lung cancers showed a 50 percent tumor reduction after only four weeks. The agent is an inhibitor of "kinases," enzymes that catalyze the transfer of ATP, the energy-storing compound in muscles.

An excellent example of an anti-angiogenic that interferes with blood-vessel intercellular material is the notorious—newly revived—thalidomide, which originally had been used for morning sickness until it proved terribly dangerous by causing catastrophic birth defects.

Today thalidomide is prescribed in low doses as an anti-angiogenic for cancer (with the stipulation that patients of childbearing age use strict birth-control measures). Thalidomide's comeback is a dramatic story of a drug in search of a disease. Developed originally by former Nazi physicians after

World War II, it was marketed by a Swiss company as a sedative that, unlike barbiturates, was thought to be "completely safe" because the scientists couldn't find a dose high enough to kill a laboratory rat. It turned out that the rats were not absorbing thalidomide; instead of entering their bloodstreams, the drug passed right through them. Not so with humans. The deformities that thalidomide caused in fetuses during the 1950s and 1960s were discovered in the 1990s to have been initiated by cutting off the blood supply to developing limbs. Anti-angiogenesis gone too far.

· · ·

The progress of angiogenesis research seems to challenge, or at least redefine, the common medical wisdom that cancer is not one but hundreds of separate diseases—malignancies of the breast, lung, prostate, skin, blood, and so on. Scientists (as opposed to most medical practitioners) define a cancer today not by where it resides in the body but by what it does to the cells. Instead of naming cancer after the organ or system it inhabits, they designate it by its molecular signature, much as we define infections. When choosing an antibiotic, what difference does it make whether a certain streptococcus is infecting your throat or your lungs or your bladder?

Why not characterize cancers by the genes and proteins that *created* the tumor cells, which just happens to be in the lung or the breast? As various anti-angiogenics are being proved effective in the current medley of clinical trials, the distinction between a cancer that affects the blood and a cancer that affects an organ is being shown to make little difference in treatment. It is the molecular mechanism of the disease that counts.

23

The Mystery of Splenectomy

THE OPERATING ROOM AT ST. ANTHONY'S IS BRIGHTLY LIT AND CRAMMED
with efficiently ordered instrument stands, digital displays, gas tanks, hoses,
sterilizers, and a host of monitors—the machinery of modern surgery. A
half-dozen green-clad nurses, an anesthesiologist, and several technicians
surround the sterile area of the operating table under a laminar-flow hood
that creates positive pressure to push microbes away. The patient lies unconscious, connected to intravenous lines, wires, and tubes.

Rade Pejic—scrubbed, gloved, masked—is in command like a battlefield
general, standing by to excise a swollen, two-pound malignant spleen, five
times normal size. Not mine. Not this time. Soon after my return from seeing the effects of Celebrex on my lymphoma, in the late summer of 2000,
Rade invited me (with the permission of his patient) to be a spectator and
to photograph a splenectomy. The patient, a woman in her fifties, has been
diagnosed with B-cell lymphoma, like mine.

The patient lies anesthetized on the table, looking bleached and impervious to manipulation as a technician turns the corkscrew deep into her
pelvis, pushing hard, his upper body well forward as he focuses his weight
on the screw until, finally inside the bone, he extracts an inch-long sample
of marrow like a bloody worm. Pathologists will determine from it the percentage of malignant cells residing there, revealing the extent of the lym-
phomatoid invasion.

Nurses drape the patient with a cutout in the sheet at her left midsection. Rade begins with a long incision, fast, deep, and steady, honed by twenty-five thousand operations in forty years of vascular surgery. The procedure is routine for him, and he starts by clamping off the splenic hilar vessels and suturing them. Nurses slap instruments into his hand as he talks quietly, directing each person on his team, showing me what he is doing and when to take pictures. He is demanding with the nurses, yet his perfectionism is contagious, and he reaches out to them beyond the natural bonds of his temperament. After only a half-hour he lifts the severed spleen with both hands out of the sleeping patient. The size of a football, the spleen is bloody but surprisingly smooth, with a sheen like the underskin of a tomato. Rade lowers the spleen into a container of formaldehyde.

Returning to the patient, he ties off the remaining pedicle vessels, makes a needle biopsy of the liver, and examines other organs while a nurse fills the cavity with a saline solution. They wait while another nurse counts the instruments, the sponges, and other materials used and unused. A nurse pumps out the water, watching to make sure it isn't pink, which would indicate a leaking blood vessel. The water is clear. Rade inserts a wide drain in the abdominal cavity, secures it, and begins the slow process of suturing, layer by layer.

• • •

Afterward, conveying only a slight hint of accomplishment, Rade walked out of the operating room. I followed, and we had a cup of coffee together. "Your spleen was the same size," he told me, "which is why I wanted you to see the procedure."

This woman's spleen and mine were not uncommonly large as lymphoma goes. John Kornet, who had served with me as a director of the lymphoma foundation, had a ten-pound spleen. (He jokes that he really vented his spleen that time.) Twenty pounders, which make the patient appear pregnant on the left side, are encountered occasionally. Rade Pejic said the tumor board at his hospital questions the value of splenectomy every time he performs one, despite the fact that he removes only grossly enlarged, diseased organs and that patients over age five or so do well without this organ. Splenectomized patients require no supplanting lifetime medication as do, for instance, those whose thyroids are excised. Instead of choosing to remove diseased spleens, the chemotherapists on the tumor board suggest chemo, the radiologists recommend radiation, the other physicians opt to wait.

That splenectomies can be life-saving is nowhere more evident than in an account from France. Eight mantle-cell lymphoma patients at the Hôtel-Dieu de Paris (a hospital dedicated to God), men in their late sixties, were diagnosed definitively with mantle-cell lymphoma via the 11-14 chromosomal translocation. All eight had enlarged spleens, but the fact that they had no diseased peripheral lymph nodes, such as in their armpits, neck, or groin, was the reason given why they were not recommended for splenectomy. All eight died after an average of only eight months.

The hospital's pathologists concluded with characteristic French understatement: "One should consider the diagnosis of MCL at presentation in leukemic phase even in the absence of peripheral adenopathies [swollen lymph nodes]."

• • •

Sure, you have a grotesquely enlarged malignant spleen, which by weight constitutes most of the lymphatic system, so your surgeon excises and it you return to normal. Right? Unfortunately it is not that easy. Splenectomy is an important beginning, not the end of your treatment for lymphoma, which may be why many physicians and others are unaware of its value. The woman whose splenectomy I observed recovered nicely from her surgery. Then she entered the care of a chemotherapist who followed the surgery with aggressive toxins. She died a year later.

• • •

The white blanket of winter covered Rochester, Minnesota, when Judy and David Cardin drove there in early 2001 to see Thomas Witzig at the Mayo Clinic. Witzig, an oncologist and scientist, led a group that authored the abstract linking splenectomy to long-term remission of mantle-cell lymphoma, and I had been trying for weeks to talk to him on the phone. After he examined David Cardin and suggested a splenectomy for him, Judy asked Witzig to phone me, since she knew I wanted more information for the MCL Group on the value of splenectomies. The three of them called me from his office.

The first thing I asked Dr. Witzig was, "Do you know why splenectomy seems to have helped *half* the patients and not all of them?"

"I couldn't give you a scientific reason," he said. "There seems to be something in the spleen, some growth factor, perhaps, that attracts the cancer cells. If you take out the spleen, the cells aren't fed, and they die or become quiescent." He added graphically, "Take the hive away and the bees die." The idea isn't exactly surprising, since the lymph nodes act as kind of sewer system for toxins and other wastes.

After Witzig and his researchers wrote their abstract on the therapeutic value of splenectomy, they followed it with a detailed paper in *Leukemia and Lymphoma.* They cited other studies showing that splenectomies were beneficial for patients with hairy-cell leukemia, non-Hodgkin's lymphoma in general, and chronic lymphocytic leukemia. Now they added mantle-cell lymphoma to the list. The Mayo study, the first that focused on the utility of splenectomy for MCL patients, was retrospective. That is, it looked back at what had happened to twenty-six mantle-cell patients who'd had their spleens excised at the clinic in attempts to remedy abnormal decreases in platelets, anemia, or both. The spleens averaged 1,488 grams, or about 3.3 pounds—bigger than mine but only a third the size of the world-class spleen removed from John Kornet. (One MCL Group member had a 24-pound spleen!)

Half the Mayo patients—of both sexes, with a median age of sixty-two—underwent splenectomies during the relapse phase following chemotherapy. After their spleens were removed, all except four were given chemotherapy when their lymphomas became aggressive—ranging from a few months to more than two years following surgery. Eight in this group remained in remission with no treatment for more than two years after their splenectomies, during which time their platelets and red blood cells had increased to normal or near-normal counts. Median survival of the twenty-six patients was five and a half years after the splenectomies. Interestingly, the four patients who received no treatment after their operations remained healthy for at least the fourteen years of the study.

Every time I hear of an attempted cancer therapy that by itself worked on some but not all patients—in this case, therapeutic splenectomy—I wonder what the outcome might have been had the patients who relapsed been treated subsequently not with toxins but with a biotherapy such as an anti-angiogenic, an immune stimulator, or a monoclonal antibody.

• • •

The value of splenectomy alone in treating blood cancers had been suspected for more than twenty years before the Mayo inquiry after an important animal study. Performed in 1980, research on mice by Brian Kotzin and Sam Strober at Stanford revealed some interesting parallels to the Mayo study. When Drs. Kotzin and Strober injected human leukemia cells in a group of mice whose spleens had been excised *before* they were injected with B-cell leukemia, they found the cancer did not progress. Yet when residual tumor cells in the blood of these splenectomized mice were transferred to a second group of normal mice, the tumors grew and killed them. A third group had their spleens removed after injection of tumor cells but before the disease progressed very far. These mice—analogous to the people in the Mayo study who (like me) did not receive chemotherapy—lived to a normal age without further tumor growth.

A fourth group of mice whose spleens were excised after they developed marked leukocytosis (a dramatic increase in white blood cells) died at about the same rate as those which had no splenectomies. In other words, splenectomy alone, with no other therapy, prevented mice from dying of injected leukemia when the disease hadn't proceeded too far.

Why? What is it about spleen removal that seems to be therapeutic?

Back in 1980 Kotzin and Strober could conclude only that the spleen provides a specialized environment for lymphoid tumor proliferation—kind of like Tom Witzig's beehive analogy portraying the spleen as a depository for cancer cells.

. . .

Jon Braun—who, remember, is not only a molecular biologist and patholo-gist but also an immunologist— commented on some of the phenomena involved. "In tumors experimentally transferred to mice," he explained, "about 99 percent of injected cells usually disappear immediately after in-oculation. In other words, the outcome in animals which are given cancer artificially could well be different from animals that would develop cancer on their own, if any could be found."

"Still, there's the Mayo study in humans," I said.

"Sure . . . and your own case as well. The spleen is an efficient site for trap-ping most anything traveling in the blood because it's designed expressly for this purpose. It is a sinusoidal blood filter." A *sinusoid* is a large permeable capillary often lined with macrophages—those "big eaters" of the immune system—found in the spleen, liver, and bone marrow.

"So the spleen can be a trap for tumors due to mechanical reasons?"

"Right," he said.

"Anything else?"

We were in his modest office, outside his small lab at UCLA, and he put his feet on a vinyl-covered chair. Jon is one of the most intelligent people I've met in this field, nicely ambiverted, enjoying his family, truly selfless. He cares nothing for the trappings of humanity: if you were to blindfold him and ask him what he's wearing, he probably couldn't guess.

"In recent years," he said, "research using mice has revealed that B cells home to the spleen. Diseased lymph cells in the spleen activate certain chemokines, along with the signaling molecules that they share." Chemo-kines ("chemical movers") are small proteins that signal neutrophils, mono-cytes, and T cells, telling them to rush to the battleground and help destroy invading organisms.

"Okay, then," I asked, "could there be a way to reproduce the favorable molecular conditions of splenectomy, kind of a biochemical splenectomy?"

"It's an intriguing idea—interfering with these soluble molecules or cre-ating a drug targeted to those that do the signaling."

We left it there. I had no way of knowing whether splenectomy alone accounted for the indolence of my lymphoma, whether it activated chemokines to help destroy the cancer cells, or whether it simply removed Tom Witzig's "beehive" and allowed the angiogenetic inhibition of Celebrex to finish the job of killing tumor cells by starvation. The mystery of splenectomy is this: why does excision of the spleen stop the progression of lymphomas and leukemias in some patients, to the point of cure, but not in others?

Only a surprisingly small handful of the six hundred people in the MCL Group have had their spleens removed. Only a handful avoided chemotherapy. And not many continued Celebrex or other anti-angiogenics for any length of time. David Cardin, who had been diagnosed with mantle-cell lymphoma in early 2000, was started on Rituxan plus a full course of CHOP. The chemo left him so weak he could hardly walk. The remedy offered him then was more-aggressive toxins. David refused and went to the Mayo Clinic, where the doctors found that the MCL had invaded his lungs. His immune system already compromised, the Mayo chemotherapists felt they had little choice but to administer more chemo, and they did. Despite Dr. Witzig's abstract on the efficacy of splenectomy having been widely published by then, and although David's spleen was grossly enlarged, surgery was still not a Mayo Clinic–approved treatment for mantle-cell lymphoma. Finally, in September, the Mayo surgeons did excise his spleen—not to treat his lymphoma, but because at a tenfold enlargement his football-sized spleen was causing him discomfort and loss of appetite.

David Cardin returned to St. Louis, where the combination of splenectomy and Celebrex restored his health to the point where he could walk without breathing hard. He went back to work at the marketing company that he and Judy own. Six weeks later a checkup at Mayo found that his lungs were clear of lymphoma cells!

Unfortunately the story didn't end there. Mantle-cell lymphoma is a relentless fiend. In the spring of 2001 it attacked David anew, this time in the form of elevated white blood cells. His local oncologist, Dr. Susan Luedke, is one of a small but growing number of cancer doctors who realize the dangers of chemotherapy in toxic doses. Instead, she supplemented his

Celebrex with a low anti-angiogenic dose of cyclophosphamide (50 mg daily). The combination was effective for another year until his adenopathy, or lymph-node swelling, began again in earnest in 2002. David's lymph node tumors are located in the same area of the body as mine: throughout the abdomen and especially along the route taken by the big blood pipeline of the aorta. In this region David's nodes had grown as large as 15 cm in diameter, the size of a grapefruit, many of them coalescing into large masses.

Witzig then treated him with more Rituxan plus interleuken-12. This powerful naturally occurring molecule, discovered and isolated in 1989, helps orchestrate the earliest in the sequence of T-cell immune responses, those that normally fight bacterial infections. Interleukin-12, or IL-12, then provokes the response of other immune molecules, including more T cells and natural killer cells. In January 2002 Tom Witzig and his group at Mayo offered data that IL-12 and Rituxan taken together augment the gradual decline of cancer cells observed after giving Rituxan, generating greater responses than those with either drug alone.

Unfortunately the combination of IL-12 and Rituxan was unsuccessful in David's case. Witzig then tried a drug that had received fast-track designation by the FDA for treating kidney cancers. It made perfect sense because the drug—called "CCI-779" by its developer, Wyeth-Ayerst Laboratories—inhibits overexpression of cyclin D1 and has been given with success to renal-cell carcinoma patients who have not done well with IL-12. The drug disrupts key signaling pathways that arrest cell reproduction early in the process.

David Cardin entered the Wyeth clinical trial at Mayo in August 2002, and within two months his abdominal tumors began to shrink. As the year 2003 unfolded, they shrank further. The Cardins have good reason to be hopeful, although David said with the acquired trepidation of MCL patients, "I hope we're not just rearranging the deck chairs on the Titanic."

• • •

If therapeutic splenectomies—with or without targeted biotherapies—are to achieve widespread currency, we ought to know a few things more

definitely. For instance, researchers could answer these questions with retrospective studies and new clinical trials:

—Do splenectomies followed by biotherapies offer a statistically
significantly better chance for long-term remission than splenectomies followed by chemotherapy? If so, which of these therapies produce the best results for specific blood cancers?

—Is chemotherapy before (or after) splenectomy harmful or helpful
in the long run?

—What is the optimum timing for splenectomies during the course of
lymphoma? Before or after other treatments? (If the Stanford mice
experiments are any guideline, the answer would seem to be "as
soon as possible.")

—What kinds of lymphoma and leukemia, besides CLL and MCL, respond best to splenectomy? (Studies of a broad spectrum of patients could reveal such data.)

—Should splenectomies be performed on lymphoma patients whose
spleens are *not* enlarged? (The Stanford animal studies seem to indicate that they should be.)

. . .

The concept of splenectomy as initial therapy for lymphoma and leukemia
raises the intriguing possibility of other surgeries to treat not only discrete
organ cancers but also blood cancers. The destruction of discrete tumors
without surgery or radiation now is being explored in hospitals around the
world.

In one new technique, surgeons image tissues by magnetic resonance and
then demolish tumors by radio frequency. The magnetic resonance imaging,
or MRI, pinpoints each tumor, allowing the surgeon to insert an electrode-
tipped needle into it with precision. The electrode transmits enough radio-
frequency energy to cook the tumor from the inside, completely destroying
it. The procedure takes only a half-hour under local anesthesia. One hospital reported success in treating a man whose kidney cancer had metastasized

to several areas. M. D. Anderson, the Weill Cornell Breast Center in New York, and others here and in Europe are experimenting with the technique for larger masses on many kinds of cancer, including breast tumors. Maybe it could be part of the treatment for some lymphomas that involve relatively few diseased lymph nodes, extending the concept of therapeutic splenectomy to destroying such nodes. Unlike radiation, there is no cumulative dose to worry about, so a patient could undergo treatment more than once.

Like every attempt in cancer therapy, no one treatment suffices for all. And yet I am reminded of a picture entitled *Vision* that hangs in Jaime Masferrer's office at Searle. It is a photograph of a nighttime lighthouse with a shoreline barely discernible in the darkness; the caption reads *Vision is not seeing things as they are but as they will be.*

• • •

Crisscrossing the country, I flew to Teterboro, New Jersey, to keep some appointments in nearby New York City. Shahid joined me during my last night there; his airplane was rented to someone else for the week, and he was looking for a ride to the Midwest. We had dinner with Michele McKenna, who had just come from work and was wearing a suit, her dark hair cut in a businesslike way. She shares her brother's affability.

I hadn't seen John McKenna since his splenectomy, but my mental image of him was of a well-built man not yet forty, a lawyer with good shoulders and a ready smile who, in a less-advanced society, might have opted to be a fisherman. He was hard to picture as anything but robust. But Michele told us he was in the hospital, weakened and taking antibiotics for a severe infection. Tumors pervaded his colon, the largest of them measuring six centimeters, the size of a small orange. John had tried to get himself into a vaccine program at Stanford, at Genitope, at the University of Nebraska, and at the National Cancer Institute. When he became too sick to make further phone calls, Michele took over and tried for high-dose Rituxan but couldn't get an oncologist to give it to him.

"Maybe it's just as well," she said, "because Rituxan would exclude him from the NCI protocol."

Holding off on a promising and approved Mab—one almost certain to do no harm—in order to get a vaccine! What kind of a decision is this for a patient to have to make?

I could recognize the emotional roller coaster John had been riding: descending into a thousand hells, picturing the cancer eating him alive from the inside, then rising to new heights with each hopeful clinical trial. Those accustomed to taking charge of their lives typically experience a brief leveling off as they separate in their minds the hinderers from the helpers in the medical-science community, finally riding the slope of stability and settling into the intense, tough work of finding their own ways. As once I had identified the bad guys in the chemotherapists, finding my heroes in the white lab coats working on tomorrow's therapies, so John and Michele were at work to save John's life. As eventually I modified my hates and loves into mere dislikes and likes, other cancer victims were trying to do the same, until they were seduced by the short-term relief of chemo, pushed into toxic therapy by their physicians, having learned as children that "doctor knows best." Regardless of the doctor.

• • •

Shahid and I took off from Teterboro on September 1, 2001, detouring a little to sightsee down the Hudson River valley before heading west as the morning mist lifted and the river mirrored the blue of sky. Far enough below to be seen as an island and yet so close, Manhattan looked like a miniature city on a model-train display. We passed uptown, then Central Park, and from our assigned altitude of only nine hundred feet we gazed *up* at the World Trade Center's twin towers glistening majestically in the sun. It was ten days before the attack, a disastrous reversal of the *Vision* photograph, seeing things as they were and will never be again.

We banked around the Statue of Liberty and passed over the Verrazano Bridge, crossing fields dressed in velvet, flying into autumn.

• • •

An onslaught of good news awaited me at home. A small Genitope vaccine trial had opened and closed the same day at Genitope that would *not* require chemotherapy. The trial, designed to test the efficacy of the vaccine alone, was discovered by one of the MCL Group (who entered the trial and wanted to remain anonymous). Michele called to say that John had been accepted into a new Kwak-Wilson vaccine trial getting started at the National Cancer Institute. While the trial protocol required chemotherapy, John could wait no longer, and his cancer might have progressed too far for the vaccine to be effective without chemo. It was too late to experiment.

More good news. The Koeffler lab at UCLA had performed an unusual assay of cyclin D1 levels in a recent sample of my blood, and the results were waiting for me on my computer. The signature 11-to-14 chromosome rearrangement that defines mantle-cell lymphoma leads to an overabundance of cyclin D1, an enzyme produced in high quantities by MCL cells. Because the overexpression of cyclin D1 is regarded to be the main pathogenic event in recognizing mantle-cell lymphoma, it becomes a proxy for measuring residual cancer cells.

"In your blood, expression of cyclin D1 is *close to the minimum detection level*," the Koeffler lab reported, providing tables showing these cyclin levels were far, far lower than when I was diagnosed originally. "In fact," wrote Wolf Hofmann, who performed the assay, "all people, especially those over the age of fifty, have *some* abnormal cells in their blood. Yours could be considered near normal."

The question, as usual in medical mysteries, is why? Was it because of my splenectomy? Or had Celebrex stopped the growth of capillaries that otherwise would have fed the tumor cells? My own opinion, shared by the researchers at UCLA, was that both were responsible, that the second continued the process begun by the first. It was only surmise, an unresolved question. As so many of the articles in my magazines had ended, "more research is required."

24

The Strep Connection

MY PERSONAL WAR AGAINST CANCER WAS BEING WAGED DURING THE first propitious moments in the historical race to a cure. It was as though I had arrived on the moon near the end of the long nocturnal darkness, only minutes before the slowly moving line separating night from day brings sudden, intense light. My fall into the abyss of cancer has landed me so close to that lunar line that I need only to step across it from the deep airless night to the cloudless brilliance of day, from the terrors of toxins to the sunshine of science. Yet in this strange landscape of cancer I am aware of the black shadows cast by craters and crevasses where the sun dawns not the same on all of us who step across the same line. We are all different. Genetically different.

For me, the effects of taking Celebrex in doses large enough to be effective as an anti-angiogenic brought an additional benefit. A full year before my first visit to the Celebrex developers in St. Louis, my ophthalmologist had detected cataracts beginning to form, especially in my left eye, and both eyes showed incipient macular degeneration, an aging disease in the macular area of the retina where fine details are visualized. "Both problems are in very early stages," he said then. "Shut out ultraviolet light with sunglasses to slow any further degeneration of the macula, and come back in a year to have that cataract removed."

A year later was the week after my St. Louis trip, and I returned to the same ophthalmologist so he could schedule the cataract operation. He examined me unusually thoroughly. "This is rather astounding," he said at length, referring repeatedly to his records of twelve months before. "You don't have cataracts now! Nor is there any indication of macular degeneration." He stood back and searched my face with an odd expression on his, not as an eye doctor now but as a detective (a "private eye," if you will). "What on earth have you been *doing?*"

I told him.

"Well, I can understand—maybe—how an anti-angiogenic could stop blood vessels forming behind the retina from contributing to macular degeneration, even though yours was mostly the 'dry' type. But how on earth could Celebrex have gotten rid of your cataracts? There *are* no blood vessels in the lens!" He gave me the standard test where you read rows of smaller and smaller letters and determined my vision was twenty-thirty—not the twenty-twenty it had been, but sufficient under federal aviation regulations to fly a noncommercial airplane.

"You don't need a prescription," he said. "Just buy drugstore reading glasses."

After taking 800 milligrams of Celebrex a day, the fortunate absence of cataracts and degeneration moved to some nether region of my brain . . . until three months later, when my biannual flight physical required another eye exam, which revealed my vision had improved in another way. It had returned to twenty-twenty.

I admit that all this could be a coincidence, that unknown factors— slower food, faster vitamins, fewer random environmental events, anything other than magic—could have restored my better vision. In August 2001 Carol and I were in Los Angeles, on our way to New Zealand with our grandson Brandon, and we spent a day with Jon Braun and his family. Jon's wife, Lynn, is the mother of their three boys, two preteens and a teen, as well as being an M.D. research ophthalmologist. Like me, Lynn doesn't give too much credence to coincidence in such close cause-effect relationships.

"In rheumatoid arthritis, especially in children," she explained, "steroids are the main pharmacologic agent against intraocular inflammation—and they *are* a known risk factor for cataracts. The topic is convoluted. We don't know whether cataracts develop because of the inflammation or because of the therapy. As for dry macular degeneration being helped by an anti-angiogenic . . . well, I'll send you some papers on the subject."

The scholarly papers were waiting for me when we returned from our vacation. I read them to discover that it is truly a convoluted and confusing subject. Both degeneration of the macula and formation of cataracts are associated with a multitude of systemic diseases, among them arthritis (usually rheumatoid), arteriosclerosis, diabetes, and oxidative stress. These diseases affecting vision are related also to a variety of medications, to smoking, to excessive exposure to ultraviolet light, to cholesterol, to diet—and to just plain *living* (widely known as a pursuit leading inevitably to death).

The lens of the eye, I was delighted to learn, seems "programmed to remain transparent under perfect conditions until age 120 or so." Why the clarity of the proteins in the lens fails "prematurely"—in other words, prior to 120 years—is pretty much unknown. Equally unknown, then, was whether the reversal of my beginning cataract and macular degeneration was due to a lowered Cox-2 level or to the anti-inflammatory action of Celebrex. What is known, though, is that most if not all of the molecular pathways in the human body are interconnected.

• • •

The caution of the often-disappointed cancer scientist infused me like some benign elixir in my bloodstream. Sure, splenectomy plus Celebrex . . . and maybe something else . . . had given me a reprieve, but would it help others? I wanted to know. The results were mixed among those in our MCL Group who had taken similar (but not the same) actions. Some seemed to have arrived at ultra-long-term remissions, but others, such as John McKenna, were nowhere near a cure. Bob Kerbel, the Toronto scientist, was right when he said that the definitive answers to anti-angiogenesis would come slowly, only after clinical trials.

I, too, was right in not waiting. I was alive.

For some time I have had an intuitive feeling about "a strep connection." Strep throats had plagued me throughout life, and I knew they figured somehow into the body's calculus of cancer, as Leslie Pejic and I often discussed. I had contracted scarlet fever (a strep infection) at age four, at which time I had both my tonsils and adenoids removed. Since then, when my dentist father looked at my throat after examining my teeth, he always described it as a "cobblestone throat." I suffered a swollen uvula and cobblestones on the walls of the throat through Army bivouac, especially after sleeping under a tank in the rain, and in the years since I have endured more than a hundred episodes. The culprit was always *Streptococcus*. Army medics, tired of shooting me up, gave me a bottle of penicillin pills to take at the first signature pain in the neck, and to this day I carry penicillin with me when traveling. Sometimes, if I mistake the bacterium for a virus and fail to take penicillin, the strep takes hold, and I require large quantities of antibiotic by injection or even by intravenous infusion. Fortunately my strep bacteria have not become resistant to penicillin, although I need more of it these spleenless days to do the same job.

• • •

In late February 2002 Jon Braun came to Chicago, where he was to attend a medical meeting the next day, and I flew him from Meigs Field to my home on the south shore of the lake. I had a sore throat at the time, and Carol asked Jon, "Is there something better Neil can take, or is penicillin still okay?"

He thought about it for a minute, glancing out at the white-capped lake doing its usual dance as winter begins changing to spring. Our two cats, always strep-free, jumped on his lap requesting attention. "Well, the doctors of tomorrow might give interleukin-10 for a strep infection," Jon said. He turned to me and added, "unless one has cancer."

"What's that all about?"

"You get a virus first, then the strep infection, right?"

"Well, it *seems* the opposite to me, that the strep comes first, and then I get a cold."

"No, you get the cold first, then the strep. Viruses take more time to be noticed. You feel the *manifestations* of the virus later—the nose blowing, sneezing, and so on."

Jon explained that the immune system is set up for regulation in both positive and negative ways. T cells and the rest of the body's combatants need to be geared for instant deployment against invasions by bacteria, viruses, fungi, or other pathogens. There are two hundred times as many bacteria in one person's colon as there are human beings who ever lived! Fortunately, most bacteria are harmless or beneficial. Bacteria residing in the colon complete the digestion of food—just as intestinal bacteria digest wood for termites—synthesize vitamins, and help us in innumerable other ways. Beneficial bacteria living on the skin or in the nose, mouth, and sinuses actually help suppress the invasion of terrorist bacteria. The immune system evolved along with our species. Over many millions of years it gradually created mechanisms to ignore or tolerate bacteria by turning down the process of immune activation in certain locations.

"*Turning down* rather than *turning off* is a critical distinction," Jon said, "because the immune system must continually be prepared to respond aggressively if a harmful species of bacteria invades us. This ancient and complex evolutionary adaptation is still only partly known. But the part we do understand is that locally produced interleukin-10 [IL-10] plays a key role at these sites in enforcing immunologic quiescence."

I thought of the interleukins as military special forces converting a generalized action to neighborhood policing. (IL-12, however, which is available commercially, is more systemic, more like the armed forces than the Green Berets.) In my case, the battleground chosen by *Streptococcus* was my throat, damaged by childhood tonsillectomy and repeated savaging of the attached adenoids, which kept growing back only for me to endure having them burned out again. They used to ravage children routinely with such surgery in the 1930s, perhaps not realizing that these tissues produce lymphocytes as well as macrophages. The control of IL-10 production at my throat or at someone else's similarly weakened site depends on genetically defined processes. The genes involved in IL-10 production take diverse forms, and this heterogeneity causes different people to manufacture varying quantities of IL-10.

I was surprised when Jon told me that Cox-2 inhibitors interfere with an important prostaglandin pathway that actually *reduces* interleukin-10 production. He thought my naturally lower IL-10 production, further diminished by the anti-Cox-2 Celebrex, could be a third explanation—after splenectomy and anti-angiogenesis—for the indolence of my lymphoma. It is always intriguing to speculate with Jon, whose mind knows no bounds.

"I suppose people like me have high IL-10," Carol said. "I *never* get one of Neil's strep throats. I never had a strep infection in my life."

"Right," Jon said to Carol. "It's a fascinating thought experiment. People who are high IL-10 producers, probably like you, can tolerate the background levels of intestinal bacteria or other insults to the system."

"Insults?"

"Sure, like allergens in the upper airway, or chili peppers in the intestine, or whatever, with few or no symptoms. That's fine, as far as it goes. The trouble is that high IL-10 phenotypes respond with less urgency to dangerous invaders—including cancer. While the idea needs careful testing," Jon continued, "it's clear that some cancers actually take advantage of this Achilles' heel by *themselves* producing IL-10."

Jon cited the lung-cancer work of Steven Dubinett, another laboratory chief at UCLA, whose group demonstrated that IL-10 is an important factor in tumor virulence. Collaborating with Harvey Herschman—the discoverer of Cox-2—Dubinett and his team have shown that the production of interleukin-10 is triggered by activation of the prostaglandins that create the body's Cox-2.

Jon looked at me, smiling in that infectious way of his. "People like you—Neil—that is, those geared to low IL-10 production—are immunologic 'hotheads.'"

"Thanks for modifying the word *hothead*."

"*Immunologically*," he stressed with a grin, "you respond with unusually strident inflammatory responses to even basic stimuli. In other words, when you catch cold, the viruses upset the equilibrium we humans have established with the billions of *Streptococci* that reside within our upper airway. You overrespond to your sometimes enemy, with the resultant swelling, pain, and mucus formation of a strep throat."

I always am amazed at Jon's capacity to wonder at unusual relationships, which must be among the higher forms of consciousness.

"The good news is that this throat problem of yours may well be *beneficial* for your lymphoma. As a low IL-10 person, your antitumor immunity is less constrained. Sure, it wasn't enough to stop the cancer in the first place, but along with splenectomy and Celebrex, it helped stop it from progressing."

"Well, if that's what happened, then why not look to see what my Cox-2 levels are now? A couple of years ago, before I began taking Celebrex, Phil Koeffler's lab had determined my Cox-2 expression was sixteen times higher than normal."

"Good idea," Jon said. "When I get back, I'll arrange for it. You can get some blood drawn locally and send it to us."

Obviously, not all high-IL-10 people get cancer, so I wondered whether low IL-10 production results in some other factor that enhances an immune response. Current research on that question is incomplete, Jon said, but one part of it is pretty well understood. He explained it as a kind of yin-yang between IL-10 and IL-12 acting on T cells and dendritic cells. Interleukin-10 guides the T cells' "decision" on whether to become activated or just remain memory cell without turning on their armaments of macrophages, killer T cells, and so on.

Conversely, interleukin-12 and the molecules it induces, such as interferon-gamma, signal the T cells to arm. Interferon-gamma, like all interferons, enables invader cells to be recognized and killed by T cells, but the gamma interferons are less antiviral than are the others, stimulating macrophages and various antigens. Signals from the IL-10 and interferon-gamma receptors thus compete with each other. The loudest win out in the T-cell decision.

It's the same story for dendritic cells: either arm for the fight or wait to gear up. In their case, a particularly important part of equipping for the battle is the expression of molecules that allow dendrites to activate T cells. Such arming, as with an army readying for combat, is a vital step in destroying the enemy tumor cells.

"Interleukin-12 comes up quite often in all this fun reading I've been doing," I said to Jon, "for instance, as an adjuvant for vaccines. If biotech companies can manufacture IL-12, why can't they make IL-10?"

"They can. In fact it was produced as a pharmaceutical by DNAX and has been in clinical trials for rheumatoid arthritis and inflammatory bowel disease. It was determined to be safe in humans but ineffective in phase-two trials. IL-10 production ought to be reassessed with better experiments, in combination with agents like Cox-2 inhibitors, and by blocking competing processes such as IL-12 and interferon-gamma."

DNAX is a biotech company involved in antibody engineering, oncology, and genomics. It was started in 1980 by several Stanford scientists in the San Francisco Bay area and quickly became part of the giant Schering-Plough Corporation. There are many biotech companies like DNAX today, profitless enterprises most of them, so far. They work feverishly to test the countless combinations accessible in tumor immunology, orchestrating responses in the body of extraordinary complexity and subtlety in a great symphony of life for the ultimate benefit of people who have cancer, arthritis, and other chronic diseases.

• • •

The strep connection became for me the interleukin-10 connection, but the interleukin story didn't end there. I ran into IL-10 again in another way. In April 2002 I returned to M. D. Anderson to see the new laboratory that Jeff Medeiros told me had just been built for research into mantle-cell lymphoma.

My flight pathway to Texas was almost as convoluted as when I had come here with Shahid in 1998, back when I had been riddled with lymphoma tumors and desperate for help. This time I flew alone, "scud running" in a staggered direction to avoid isolated thunderstorms, then heading south to Mississippi to avoid the solid line of aggressive lightning that covered the western half of my stormscope. On the screen the storms looked like a single malignant lymph node. I refueled at Jackson, crossed the great snaking, muddy river that divides Mississippi from Louisiana, and headed west into the sun, landing at Houston as night fell.

The following morning, a Saturday, all was quiet. The Anderson campus seemed changed, the trees more alive, the buildings brighter in the sun that shone through a clear blue sky. The arrival of spring seemed appropriate to the new cancer therapies coming on stream in the country.

Jeff Medeiros's office betrayed the clutter usual for a chief of pathology: papers piled high, opened reference books, boxes of slides, and the same microscope through which four years ago I first encountered my personal enemy, my blue-stained mantle cells. I hadn't seen Jeff since then, but we had spoken frequently on the phone about new research, and I had talked to a patient he asked me to call, a young man worried sick about his lymphoma.

Jeff, in his late forties, has the good looks more typical of a movie actor than a medical investigator. He had just been promoted to chairman of hematopathology, the department that diagnoses blood diseases, and one of his first jobs was to hire Raymond Lai to direct the new MCL laboratory. Jeff introduced me to Lai. A tall, thin, intensely serious man, he impressed me as having the amiable restlessness of the gifted young. Ray Lai, thirty-five at this time, had emigrated from his native Hong Kong to Canada when he was fifteen. He earned M.D. and Ph.D. degrees and then worked in Jeff's former pathology lab at City of Hope (the Los Angeles hospital where Ellen died).

The new laboratory was spotless. White countertops gleamed in an area the size of a small house, supporting incubators, microscopes, glassware, the latest in instrumentation . . . but no people. At first I thought it strange that M. D. Anderson could spend almost a million dollars to build and outfit a lab but not to hire staff until I realized that, although Anderson is a federally funded cancer center, it is also a branch of the University of Texas. For better or worse, it is the norm for a university to have its scientists and faculty apply for grants. The center pays 100 percent of Lai's salary as a pathologist while allowing him to do research half the time, and it also pays for supplies, equipment, and overhead for the lab.

I asked Ray Lai about M. D. Anderson's sacrosanct reliance on aggressive chemotherapy, such as hyper-CVAD. I really wanted to know. But I was asking the wrong person.

"What we need is more molecular science," he said, answering my question obliquely, "to find prognostic markers so we can give . . . more-appropriate therapies."

Ray and Jeff are studying the pathogenesis—or progression of a disease—of mantle-cell lymphoma, trying to determine the significance of cyclin D1 and various genes in controlling cancer-cell proliferation. They are using both mice and laboratory cultures of human cell lines.

"The research is progressing here and elsewhere in understanding the mechanisms and in finding prognostic markers," Lai said. "The problem is that there is virtually no work being done to translate this research into actual clinical trials."

During the previous two years Ray and Jeff had concentrated on the biochemical defects that result in mantle-cell lymphoma, gathering and using cell lines—those immortal cancer cells that can be propagated in tissue-culture flasks. Despite MCL's being characterized by an excessive production of cyclin D1—a protein that results in increased cell proliferation—cyclin D1 overexpression is insufficient to form the disease. Therefore, Ray began focusing on a signaling pathway formed by proteins called STATs—an acronym for "Signal Transducers and Activators of Transcription." He has found that one of these proteins, STAT-3, is consistently activated in mantle-cell lymphoma and that interleukin-10 leads to STAT-3's abnormal activation.

In fact, other scientists have shown the converse, as Jon Braun had indicated, that STAT-3 produces IL-10. They suspect a vicious cycle takes place in mantle-cell lymphoma, in which interleukin-10 and STAT-3 stimulate each other in a positive feedback loop. If this is proven to be the case, Ray and Jeff will strive to interrupt the loop with highly specific inhibitors for STAT-3. They now are testing various agents on their cell lines to accomplish such a disruption. One agent in particular, called "piceatannol," occurs naturally in grape skins and red wines and has been found to arrest cell proliferation at low doses. At higher doses it kills the cancer cells.

During lunch and through the day, and over a few beers that night, Ray and Jeff made their case for a "translational" project in which they would need first to test these agents in STAT-3 "transgenic" mice—that is, mice that have been given a disease. The realization that not all mantle-cell lymphomas are aggressive, at least not in the beginning, points to the idea of correlating STAT-3 and interleukin-10 levels with the aggressiveness of the disease.

As I had learned in my earlier days, scientists involved in industrial research typically need not do much to transition from basic to applied research. The former segues automatically into the latter, as in solid-state physics developing into semiconductor research. But cellular science is so infinitely more complex, it requires the intermediate step of *translational research*. It was a term I had begun to hear more and more, sounding almost like fad words. Translational research is a bridge between basic research (to understand the complexities of systems) and applied research (to create a drug). The need for this kind of activity is no fad, however. It is a contagious force, born of the new biological approaches, the compelling new symphony of therapies that can lead to a cure for cancer.

When you find someone doing significant science, someone like Ray Lai—young, highly educated, aggressive, enthusiastic about ideas, working under the tutelage of someone as experienced as Jeff Medeiros, and trying to translate basic research from various fields so they can be applied to cure lymphoma—you are inspired to help. If you are the management of a cancer center lucky enough to find people like that, you encourage them to the hilt with a laboratory and collaborations, hoping they will stay and not return to their native lands. If you are only a patient who wants to help other cancer victims, you decide to help fund his project.

• • •

Back home, I e-mailed those in the MCL Group, telling them about this specific MCL project and asking them to contribute to it with me (being careful to direct the request only to those who could afford it). Although many in the group responded with donations to the Ray Lai laboratory, I was surprised and disheartened at some of the answers. "M. D. Anderson has no shortage of money!" said one. "I had a transplant in their hospital, which is full of grand entrances and marble-lined hallways. Everything is state of the art! I take offense that you use this post to solicit for your favorite program!"

In selling shares in my start-up companies so long ago—the magazines and later the Island for Science—I discovered that there are different kinds of money, just as there are different kinds of snow to an Eskimo: old money that frowns on start-ups, new money inseparable from its owner that you'd never attract in a zillion years, bank loans, the mortgage of your house, venture capital, and so on. In the case of funding Ray Lai's project at M. D. Anderson, there is money designated for philanthropy. Most of that kind of money, however, is directed through the American Cancer Society and similar foundations toward the general "war on cancer," a war in which charities join the government in efforts toward preventing the disease, building and operating cancer hospitals, gathering statistical data, funding beginning scientists, conducting clinical trials . . . and somewhere at the bottom of the list, funding explicit basic research projects with short time horizons. M. D. Anderson and similar institutions derive billions from the government for running their facilities, teaching units, *and* research. But they go begging for money to translate that research into a form pharmaceutical companies can use to make next-generation wonder drugs.

In order to fill a minor part of that need, I incorporated the Ruzic Research Foundation as a nonprofit scientific organization. It is small but has one characteristic unique among nonprofits: it spends no time or money on fund-raising. Its purpose is to encourage collaborations among scientists of different disciplines in different institutions and to sponsor a few vital, cutting-edge projects that are unfunded, as had been the Ray Lai research at Anderson or Project Indolence at UCLA.

I decided to use my own moderate but not absolutely needed savings plus whatever might be contributed by friends or cancer victims who hear about it and want to help. No staff. No advertising. No mailings or other solicitations. My volunteer scientific advisory board consists of Jon Braun, Phil Koeffler, Jonathan Said, Wolf Hofmann, Mike Blend, Rade and Leslie Pejic, and Jeff Medeiros. The nonprofit foundation is incorporated in Illinois, where my son David lives, and he will continue it after I am gone. (See <www.ruzicresearchfoundation.org>.)

Our plan is to catalyze the efforts of scientists, to help smooth their way with information and seed money, and to make funding suggestions to the established large foundations and societies. When I say "catalyze," I include cross-fertilization, finding in one compartmentalized science the answer to questions posed by another. Not being a cancer scientist may have its compensations, for when you avoid the pigeonholes, the pigeon can fly.

25

Patient Rage

FLYING BACK FROM HOUSTON, I LANDED IN OKLAHOMA CITY TO SPEND
an evening with Bill Hawley and his wife, Carol. Bill—early sixties, reddish
brown hair, short matching beard—was one of the surgeons who helped save
victims of the 1995 Oklahoma City bombing. I had met him at meetings of
the lymphoma foundation's board, on which he still serves. Bill has follicular lymphoma, the least aggressive of lymphomas, but he was more concerned
about Carol, never a smoker, who had developed an adenocarcinoma (gland
cancer) of the lung. In fact, he was so worried that he retired early from thirty
years of heart and other thoracic surgery to work full time learning about
better scientific treatments for Carol's "non-small-cell" lung cancer. As we
sat in their new home, the Hawleys told me of their ordeal. Carol, a thin but
cheerful and robust mother of three, had undergone surgery to remove some
of the five lobes of one lung, followed by radiation and a clinical trial using
agents that inhibit a protein strongly implicated in lung cancer.

About a year before this visit, in early 2001, the Lymphoma Research
Foundation of America and the Cure for Lymphoma Foundation had
merged to become the Lymphoma Research Foundation. I asked Bill whether
the LRF had gotten around to sponsoring research projects. His answer was
a disappointment. "The combined organization," he said, "sponsors young
postdoctoral fellows with considerably larger grants. The board is still *planning* to fund specific research projects . . . at some point. My main job right

now, though, is trying to find something better for Carol than chemo or radiation. In the process I've become a full-time patient advocate."

If you get the impression that people like Dr. Hawley, the MCL Group, and other clusters of patients are running around the country and the internet trying to find scientific cures while their chemotherapists cede them the initiative, you have correctly assessed the dizzying state of cancer therapy as it perches today on the crest of the onrushing wave of science. Chemotherapists hold that their brute-force toxins extend lives for some years, and they doubtless are correct, as far as it goes. Whether other therapies would extend them considerably further never seems to enter their minds once a chemo proves "efficacious," especially over a long period for relatively easy-to-cure cancers such as Hodgkin's disease.

Some MCL patients aren't as complacent as their doctors. "I'm so mad I could scream!" Nancy Marx yelled through cyberspace to the MCL Group when her father-in-law's scans showed a mass in his colon ignored by his chemotherapist, who thought it was unrelated to his MCL. Wrote another, "My husband died from the relentless chemo they gave him." These are not isolated notes from disgruntled patients. They are the norm. I personally have received hundreds of e-mail messages like those.

Dr. David Granet, the founder of the MCL Group, is still angry about how his father died of a fungal pneumonia after being denied then-unapproved monoclonal antibodies in favor of chemo for his mantle-cell lymphoma. "We just can't keep throwing toxic chemicals into our bodies in the hope the cancer dies before we do," he said recently.

For the past sixty years it has been set in concrete that the optimal way of using chemotherapy is to hammer tumors as hard as possible as soon as cancer is detected. After your hair falls out, and you suffer intestinal damage and severe diarrhea, and your bone marrow deteriorates sufficiently to reduce natural immunity, *then* your chemotherapist spends the remainder of your life dealing with the problems he has caused.

There used to be no alternative. It was chemo or die. And there are many, many cases where chemo has worked admirably. But instead of *leading* the way into better biotherapies, tens of thousands of research projects and clinical cancer trials over the last half-century—their numbers increasing year by year—have *followed* clinical practice. Mostly they have attempted to develop toxins, steroids, antibiotics, and other drugs that will kill or shrink tumors with fewer side effects or repair the damage caused by previous chemotherapy. Among countless clinical trials involving chemo over the last two decades—when Mabs, vaccines, and immune stimulators have been developed, announced, and tried—virtually none of them has been conducted to compare chemo as first therapy with biological agents as first therapy. It is one thing to conduct a scientific trial. It is another to hold a *fair* trial.

• • •

Being busy helping others find their ways into clinical trials of biological drugs, I hadn't paid a lot of attention to "chemo brain." By this time it had become evident that some of the chemo poisons traveling throughout the body penetrate the blood-brain barrier and wreak havoc on brain cells. The Dartmouth Medical School study mentioned in chapter 7 reported that people who take ordinary doses of chemotherapy drugs are twice as likely to suffer brain impairment as cancer patients who have had only surgery or radiation. The Dartmouth psychologist who conducted the study tested people ten years after they underwent chemotherapy. He found that they thought more slowly, had a harder time comprehending what they read, forgot more easily, and did mental math with considerably more difficulty than those in a group of nonchemo cancer patients who were tracked over the same ten years.

MCL Group members know chemo brain firsthand. One wrote to the group: "After hyper-CVAD, I have to keep telling myself what I intend to do from moment to moment; I've had to forget trying to do two or three things at once." Another: "Three years after eight rounds of my CHOP (the only treatment I've had) my head is tilted slightly to one side, rooms spin, and I frequently hit the jamb walking through doorways. I have to hold the handrail going downstairs. I sleep ten hours a night and am always tired. My mouth is dry, my sense of smell is almost gone, and I get a lot of colds."

Even those who respond well to chemo and see their cancers regress for long periods are not entirely symptom free. The toxins' massive kill-off extends everywhere in the body, including the mouth, nose, and eyes, where it curtails production of bodily fluids such as saliva, mucus, tears, and semen, leading to caries in the teeth, infections in the nasal passages, cataracts on the eyes, and decreased sexual function.

Less concerned about my own lymphoma, I found myself in the enviable position of helping others with information. Questions came in a steady stream from the MCL Group, from friends, from friends of friends, even from patients referred to me by doctors. A common concern was whether a biotherapy such as a Mab or vaccine is working if it doesn't shrink the tumors as fast as chemotherapy usually shrinks them.

Chemotherapists believe that the only good lymphoma is a shrunken lymphoma, a view unsupported by anti-angiogenesis and other biotherapies that aim instead for stability. As Giannoula Klement had told me in Toronto, tumors mutate both on their own and in response to chemo drugs. The cancer cells carrying the mutations that allow them to survive chemo continue to multiply. Thus, if you attempt to kill the tumors fast with the usual aggressive dose of standard chemotherapy, some cells die, but others soon take their place to evade the poison. That shrinking tumors do not equate with survival has been known for more than a decade. In 1990 the German biostatistician Dr. Ulrich Abel, at the University of Heidelberg, found that reduction of tumor mass does not prolong expected survival. Instead, *reduction of tumor size by chemo actually can cause the cancer to return more aggressively.*

Why?

Because killing off most of the tumors allows drug-resistant cells to increase. There is no direct evidence that the brute force of chemotherapy prolongs survival, said Abel, who called its use "ethically questionable."

Using chemo to shrink the tumor load before administering an idiotype vaccine emerged as standard practice because of the FDA's reliance on comparing new treatments to old treatments, not because it was good medicine. Two questions arise concerning vaccines. Do the tumors need to be shrunk for the vaccine to work? If so, are there better ways to reduce the tumor load, for instance, with naked or radioactive monoclonal antibodies? Some stem-cell-transplant trials are using the radio-Mab Zevalin instead of chemo-therapy or radiation. Why couldn't the same be done with vaccines?

While these questions need to be addressed, patients take what they can get. John McKenna enrolled in a phase-two vaccine trial at the NCI. Fortu-nately, there are no control groups in phase-two trials; he would receive the vaccine, not something else. Unfortunately, the vaccine was preceded by six courses of an aggressive chemotherapy designed to shrink his lymph-node tumors under the conventional supposition that the vaccine would work better that way.

John had to drop out before the last of six rounds of inoculations when it became clear that, for him, the idiotype vaccine was ineffective. In the fall of 2002 John entered a trial of another biological agent—antisense—which also failed to help him. Had the chemotherapy weakened his ability to mount an immune response? No one knows. It is conceivable that the reverse could be true, that in his extremely refractory condition, he might have been even worse off without the chemo. Again, no one knows that. Now, after his im-mune system has been compromised with chemo, John is trying high doses of Rituxan. If that fails, he may reach his last resort—a stem-cell transplant in order to endure even more aggressive chemo.

· · ·

Patient rage over the indiscriminate use of chemotherapy—which includes using it first without even trying benign biotherapies—leads to patient ac-tion. As cancer therapy becomes more rooted in molecular science, patient advocates have been forming into groups to fill the vacuum abdicated by the nation's cancer doctors. They have names such as the Cancer Information Network, the National Coalition for Cancer Survivorship, and scores of oth-ers denoting alliances specific for each type of cancer.

Some advocates don't bother with organizational names other than their own, such as Bob and Lynn Bennett, who are lymphoma victims in New York City. The Bennetts responded to a televised *Nightline* program in the fall of 2002 featuring NCI vaccine-maker Larry Kwak, who lamented that he had only a hundred patients for his idiotype vaccine trial after two years of promoting it. "Dr. Kwak's vaccine trial is shunned by patients because it is flawed and anti-patient," the Bennetts wrote to CBS. "All subjects in one of the Kwak trials must take up to eight doses of PACE, a powerful and toxic chemo cocktail." The Bennetts, joined by others, were angered that not one of the established nonprofit lymphoma organizations *ever* had requested accelerated approval for lymphoma vaccines. In 2003 the Bennett group gathered ten thousand petitions and sent them to the commissioner of the FDA, pleading on behalf of thousands of dying patients that idiotype vaccines be approved without further delay—and without the chemotherapy requirement when unwanted.

Another patient advocacy group, the one that Bill Hawley and I have come to know best, is Patients Against Lymphoma, run by Karl Schwartz. Karl—tall, thin, curly haired, middle-aged—is a computer consultant who lives on Staten Island, N.Y., with his wife, Joanne, a follicular lymphoma patient since 1996. His acute computer literacy makes it relatively easy for him to store answers from scientists to frequently asked questions and to share the information with patients. He is doing what Ron Edwards did from England and what Ron's son Vince continues to do after his father's death. Both the Edwards and Schwartz Web sites are invaluable to lymphoma victims and anyone else exploring cancer options. Living in the United States and being in good health have allowed Karl Schwartz to go beyond Ron, moving into the realm of questioning protocols and clinical trials.

"When standard treatments—chemotherapies—do not cure or improve survival, it's not in the patient's best interest to use them when less-toxic agents are available," Karl wrote. "Patients have *one life* to experiment with."

Trying to get a vaccine without chemo hasn't changed much over the four years I was attempting to have one made one for myself. In 2002 there was *one* quick and inconclusive trial of only twenty patients who received customized vaccines without having to take chemotherapy first. At the same time, Genitope, the company allowed to conduct that trial, and the NCI each began separate five-year, large-scale, phase-three clinical trials at dozens of hospitals and cancer centers. These involve about a thousand volunteers for

whom chemotherapy continues to be requisite as the first stage of the protocol. One patient, a Ph.D. biochemist who asked for anonymity (because
he is looking for a job and does not want cancer to appear on his résumé),
asks, "Why can't we try a personal vaccine *without chemo* and see if it works
for us? If we wait until all phases of these trials are complete and the vaccine is commercialized five or more years from now, we will have absorbed
too much poison to retain the same chance of success we have now."

It's true that many if not most lymphoma vaccines work better when preceded by chemotherapy. One reason for that, however, could be because almost all lymphoma patients have had multiple rounds of immune-defeat-
ing toxins long before they get to the stage of entering a vaccine trial.
Research suggests that the more chemotherapy a lymphoma patient has had,
the less likely he is to mount an immune response to a vaccine.

"But if the vaccine does *not* work, what have we lost?" the anonymous
patient advocate continued. "We haven't hurt our immune systems. We
haven't risked organ or brain damage. And it wouldn't prevent us from trying another custom vaccine, or from using any other therapy."

At this stage in the evolution of targeted biotherapies, few treatments are
as effective for non-Hodgkin's lymphoma in the long run as an idiotype
vaccine. I have yet to hear of many patients who mounted an immune response to an idiotype vaccine who were not still cured ten years later. The
scientists who make these vaccines employ several techniques to enhance a
response. The simultaneous and virtually identical Genitope and NCI trials, to be conducted between 2002 and 2007, employ a valuable technique
that could be called the "sheep-in-wolf's-clothing" procedure. A sample of
a patient's diseased tissue is attached to a molecule called KLH, or "keyhole
limpet hemocyanin," which the body recognizes as foreign and so fights back
with an immune response.

Keyhole limpets are mollusks, like snails or whelks, but possess flat, coni-
cal shells that are open on the bottom and have a hole (the "keyhole") on
top. We often see limpets, which are about the size of your hand, at the Island for Science, browsing around the shore with their single foot, eating
algae, or if disturbed, stuck to rocks. Hemocyanin is a copper-containing

protein extracted from the animal's blood and used to induce both antibody and T-cell responses in vaccines.

Both the vaccine-inoculated and the control groups in the large, randomized, phase-three trials receive the same adjuvant (helper drug) to boost the immune system, which is called "granulocyte-colony stimulating factor." However, the control group, instead of receiving the vaccine, gets only the keyhole limpet hemocyanin unattached to tissue from the patient's diseased cells. This system allows perfectly controlled scientific experimentation. But how about the patients? Control-group patients are told they are getting "a nonspecific vaccine," but researchers don't spell out what that means. It is an excellent scientific trial, but again, is it a fair trial?

Schwartz's group wants patients warned, because those used as controls may risk developing an anti-KLH response that could interfere with future vaccine treatments. He adds, "First treatment is vitally important because it offers the patient the only significant chance, with available treatments, of improving survival."

Not only will half the participants in the trials mentioned be denied the active vaccine, but far worse is the holding back of these vaccines to other lymphoma victims. Over the five years of these trials, 125,000 people will die from lymphoma, an untold number of whom might otherwise have had an excellent change of survival. (Devastating as is the FDA-required withholding of vital therapy for lymphoma victims, it is important to recognize that we would have gotten nowhere near this far had it not been for Ron Levy and his many protégés, such as Dan Denney and the NCI's Larry Kwak, who paved the way with these life-saving immunotherapies.)

The tragedy of denying modern treatments to patients is a prelude to the dramatic changes in FDA regulations that the emergence of new biotherapies will require. Cancer vaccines have been around for twenty years with fantastic safety and efficacy records, yet none has been approved by the FDA. Although monoclonal antibodies have existed for more than twenty years, only eighteen Mabs have been approved; an additional hundred Mabs are being tested in clinical trials. In the eighteen months prior to September 2002, the FDA stalled twenty-five biological drugs at the application stage.

Placebo-controlled trials for biotherapies, especially for personalized immunotherapies such as cancer vaccines, make no sense. Volunteers for such trials who take the risk of getting a placebo instead of the vaccine are the most-desperate, most-refractory patients, close to death, holding few options. Patients who have had their immune systems compromised by chemotherapy are hardly the ideal candidates for immunotherapy.

The FDA requirement for phase-one studies to establish the maximum-tolerated dose and phase-two studies to prove efficacy are meaningless when it comes to vaccines and other molecular-targeted therapies. Vaccines are incapable of causing serious toxicities at *any* feasible dose. And neither toxicity nor efficacy can be determined in patients whose immune response is blunted, because both safety and effectiveness depend upon the response. When it comes to anti-angiogenics, the idea of maximum tolerated dosage is worse than meaningless: the entire concept is to use tiny doses of an agent for the slow killing of capillaries that feed tumor cells.

Instead of mere informed consent, what we need are informed options—a clear understanding by each patient of every conceivable scientific therapy, whether FDA approved or not, along with an assessment of potential risks and benefits.

• • •

To say that the FDA has a bias toward chemotherapy is like saying that armies have a bias toward guns. The Chemo Culture is a classic case of "cognitive dissonance," the difficulty in holding contradictory ideas simultaneously. According to this theory in psychology, individuals tend to seek consistency among their beliefs and their actions. When an inconsistency (dissonance) arises between the two, one of them must change. In the case of a discrepancy between attitudes and behavior, the attitude usually changes to accommodate the behavior. In other words, it is a lot harder for oncologists to change their behavior, such as administering chemotherapy, than to change their beliefs and accept that new therapies have arrived to replace the old.

The longer the Chemo Culture remains unchallenged, the more obsessed it becomes with its own cohesion. Shahid and I attempted to update the National Cancer Data Base by extrapolation and estimated that more than one million people in the United States are currently receiving chemotherapy. Our estimate of the worldwide market for chemotherapeutic drugs comes to about $22 billion for 2003. Clinical trials of cytotoxic drugs remain rampant: in 1995 some *three hundred thousand papers* referred to chemotherapy trials, of which the NCI itself sponsored several thousand. In one year alone some forty-six hundred clinicians tried out various combinations on more than twenty-three thousand cancer customers. Very few cancer patients refuse chemotherapy when their doctors recommend it—including those who have mantle-cell lymphoma, for which chemo usually does at least as much harm as good even in the short run. As Schwartz points out, "Many patients feel disloyal to their oncologists when they investigate trial options on their own."

Dr. Ulrich Abel, the German statistician mentioned earlier, asserts that the "almost dogmatic belief in the efficacy of chemotherapy is generally based on false conclusions drawn from inaccurate data."

Samuel Epstein, a widely known M.D. at the Chicago branch of the University of Illinois, points out there has been no significant improvement in treatment or survival rates for most common cancers. Epstein says that M. D. Anderson's claims of curing half its cancer patients are nonsense and unsubstantiated. He believes the cancer establishment remains myopically fixated on damage control, such as diagnoses and unreliable treatments.

The science writer Ralph W. Moss, a Ph.D. who wrote *Questioning Chemotherapy*, goes so far as to suggest collusion between oncologists and the drug companies. Like Moss, I seethe over the continued use of chemotherapy as first therapy . . . but collusion? No. Conspiracies work only if kept secret, which is virtually impossible with a handful of people, let alone some seventeen thousand oncologists and hundreds of manufacturers of the various chemo drugs. In our capitalistic system, the first pharmaceutical companies to produce better agents and the first oncologists to use them would earn far more money and greater reputations as desperate cancer patients stampeded in their direction.

While it is true that high-priced chemotherapy is a major source of income and the main commodity sold by oncologists today, as Moss and others have charged, the cost of biotherapies is at least as high. Bias toward chemotherapy is not the result of money-grubbing chemo benefactors. It is simply the way these people view their jobs. Don't forget, it hasn't been that long since physicians in the first half of the twentieth century routinely lied to their patients who had cancer. When I was growing up, my physician uncles explained that withholding cancer prognoses was in the best interest of the patients, who were going to die anyway.

These days medical and radiation oncologists complete at least a four-year residency after earning their M.D. or D.O. degrees and certainly know about new biological treatments. What is their excuse for not leading their patients into the new era beyond chemo? And what are leaderless patients supposed to do when they read about new biological therapies?

• • •

I can answer only the second question. Cancer patients who want to live are supposed to do their own investigating. They are supposed to read scientific papers on the efficacy of various treatments for their own disease. They need to join groups of other patients who share information on their kind of cancer. They are supposed to find clinical trials open to them (see the notes section). The patients then are supposed to become salesmen for what they discover—with all the tenacity, communication skills, and tactics of "asking for the order"—to convince their doctors to help them directly or to help them qualify for an appropriate clinical trial. Ours is not a perfect world.

These days only 3 percent of cancer patients in the United States—about 381,000 people, based on an estimated 12.7 million Americans living with cancer—participate in cancer clinical trials annually. It is a mind-numbing ratio. (The big cancer centers, such as Anderson or Sloan-Kettering, place more than a hundred times more patients in trials than do private cancer doctors.) Meanwhile, noncancer trials for everything from dermatology to psychiatry have tripled over the last decade and are expected to grow astronomically in the next. In 2001 some twenty million Americans participated in some eighty thousand medical trials unrelated to cancer, according to

Center Watch. Before this patient advocacy group began monitoring clinical research, reporting by various government agencies of noncancer and cancer-related trials was piecemeal and haphazard, making it next to impossible to find out what is really happening. Now we know.

Cancer trials: 381,000. Noncancer trials: 20,000,000. Why the tremendous difference at a time when cancer is largely incurable with conventional methods and patients are desperate?

One of the scientists described in this book (who requested anonymity) offered a reason for the disparity: "Private oncologists ignore cancer trials for the same reason stockbrokers don't put you into bonds. It takes a lot of time and they don't get paid much for it because usually it's universities or small biotech companies that start cancer trials. Large pharmaceutical companies, which are involved primarily in trials for noncancer diseases, pay more to doctors." Others say that money has nothing to do with it, that chemotherapists are distrustful of anything experimental, and that they give chemo because they see immediate results in many cases. In other words, they pay far more attention to short-term benefits than to the deaths of the same patients years later.

• • •

Happily a growing number of oncologists are resorting to chemo only in a last desperate attempt to save lives, usually of patients whose immune systems already have been wrecked by past chemotherapies. Among those leading the way into the new paradigm is the famous NCI researcher Steven A. Rosenberg. Starting as a surgeon, Rosenberg has braved an enormous amount of criticism over the past thirty years in pushing new immunotherapies for cancer patients considered hopeless.

The history of drug development is the history of trying a drug meant for one disease on a related disorder—like aspirin, which was originally meant for headache and then used to reduce the effects of platelets, or "thin the blood," for patients with dangerous plaque in their blood vessels. Or like thalidomide, which was dismissed as too dangerous (as it certainly was) for morning sickness but is now used as a powerful anti-angiogenic. Or Gleevec, first developed for myelogenous leukemia and then found to be useful against chronic lymphocytic leukemia and gastrointestinal stromal tumors.

The neuro-oncologist Henry Friedman co-directs a team of two hundred brain healthcare professionals and scientists at Duke's Brain Tumor Center who routinely try drugs developed for other cancers. Friedman's group regularly treats some of Duke's two thousand brain-cancer patients with drugs approved for colon or other cancers.

"It's all well and good to do phase-three trials to give you strong data that something increases survival," Friedman says, "...unless you're a patient waiting five years for these trials to be done! Use of drugs in off-label single arm situations is appropriate if data exist (lab or clinical) supporting their use."

• • •

Chemotherapists argue that chemo works for some lymphomas and for some other cancers for long periods. That may be true, people being genetically different. Dirigibles worked too, but the rapid development of the airplane made it far better for air transportation. Something similar is happening in cancer therapy. Is there anyone in the cancer field today who seriously believes that chemo toxins will continue to be given as first therapy ten years from now? Or for that matter, that they will be used at any stage except in the most refractory of patients or those so raved by toxins that nothing else can extend their lives?

James Watson and Francis Crick wrote the most important scientific paper since Darwin (on their discovery of the double helix), sparking the worldwide revolution in DNA and genomics. No less an authority than Watson has said that chemotherapy has outlived its time, not because of misspent funds, but because of an inherent problem underlying previous basic biological research. "There is no way," said Watson, "that molecular procedures could have been worked out by applied scientists without prior intense development of pure molecular and bacterial genetics."

Reading that, I was reminded of instances in the history of technology where one development must await another. Leonardo's helicopter could not possibly work until small high-powered engines were invented centuries later.

Spaceflight could not have come about without the development of computers (of which there are today more than a half-billion on the planet). Similarly, computers are making breakthroughs in genomics possible by allowing the simultaneous analysis of the complex equations in a human being.

The genomic revolution is heralding the new era of cancer biotherapy. The sixty years of chemotherapy are typical of great but flawed periods in history (such as the seventy years of communism): until those epochs end, their adherents are impervious to the fact that something better has arrived.

26

The Biotherapy Revolution

IN OUR TOWN WE SEE NEIGHBORS AT THE POST OFFICE, SINCE THERE is no door-to-door postal service. People whom I haven't seen for a long time approach me gingerly, with earnest looks, and say in voices that have been cancer-shaped by our culture, "How *are* you?"

"I'm fine. How are *you?*

"But you had . . . cancer. Didn't you?"

"Yes," I say, "but for the last four years, I've been in complete remission."

"Oh!" they say, clearly in awe that I am still alive—and have hair. "How did you do that?"

Some of these neighbors are aware of the revolution in cancer biology. A few are scientists contributing to the revolution. Others are lost somewhere in the thirteenth century. If I make the mistake of telling the latter about anti-angiogenesis and progress in biotherapies, I have to listen to their own cures for cancer. For instance, an artist friend proceeded to tell me about a miracle cure in which a large tumor disappeared after the patient switched to a raw-vegetable diet rich in carrot juice. Was the tumor malignant? Was the patient's blood or tissue tested for different gene expressions before and after the "cure"? The artist didn't know, but he drank a ton of carrot juice every day.

In April 2002 Jon Braun arranged for his own laboratory and for the Phillip Koeffler lab at Cedars-Sinai to perform the definitive tests to determine whether I still had cancer. I went to the local hospital to have 50 milliliters of my blood drawn. The technician on duty, Patricia, remarked that it was "somewhat" unusual for a patient to show up with two styrofoam shipping containers full of wet ice, so I told her what I was doing.

"My father had lymphoma too," she said after she heard of my experience, "all over his body. It killed him."

Something clicked in the back of my mind. "Was it cutaneous T-cell lymphoma?"

"Why, yes," she said.

"His name was George, and he had a biopsy taken by Dr. Pejic?" With so many tragedies in the MCL Group, I had all but forgotten about George Farley, the emaciated man with advanced T-cell lymphoma whom I had gone to see at Rade's request.

She looked at me curiously. "Yes," she said.

"I knew your father. I tried to get him to see Dr. Duvic at M. D. Anderson."

"Oh, I know Dr. Pejic urged him to see her. We offered to drive or fly Dad to Houston, but with those lesions all over his body, he was in such pain he refused to go."

"What did he do?" I asked.

"He went to the University of Chicago hospital," she said, "where they gave him chemotherapy. He died shortly afterwards."

Patricia wiped a tear from her eye, smiled, and placed five vials of my blood in each container of ice. I brought them to the express office, shipping half to the Braun laboratory at UCLA and half to the Koeffler lab at Cedars-Sinai.

Hearing about Patricia's father and knowing about my friend Thayer's successful outcome with the same disease, I thought of my own case and what might have happened. Had I followed the advice furnished me at the first four institutions where I sought help in the fall of 1998, I would have received aggressive chemotherapy and a bone-marrow transplant. At that time, fatigued and exhausted with pain, I had not expected to live into the new millennium—let alone be in full remission for the ensuing four years.

Now I imagined a scenario of the biotherapy revolution unfolding in the future, how it *should* be by 2010 . . .

The local oncologist visits me at St. Anthony's Hospital armed with the latest in the research race, which she follows closely, automatically incorporating new science into her practice. She says to me at my hospital bed, "We've made tests of your excised spleen, which was five times larger than normal. The bad news is that you have the chromosomal translocation confirming mantle-cell lymphoma. The good news is that your interleuken-10 level is low. We did an expression profile of your genes and know which ones have mutated. Your Cox-2 level is sixteen times too high. We're going to give you a Cox-2 inhibitor, both to inhibit angiogenesis to the tumor cells and further to lower your IL-10. After that, you can get CAT scans every once in a while, and we'll also check your genes periodically to see whether you need anything else. In the end, you'll be fine."

· · ·

At their laboratories in Los Angeles, the scientists used polymerase chain reaction (described in chapter 16) to proliferate DNA fragments in my blood and then affixed the resulting RNA to microchips. The Koeffler lab reported that my Cox-2 level was no longer detectable. In other words, it had fallen sixteenfold since 1998 following daily 800-mg doses of the Cox-2 inhibitor Celebrex. Using the same technique, Jon Braun's lab showed that my cyclin D1 level had increased from the year before but was nowhere near the ranges seen in active mantle-cell lymphoma.

An unbridled lifelong optimist, I didn't worry—enough, as it turned out—about the elevated cyclin D1. "Don't forget," Jon said, "these assays are a snapshot in time. They could show different levels at different times." In my mind, the tests seemed to confirm what I had believed for the past few years, that I was cured . . . almost. Finding you are cancer-free or almost cancer-free is one of those privileged moments of life, and the news flowed into me like ocean waves, which seem always the same, but never quite the same.

Others were not so fortunate. They were dying. During the first four years of my cancer education, about a hundred members of the MCL Group had lost their battles with lymphoma. In the summer of 2002 Bill Hawley, my surgeon friend from the board of the Lymphoma Research Foundation, saw his wife, Carol, die of lung cancer.

We can do nothing for friends after they die, but we can help the 12.7 million of us in the United States who are living with cancer. Certainly progress was being made. An announcement of a new clinical trial crossed my desk recently, offering two Mabs in synergy—with no chemo required! You can't pick up a scientific journal or even a good newspaper these days without reading of new treatment options on the horizon through research at the molecular level. More patients, the government—everyone—ought to advocate increased research into molecular biology. If we don't know how we work, how can we possibly hope to fix ourselves?

. . .

As I traveled the country, continuing my dialogue with scientists with no urgency on my own behalf, I kept hearing about impediments that struck the heart of the biotherapy revolution. Compliance requirements for NCI projects resulted in a torturous overload of paperwork. Even worse were the FDA's Byzantine procedures and oversight, which would have put the Politburo to shame. One scientist had told me how FDA assessors of clinical-trial data for a new biotherapy convened a panel of outside experts to review the company's data—and then watched the proceedings from behind one-way mirrors.

Deregulation has benefited so many industries in the United States, it would seem that the most creative industry of them all—scientific research—should be somewhere on the government's agenda. Deregulating cancer research is vital, but it won't be easy. Ronald Reagan once said, "A government bureaucracy is the nearest thing to eternal life we'll ever see on this earth."

In my efforts to catalyze cancer research, I wanted to add an outsider's voice to the silent agonies emanating from the laboratories, maybe writing articles or meeting with cancer societies to suggest the unfettering of research. The first step in solving a problem is to understand it, and the best way to find out what people are thinking is to ask them. Having met with some sixty cancer researchers in the last few years, one day I sent them all the same two questions by e-mail. (What did we ever do without e-mail?)

1. What changes in regulating cancer research or clinical trials, if any, would you recommend for the FDA?

2. If you could have the NCI change its funding emphasis, what changes would you like to see?

The scientists hold the NCI in high regard, but an implacable fault line runs between them and the FDA. Many of the researchers, in universities as well as biotech companies, attacked a bedrock FDA decree: the randomized clinical trial to prove that a new therapy works. Random clinical trails, double-blind where possible, were designed to prove safety and efficacy for mass-marketed drugs. It was a prudent idea in 1962 when it was amended to the federal Food, Drug, and Cosmetic Act.

In the twenty-first century, however, those rules no longer make sense. Today's molecular-targeted therapies are not oriented toward the masses of cancer patients, as no one knows better than the nation's thirteen hundred biotech companies, which have pumped $100 billion into research in the last ten years. Their therapies are customized for small groups of patients with similar phenotypes or, as with vaccines, made specifically for each person. It's as though we had to endure clinical trials for new surgical procedures; obviously, no one in his right mind would suggest "surgical placebos"—cutting open and sewing up people in control groups.

In regulating biological therapies as it does conventional drugs, the FDA suffers from institutional sclerosis. The agency should ensure the safety of the procedures involved but not try to prove the efficacy of a treatment as though it fit the same huge mold.

Other suggestions for improving the FDA centered on combination therapies. For instance, John Reed, scientific director of the Burnham Institute, one of the world's leading experts on apoptosis (programmed cell death), feels that clinical trials ought to be conducted on two or more new agents at the same time; the present practice is to compare one new therapy against chemo. He pointed out that "many of the molecularly targeted therapies lack activity as single agents but work synergistically in combination."

Alane Koki, chief scientific officer of Ipsogen Laboratories, echoed this attitude: "There must be a way we can be allowed to test multiple combinations of agents—multiple approaches—right from the beginning. Patients with AIDS did it themselves, by mixing various drugs into 'cocktails.' The single-bullet approach we use now takes way too long."

Ann Mohrbacher, of USC in Los Angeles, argued that effective new therapies are stymied because only 3 percent of U.S. cancer patients participate in clinical trials. (You have to wonder about the other 97 percent—more than 12 million cancer victims. They must be doing what their chemotherapists tell them to do or else devising their own cures out of alternatoid medicines—or both.) Ann would increase participation in cancer trials by moving the studies from academic centers to local communities. She recommended a big public-awareness campaign, as well as major efforts to standardize study forms and data requirements, to break the stranglehold of oncologists in private practice resisting clinical trials for their patients.

Researchers in England and Canada, as well as Wyndham Wilson, who works with Larry Kwak at the NCI, emphasized how lack of coordination among governing drug regulatory agencies in the United States and other nations slows progress, because too many of the same experiments have to be repeated. Billions of dollars are spent on redundant research and trials, and many lives are lost in the process, said another scientist (who wanted to be anonymous). It reminded me of the methylglyoxal therapy in India, which had been bouncing around in laboratories since the Nobel laureate Albert Szent-Györgyi suggested its use in fighting cancer back in 1937.

The head of a biotech company (who also requested anonymity) recommended inaugurating an appeal process for drugs the FDA refuses to approve—provided there is a reasonable likelihood of safety and efficacy, as determined by an independent board of scientists.

Carl June, the T-cell co-stimulation pioneer, said, "Promising findings at the [lab] bench are going nowhere because of barriers in translating them into clinical trials. FDA oversight needs to foster early-stage concept trials instead of hindering them."

Mike Blend, the nuclear biologist at the University of Illinois, was even stronger in his condemnation of the FDA's intransigence. "They are unwilling to sit down with researchers and agree on a set protocol for a combined phase-one, -two, and -three trial. There is no need for the adversarial relationship between the FDA and the rest of the world."

. . .

By contrast, the researchers generally feel the National Cancer Institute is on their side and doing a good job in supporting and conducting good basic and clinical research. Ron Levy, of Stanford, spoke for them all when he said, "The peer-review system is incredibly good."

That doesn't mean the scientists don't see ways for NCI to improve. With the dramatic recent increases in funding, no one thought that the NCI or the other twenty-six agencies in the National Institutes of Health weren't spending enough. *How* they spend it is a different story. One person's basic research is another person's lack of funding.

Phil Koeffler, of Cedars-Sinai, feels that comparatively too much is delegated to research on HIV, which infects 900,000 people in this country, whereas the NIH spends $6 billion for cancer, which claims 12.7 million Americans. He added, "Ideally, the entire NIH should try to fund at least 25 percent of submitted cancer-research grants; with the NIH running at only a 16 percent funding rate, it is almost impossible to discern a difference in the excellence of the grant that gets funded and the one that does not."

Carl June agrees and warned that "we will have a dearth of young scientists and an excess of great academic career opportunities if we don't stop year-to-year funding whims."

Giannoula Klement, now at Harvard University, suggested establishing some sort of tenure system to accommodate scientists with longer-term visions. "If Dr. Folkman was to begin his career today, with the emphasis on applied research and drug testing, he would never get funded," she said, "and might never have been able to develop anti-angiogenesis."

UCLA's Mike Teitell argues that the NCI prefers safe projects that push science one slow step at a time. "At least occasionally, they ought to try for breakthroughs with an uncertain line of research. Sure, risky projects are usually doomed to fail, but you only need a few successes to open new fields of inquiry in ways we can't even imagine prior to their discovery."

Many of the suggestions involved translating basic research to a form usable by drug developers. "The biggest hurdle to progress," according to a biotech scientist (who, like so many others, requested anonymity), "is the convoluted regulatory procedures to move research from bench to bedside. Countless committees require separate paperwork for biosafety, animal use, radiation safety, use of human subjects . . . forms to document ethnic diversity, ethics, and other concerns in reaction to some lawsuit or spectacle in the press, rather than reasonable risk and benefit. These committees operate in a punitive-defensive cover-your-ass mode. We're swimming in mud."

Ollie Press, of the Hutch in Seattle, said, "A lot of the fun has gone out of clinical research because we spend most of our time filling out forms rather than in the lab or seeing patients." Press and Raymond Lai, of M. D. Anderson, both feel that the lack of translational research is the bottleneck in developing new cancer therapies. "A lot of promising findings gather dust at the bench," Ollie Press said, "because of difficulties in translating them into phase-one trials."

Another way to advance biotherapies is for the NCI—and cancer societies—to sponsor *hypothesis-generating* inquiries, not just *hypothesis-testing* projects. Almost all science proceeds from the top down, testing hypotheses. You start with a theory and try to prove it. Both David Mason, of Oxford's Radcliffe Hospital, and Jon Braun pointed out that almost all NCI research fits this model—for example, the testing of hundreds of toxins to find some that will inhibit angiogenesis. "It's usually a fruitful pursuit," said Mason. "On the other hand, preconceived hypotheses often lead researchers down murky alleys to dead ends. In addition, we ought to aid discovery by pure observation. Do something and see what happens."

That was the way Priestly discovered oxygen. He put a mouse in a closed chamber and noticed that after awhile it used up "the kind of air" it needs for respiration. In more-modern times, my magazine *Industrial Research* advocated hypothesis generation. It consists of unadorned inquiries into a mechanism of nature, such as "how does a prism split white light into colors"—leaving for applied research to determine from that spectrum the distance of stars or how to make sunglasses. Similarly, discovery science provided the impetus to the Human Genome Project, which began by saying, *Let's look and see what we can find, without cramming our assumptions into a preconceived mold.* It's not so different from the journalist's or detective's approach: *knock on some doors and see who has something to say.*

"Thanks to new technologies such as microarray screening and gene-expression profiling," David Mason said, "the quantity of information available today far outstrips anything in the past by an enormous factor that many funding agencies don't seem to grasp. The mountains of data already painstakingly gathered *should* shift the balance of research towards analyzing relationships and correlations. But that doesn't seem to be happening. At least not yet."

Jon Braun came to the same conclusion from a slightly different perspective. "The cell is a huge center of activity," he said, "with thousands of processes that may be useful to understand. How should we proceed? If we do it one hypothesis at a time, such as activating gene-1, or deleting gene-2, we're going to need thousands of man-years before we hit on an answer."

It made me think of the early days of aircraft development—men flapping their wing-sheathed arms or tying themselves to giant firecrackers —before someone designed an airfoil for a propeller or a rotor blade. Evaluating ideas one at a time worked with airplanes, but it's too slow for cancer research because cells and their interactions are infinitely more complex.

"The solution," Jon told me, "is parallel-processing, looking at many factors at the same time, looking at people like you, Neil, who violate the norm. For instance, those whose indolent cancers don't become aggressive. We think we know how you yourself have beaten the odds—at least, so far— and now we need to look at other successes too."

The idea of interdisciplinary research, which has become almost conventional in industrial research, ought to enter the lexicon of cancer science. If we're going to cure cancer, why not draw from fields in addition to medicine and biology? Immersing postdocs in more than one discipline and designing projects that involve different kinds of laboratories could induce young physicists, chemists, and research engineers to study the biology of cancer. Biologists and other scientists are apt to ask different kinds of questions. Biologists, trained in observation, might ask why certain proteins are switched on or off in a network. Physicists might ask, more fundamentally, Why are we looking at proteins instead of some other system? Interdisciplinary research would foster unusual and surprising innovations.

Giannoula Klement said, "One rarely thinks on a day-to-day basis of the hypothesis that triggered the experiment being conducted. The good scientists are those who can make unexpected connections between fields that seem unrelated or into areas not even within one's expertise."

She said anti-angiogenesis discoveries were made that way when researchers looked outside the boundaries of their expertise to find that capillaries could be killed without developing drug resistance. They got there (and she was a principal in the endeavor) by thinking first of the side-effects of chemotherapy, to which the patient never becomes resistant. Since it was not the cancer cells of the capillary linings that were being attacked by anti-angiogenic drugs but rather the normal cells lining those microvessels, Giannoula knew these cells had no evolutionary way to evolve resistance to the drugs and therefore were likely to *stay* killed.

Karl Schwartz, of the Patients Against Lymphoma group, also answered my questions. Working with the NCI's progress review group, he is advocating a new initiative to bring together experts from multiple disciplines, institutions, and governmental agencies for the rapid discovery and development of cancer therapies. The goal of their organization, the Cancer Translational Research Allied Consortium, is to shorten the time lag between discovery and development from ten to two years.

• • •

A few renowned scientists (the heads of well-funded cancer laboratories) elaborated their answers to my questions by saying that you can not mandate discovery. "What we need are better ideas, not just more money."

They may be correct in an individual laboratory at a given time, but directing the goals of thousands of research scientists is hardly fruitless. Anyone who has directed research and development—in any field—knows that you *can* mandate the projects on which scientists work. It's done in industry routinely. As a nation we mandated development of the atom bomb during World War II and mandated landing men on the moon (twelve in all), massive projects involving multiple research projects and coordinating enormous numbers of scientists and engineers.

When you mandate the projects on which researchers work, you find (not too surprisingly) that it is *there* that they make their breakthroughs. It is how we discover tomorrow, which grows out of our yesterdays, deciphering what we have learned step by step, theorizing, tearing down hypotheses, learning from mistakes, observing . . . and in the process building the future. We can and do mandate discovery. Every day. Viewed in that light, curing cancer, like any other human endeavor from the pyramids to spaceflight, is primarily a matter of national commitment.

27

Detour

OVERREGULATION AND THE PERSISTING CHEMO CULTURE WERE BROUGHT home to me in September 2002 in an explosive way. A routine blood test showed my white-cell count had increased to 65,000.

Blood, our most valuable juice, run amuck.

The disease-fighting portion of mine was ten times higher than normal. A CAT scan revealed lymph nodes throughout my abdomen packed so densely they had melded together in large masses. Those that could be seen separately were ovals I measured as large as three by six centimeters. In the countless CAT scans I'd had taken over four years, I had never seen my lymph nodes this big or plentiful. Oddly, I felt no pain. A PET scan, which reveals metabolic activity, showed the tumors growing only moderately fast. Suddenly I was back in the survival business, my thoughts plunging, the shock of it bloodcurdling in an almost literal sense.

Why hadn't I become more of a hypochondriac? Why had I been so convinced of my invulnerability? I was mad at myself for not realizing that you reach a tolerance level with any drug, angry at being such an optimist and not having acted over the past few years to find another anti-angiogenic that would work in synergy with Celebrex. How many times during those four years had I read that human cells develop resistance to drugs, the major reason for combination drug therapy? As one pharmacologist put it, "I have never seen a drug that didn't become less specific with time." Over four years, my cells had become at least partially resistant to the anti-angiogenic effects of Celebrex.

Why hadn't I taken a combination of anti-angiogenics? It wasn't as though I had known nothing about them.

Now I revisited the subject. One problem was that most of these drugs were harmful in one way or another to the immune system, which I was determined to preserve. Vinblastine and cyclophosphamide, even in small metronomic doses, could deplete the white blood cells over time. Others, such as green-tea extract and shark cartilage, had been compared to pipe dreams. Thalidomide might have been a good choice because it doesn't alter the ratios of various types of immune cells or change the expression of molecular surface markers, as do the chemos, even in low doses. On the other hand, while thalidomide is effective in stopping the migration of white blood cells to produce anti-angiogenesis, it can cause rashes, nausea, muscle weakness, impaired reflexes, and loss of feeling in the arms and legs.

These considerations lessened anxiety over my own inaction. Anyway, I never stay mad at myself for more than five minutes (although it sometimes takes as long as six minutes to forgive others.) When I became accustomed to breathing again, I soon realized that the customized learning I had done could rescue me yet. And that Celebrex, having kept my cancer in remission for four years, was still remarkable, since survival of MCL patients after diagnosis is normally eighteen to thirty-six months.

I knew my way around now. It was my turn to do what I had advocated for others and had attempted to do for myself four years ago—to get a vaccine, somehow without chemo. I called some scientists, friends by now, to see whether any vaccine trials were looming on the horizon. If I could enter one, it would constitute long-range strategy. For the short term, I brought myself up to date on monoclonal antibodies and other biological agents. It was time to take Rituxan. If that proved insufficient, choice two would be high-dose Rituxan. From there I would move down the line into other Mabs, antisense, co-stimulation of T cells, and whatever else I could get. Meanwhile, if I could delay any of these therapies for a few days, I would have time to bank my "dirty" white cells, thus avoiding surgery to get tissue for making a vaccine.

I called Carl June at the University of Pennsylvania and asked him whether his T-cell co-stimulation procedure was ready yet. He said there was a clinical trial he was trying to get started involving both his process and an NCI idiotype vaccine. Carl suggested I come to U. Penn. not only to learn more about the trial but to have a billion or so of my white cells removed, both to save them for a possible vaccine and also as the first step in therapy to reduce their number.

In the week before going to Philly, I worked late every night writing e-mails to dozens of scientists, including Jon Braun and Phil Koeffler at UCLA and Ron Levy at Stanford. Giannoula Klement had just moved from the University of Toronto to Harvard's Dana-Farber Cancer Institute, where she was continuing her angiogenesis research as part of Judah Folkman's ever-expanding group. I e-mailed her asking for her latest thoughts on adding another anti-angiogenic to Celebrex.

She and some of the other scientists were traveling. Others responded immediately. Phil offered to make a microchip of my RNA for a gene expression analysis so he could compare it with the one he had done three years before. Jon arranged to have my blood banked at UCLA in case a vaccine trial opened up there.

"Don't forget," Jon said, "your immune system is intact. Supplementing it is always a good idea."

Carol bought a bunch of insulated picnic containers—small ten-inch cubes of the type that in an earlier life we used in the spring to transport wild morel mushrooms, which we hunted as far as upper Michigan. Now the containers would be used to insulate blood. My blood. I felt like a donor (as once I had been), bringing the containers with me to the lab in Michigan City. Here I was again, having my blood drawn, packing the tubes in insulating material, and bringing the preaddressed boxes to FedEx for next-morning delivery. I sent blood to UCLA, to Cedars-Sinai, and to UC San Francisco, where they had offered to check whether I was still a candidate for Oncolym should I need it. (I was.)

Another sample went to Jeff Medeiros at M. D. Anderson to make sure I didn't have some other blood cancer, such as CLL, in addition to mantle-cell lymphoma. (I didn't, thankfully; MCL was enough to handle.) Jeff grew a culture from my blood and confirmed the MCL with translocations beyond those of the 11 and 14 chromosomes, this time including translocations of chromosomes 1, 4, 5, 8, 9, 13, 19, and 20, plus defects in 14, 15, and 21, "indicating highly advanced disease activity." I was back in hell, and it looked like it would be an extended visit.

My step-by-step plan of action, forged in the heat of those anxious days when I had first been diagnosed with cancer, started with Rituxan, the anti-CD20 monoclonal antibody. But it was not too early to consider a second step, because Rituxan alone was still considered to be insufficient in advanced mantle-cell lymphoma. I had known of human trials going on to test a (non-radioactive) anti-HLA-DR antibody called apolizumab and tradenamed Remitogen by its developer, Protein Design Labs, in Freemont, California. I wanted to avoid radiation for as long as possible, even in the targeted doses that Oncolym delivers. The developers of Oncolym had coupled their antibody, which uniquely attaches to various HLA cell-surface markers, with the radioisotope iodine-131 because the naked Mab had not proved effective alone.

The naked anti-HLA antibody of Remitogen would be a safe option should my first-choice Rituxan prove insufficient, but whether I could take it depended on two events. First, tests would have to show that my blood cells were expressing the particular HLA markers attacked by Remitogen. Second, I needed to determine whether Remitogen's manufacturer had extended its current trials to include mantle-cell lymphoma. I found out that expressing the HLA markers attacked by Oncolym is not predictive of the antigens for Remitogen. Another blood test would have to be given, but I couldn't find anyone to give it to me without appearing personally in Omaha, Houston, or some other place where trials were being conducted. There wasn't time for that right now.

I know of Genitope's large ongoing clinical trial to test idiotype vaccines in MCL patients, but the protocol required chemo first and was a phase-three trial. In late-phase trials like that, I had an equal chance of falling into a control group, which would receive only an adjuvant instead of the vaccine. Since it was a double-blind trial, no one—not the doctors, nurses, or patients—would know.

Other scientists echoed the refrain of chemotherapy plus Rituxan that I had heard for the last few years. The grand pioneer of lymphoma vaccines, Ron Levy, returned from a trip and answered that he had no vaccine trials running. "Take CHOP plus Rituxan," he said. Coming from Levy, the siren's song was seductive, even after my four years of deploring toxins, because I knew chemo would bring down my white-cell count in a hurry and shrink the lymph-node tumors temporarily. But I also knew chemo was a road I didn't want to travel, a relatively short road only a few years long.

• • •

Dan Longo, the remarkable scientific director at the NIH who somehow keeps his pulse beating in synchrony with absolutely everyone in the world doing research in lymphoma, agreed that I ought to start with Rituxan as a single agent. Then, without much hope for a positive response, I asked him, "Do you know anywhere that I can get an idiotype vaccine without chemo, maybe without even entering a clinical trial?"

"Yes!" he said surprisingly. "From Maurizio Bendandi. Dr. Bendandi learned idiotype vaccine making here—at the NCI—and now is in Spain. He is a superb physician and scientist, and I can recommend him to you enthusiastically and without reservation."

Meanwhile, I heard back from Giannoula Klement. She confirmed my supposition that I had become resistant to Celebrex. "Here at Harvard we've been working with common chemo agents to inhibit angiogenesis," Giannoula said, "delivered, of course, in low metronomic doses that cause no or minimal harm to your immune system. We've narrowed our focus to vinblastine, Taxotere, and cyclophosphamide. I prefer vinblastine or Taxotere," she said. "Bob Kerbel, still at Toronto, likes the idea of cyclophosphamide [Cytoxan] because it can be given orally. Of course, that's an important consideration when you take it daily, or almost daily."

She sent me the preferred doses. *Cytoxan:* one 50-mg pill daily. (Giannoula explained that the Italians had arrived at this dosage in breast-cancer studies.) *Vinblastine:* 0.5 mg per square meter of skin surface, administered by injection twice weekly. *Taxotere:* somewhere between 10 and 20 mg per square meter weekly, depending on bone-marrow suppression. Such small amounts had been sufficient to kill the microtubules—microvessels feeding the tumors. "The hope is to have minimal to no bone-marrow suppression," she said, "in order to be able to continue indefinitely or until a tumor regression is seen."

My problem was that I had to do something fast. Any anti-angiogenic, I knew from taking Celebrex, would require a minimum of three months to starve any appreciable quantity of cancer cells, if it worked at all. Failure to bring down my white-cell count soon could result in damage to my brain or other organs.

Carol flew with me in Papa Whiskey across the south end of the lake to Chicago for a flow-cytometry test to determine the percentages of my white cells in various stages of development. Unfortunately, many of mine—too many—were "blastic," or immature cells. That count could mean that my bone marrow was heavily involved, churning out white cells like crazy to fight an enemy cancer they could not find.

The doctor who took my blood for the flow test offered to be my oncologist. I talked to him at length and made another appointment. Back home I e-mailed him my chapter on anti-angiogenesis and some recent scientific papers on Mabs and other biotherapies. He called me and said, "Neil, *you need chemotherapy,* but you don't want to take it!"

"I apologize for being a difficult patient," I said. "But why not try Rituxan first . . . ?"

He interrupted in a turgid voice. "Rituxan won't work alone for MCL. Take chemo *and* Rituxan together."

When I didn't reply immediately, he added, "*Forget* these scientists you talk to. All those guys ever do is take your money and give nothing in return!"

"Dr. E," I would call him. One more in the alphabet soup of chemotherapists doing their jobs, knowing they are helping cancer victims live, albeit for only a few more years. Did I have to put up with this recurring nightmare once more? As before, I reminded myself that I was the customer and that my private war on cancer was too important to leave to the generals. I had gone to see Dr. E only for a flow test, not for his advice. Later in the day I called his office and canceled my appointment.

• • •

Philadelphia, with the Schuylkill River running through it and its mix of old and new buildings, appeared the same as when I used to come here to work with my magazine's advertising-space salesmen. It had been more than three years since I'd been to the University of Pennsylvania with Shahid. That was when we met David Liebowitz for the first time, and I had made my first contribution to cancer research: the T-cell co-stimulation project that became so enriched by dollar megadoses from the Gates Foundation. David Liebowitz was no longer here; he had moved to Amgen/Immunex, in Seattle. But Carl June, who originated the co-stimulation research at the Naval Medical Research Institute, had joined the university the year before. Carl and I had spoken by phone for years, but I had never met him.

The night we arrived Carol and I met Carl and his fiancée, Lisa, for dinner, and we listened to Carl describe his upcoming combination vaccine and T-cell protocol. The clinical trial wouldn't start for at least six months, and it would take more months after that to make my vaccine. If I could keep my white-cell count down to safe levels until then, I could enter the trial, which would include not only the NCI vaccine developed by Larry Kwak but also June's co-stimulation. Unfortunately, FDA intransigence on requiring chemo was unbending. Even worse, the first part of the trial consisted of a minimal allogenic (donor) stem-cell transplant coupled with a nonlethal— yet high—dose of chemotherapy. Carl said that his university could search the various donor registries around the country for stem-cell blood that would match mine.

Carl June is fifty and slim, with a ready smile and the slightly stooped posture of the very tall. He carries an unusual load of compassion born of life's tragedies. Carl had served nineteen years in the U.S. Navy, rising to the rank of captain, and gave up the opportunity to make admiral, a promotion that would have forced him to leave research for wider administrative duties. Fortunately for cancer research, he declined the chance. Instead he came to the University of Pennsylvania to become its director of translational research. His wife died of ovarian cancer one year before our meeting, despite his heroic attempts to save her. Now he had met Lisa, an attractive Ph.D. in cell biology and the director of experimental medicine at nearby Wyeth-Ayerst Laboratories, in St. David's, Pennsylvania. Our dinner with them took place on a Tuesday, and they were to be married the following Saturday. But Carl June had suffered another calamity: the day before, on Monday, his brother had drowned while swimming.

The day after our dinner, Carl—whose research leaves no time for him to take patients except in trials—turned us over to Dr. Stephen Schuster, his clinical collaborator and the director of lymphoma research at U. Penn.'s cancer center. One of the first things Steve Schuster said to me was, "I have no ego, no preconceptions. I'm open to learning."

After spending a couple of hours with Steve discussing my history and his approach to therapy, I discovered he was a rare, modern bio-oncologist and hematologist, not just a chemotherapist. That is not to say that he doesn't use chemo. He has used it and still does, when necessary, and believes he has extended the lives of many lymphoma victims that way. With Steve, however, chemo would be my *last* resort, not the first, and if we worked it right, we'd never get to that point.

We would try Rituxan alone. If that proved insufficient to lower my white-cell count and stabilize my lymph nodes, we could try other biological therapies, such as interferon-alpha or interleukin-2 to stimulate my immune system, in conjunction with larger doses of Rituxan. For the long term, assuming I could achieve remission, the best idea was to get a vaccine made from my own diseased blood: an idiotype vaccine.

I hadn't had an oncologist since John Ultmann in Chicago, who himself had died. I readily accepted Steve as my oncologist. Stephen Schuster, in his late forties, is perfectly weighted, with dark brown hair flecked gray at the sides. His light-blue eyes are penetrating. Steve and his wife, Barbara, have two sons, a teenager and a preteen, and Steve's hobby is fresh-water fishing. He received his M.D. degree at Philadelphia's Jefferson Medical

College. Later he directed research at an NIH-funded laboratory, but he soon became bogged down in regulatory paperwork, mired in bureaucracy, and longed for patient care. Steve joined the University of Pennsylvania four years ago, treating lymphoma and conducting clinical trials. Earlier in the year he'd won a prize for teaching excellence and was included among the "Top Docs of 2002" by *Philadelphia Magazine*. In addition to maintaining a close collaborative relationship with Carl June, Schuster confers frequently with Dan Longo and Larry Kwak at the NIH.

I asked Steve why he thought Celebrex had stopped inhibiting the microvessels to my tumor cells after having worked for four years, mentioning what I had read about drug activity diminishing over time.

"It's not only that the drug loses its activity," he said. "Our cells have a built-in redundancy that resists single-pathway inhibitors. Alternate pathways emerge. In other words, resistance. Think about it. If our ancestors hadn't evolved redundant mechanisms to overcome fragile pathways, we'd be killed by the first cosmic ray to come along and wouldn't have evolved in the first place."

• • •

Under Steve's direction, I underwent apheresis the same day. An old and still widely used technology, it is somewhat like having a blood transfusion—from yourself. Blood is pumped out of your right arm and reinfused back into your left arm. In between, it passes through a continuous-flow separator consisting primarily of a centrifuge that separates a few billion white cells from the blood. These "dirty" cells then are banked for future use in making a vaccine. Of course, removing a few billion white cells is also therapeutic when your count is so high. As I sat on my hospital bed with tubes in both arms, it seemed strange, after four years of mantle-cell lymphoma, to be receiving treatment.

As my primary oncologist, Steve Schuster consulted with both Carl June and Dan Longo. But the rules of the game were such that I would have to hire a local oncologist to carry out Steve's instructions closer to home. Carol and I flew home that night, an odd sensation for me to be on a commercial jet instead of Papa Whiskey. The next day I chose the oncologist at the cancer clinic in Michigan City where I'd had a bone-marrow core taken the week before. The oncologist there was expert at taking these cores, unlike many others who had applied their corkscrews to my pelvis, and I barely knew it was happening. The involvement in my marrow turned out to be not much worse than four years earlier, less than 10 percent, despite the high white-cell count.

At Steve Schuster's suggestion, Rade Pejic got me into St. Anthony's Hospital for two nights to monitor kidney, liver, and heart functions while the first doses of Rituxan dripped into my veins. Patients with high levels of circulating lymphoma cells have been known not to tolerate the quantities of Rituxan that others can take with ease. So Steve ordered separating the first full dose—700 mg for my six-foot, two-hundred-pound body—into three, infusing the Mab slowly over three days: just 50 mg the first day, 150 the second, and 500 the third. Premedications included an antihistamine, Tylenol, and a "glucocorticoid," a naturally occurring hormone that protects against stress. The one used for me was dexamethasone (tradenamed Decadron), a synthetic steroid generally used in the treatment of allergic reactions. It has been shown to work synergistically with Rituxan.

The principle guiding Steve Schuster is partnership, working together with his patients. He uses the word *we* a lot. If I could tolerate Rituxan and if we could bring down the white-cell count, I would continue receiving a full dose weekly as an outpatient at the cancer clinic in Michigan City. If it failed to bring down the white count, yet I could tolerate it, we would step up the Rituxan infusions to three times weekly, as Dan Longo had recommended.

"Despite Rituxan's common use now," Dan told me by phone, "we have little understanding of the best way to give it. Once a week doesn't usually work well in mantle-cell lymphoma—or in chronic lymphocytic leukemia—and it may have greater activity when given faster."

Dan's comments came as a revelation to me. After four years of studying everything from alpha emitters to Zevalin, I realized I had bypassed a comprehensive understanding of how Rituxan works. At the time of my

MCL diagnosis, the same year as its FDA sanction, Rituxan was widely believed to be of little or no benefit for so aggressive a cancer as mantle-cell lymphoma, and at the time, David, Carol, and I had written it off in favor of the more-powerful radioactive monoclonal antibodies. During the ensuing four years, oncologists, scientific papers, results of clinical trials, popular articles, and even brochures from its manufacturer had continued to specify Rituxan as a drug to be used as a *second-line therapy* or in combination with CHOP—not as first treatment, and certainly not for mantle-cell lymphoma. In fact, in mid-2002 I called the author of a paper describing a clinical trial using Rituxan against various lymphomas, who told me he doubted whether that or any other Mab used alone would do much for MCL.

In spite of timid attitudes toward new therapies (while doctors cling tenaciously to their toxins), it should have dawned on me that a manmade antibody specifically attaching to the ubiquitous CD20 cell marker would find its way in treating cancers far beyond those first hesitant steps authorized by the FDA for use against only the easiest-to-repress lymphomas. But at that stage of my renewed learning experience, I wanted to consider all biotherapy possibilities. I wondered whether my second-choice Mab, Remitogen, was available yet.

Dan provided the answer. "Remitogen is now in phase-two testing for lymphoma, including MCL," he said. "If Rituxan doesn't work, you could try that. I am unenthusiastic about radioactive Mabs for the same reason you are unenthusiastic about chemotherapy. Radio-immunotherapy burns the marrow in irreversible ways and compromises the capacity to give other therapies later, should they be necessary. Be cautious about thinking that the antibody targeting of the radio-Mabs protects tissues that don't express the antigen. It simply isn't true."

Mike Blend, who has spent a good deal of his life conducting clinical trials on radio-Mabs, is certainly aware of those dangers. He will not administer a radioactive antibody unless you have less than a 20 percent involvement of cancer cells in the bone marrow.

Dan Longo gave me the leads to clinical trials for Remitogen, and I followed up. There was an ongoing trial at the University of Iowa and elsewhere combining Remitogen and Rituxan. It sounded like the best bet if Rituxan wasn't sufficient, provided my blood expressed the proper antigens. Then, if *that* didn't work, I'd try for Genta's antisense therapy called Genasense.

Antisense describes the regulation of genomic information in DNA by pairing of sense and antisense nucleic-acid strands. Antisense knocks out the sense protein that carries the message to create immortal cancer cells inhibiting Bcl-2, or B-cell lymphoma number 2 (see chapter 18). Despite its name, Bcl-2 is expressed in most human malignancies—one more example of why the study of a systemic disease like lymphoma can lead to therapies for other cancers. Fortunately, antisense cleaves the Bcl-2 protein without affecting other proteins in the body, making this biotherapy extremely well-tolerated.

By fall 2002 Genta scientists were conducting phase-two trials around the country for melanoma; multiple myeloma; chronic lymphocytic leukemia; non-small-cell lung cancer; cancers of the prostate, lung, colon, and breast; and mantle-cell lymphoma. Genasense does not work for everyone. For example, it had been of no benefit to John McKenna, who had proved impervious to the NCI vaccine—after chemotherapy. I felt in my case, however, it could do no harm and would constitute a good option if I could not tolerate enough Rituxan to do the job.

There were good reasons, however, why Rituxan alone *would* bring down the white cells and tumors. Rituxan attacks the CD20 surface antigen of MCL cancer cells, and my flow test had shown that the cancer cells in my body were tremendously overexpressing CD20. In fact, 96 percent of these cells were positive for CD20. If I couldn't tolerate sufficient Rituxan, though, and if the HLA-targeted antibody Remitogen and then antisense proved ineffectual . . .

There were lots of ifs. But it meant that I had a whole arsenal of biological therapies to choose from. For instance, natural infection-fighting agents, such as interferons or GM-CSF (granulocyte macrophage-colony stimulating factor). Or a telomerase inhibitor to short-circuit these enzymes on the ends of the chromosomes, inducing apoptosis. If all else failed, there was always methylglyoxal (as being used in India, described in chapter 21). Any or all of these biotherapies could keep me healthy, possibly indefinitely, certainly long enough until I could get a vaccine made. Afterwards there were other anti-angiogenics, including thalidomide, to be added to Celebrex for the long term. With so many choices, I doubted whether I ever would need to consider chemo or, for that matter, a radioactive Mab.

. . .

At St. Anthony's hospital—even though I was being infused with a benign antibody—the nurses posted a large red label over the IV bag containing Rituxan:

CHEMOTHERAPY DRUG
TOXIC
BIOHAZARDOUS MATERIAL

What was that all about? What on earth is toxic about Rituxan? Oh, I get it. Rituxan is a chemical, so the hospital personnel call it *chemotherapy!* They don't understand the difference. Even as hospitals forge ahead into twenty-first-century medicine, if it hangs from a bag and drips into a cancer patient's wrist, it's all the same stuff. Just another chemical. Obviously hospitals should fine-tune their terminology, distinguishing between the toxins of chemotherapy and targeted nontoxic treatments. Call one Toxic Therapy and the other Biotherapy.

And then it occurred to me how the revolution in biotherapy would likely unfold in the real world of doctors and patients. There would be no comparable revolution in cancer therapy, as there has been in cancer science, no insurrection led by patient rage. No sudden epiphanies by chemotherapists, no bells tolling the end of an era. Instead, the festival of biotherapy would enter the culture by gradual evolution. Biotherapy would replace chemotherapy over the years without the kind of dramatic media attention given to, say, the end of slavery or the fall of communism. Rituxan and other Mabs already are replacing toxic chemos little by little, without fanfare, because they are considered by the chemo-honed medical community to be *merely better chemotherapies.*

. . .

Yet when medical historians look back on the fin-de-siècle, biotherapies will be analogized to antibiotics. The first manmade antibody to achieve widespread use, Rituxan (as Steve Schuster predicts), may well go down in history, alongside penicillin, as one of the two major wonder drugs of the twentieth century. Both spurred a flurry of comparable agents: additional antibiotics midcentury and additional monoclonal (and polyclonal) antibodies at the end of the century as therapy for cancer, heart disorders, AIDS, organ transplants, arthritis, and other diseases.

In fact, the biotech company Applied Molecular Evolution was in the process of preclinical animal trials of its "AME-133" anti-CD20 Mab, said to have even greater efficacy than Rituxan. Success building on success. Later the company announced that AME-133 "exhibited a tenfold higher affinity than Rituxan and a tenfold improved killing of human cancer cells" (*in vitro*) and also revealed development of a similar Mab for arthritis.

Meanwhile in 2003, IDEC was proceeding up the chain of clinical trials, testing the combination of Rituxan and an anti-CD80 monoclonal antibody called "114" for use on lymphoma patients who do not respond to Rituxan alone. Originally developed for psoriasis, it was found in phase-one trials to be far more effective against lymphoma because CD80 is expressed on malignant B cells and facilitates the T and B cell interaction. One more target.

Although Rituxan had been in clinical trials for a decade prior to approval in 1998, its action is still only partly understood. Steve Schuster told me more and more about this wonder drug, beginning by describing the steps in making it.

First, mice are immunized with human B lymphocytes. Second, scientists isolate that portion of the mouse B-cell antibodies found to bind exclusively with human B cells. Third, they graft the mouse CD20-antigen-binding portion of the antibody to a human antibody, creating a "chimeric" molecule, that is, one that combines features of two species. The *mouse portion* of the antibody structure binds to CD20, while the human portion interacts with other human cells and proteins that stimulate an immune response against malignant B cells. By so doing, the danger of human anti-mouse antibody (HAMA) formation is greatly reduced. Since the body recognizes the mouse portion as foreign, the HAMA reaction decreases the functionality of the mouse antibody and can induce fairly severe symptoms in the recipient.

The immune stimulation of Rituxan doesn't stop there. The *human portion* of the Rituxan molecule activates a group of about twenty plasma proteins called the "complement" system, which organizes a protein attack on the surface of malignant B cells. This complement of proteins literally punches holes in the cell membrane to get inside and kill the cancer cells. The addition of dexamethasone (Decadron) to Rituxan significantly increases cell sensitivity to complement-system cell killing.

There are additional therapeutic triumphs of Rituxan, some known, some unknown. One known mechanism is the Mab's interaction with natural killer cells. These are large cells whose action is enhanced by interferons, interleukin-2, and other immune-stimulatory molecules. The interaction occurs through the cell-surface receptors for Rituxan (and other Mabs), called "Fc receptors" (for "fragment crystallizable"), which appear on the surface of natural killer cells. Thus, combining Rituxan with interferon helps stop lymphoma in many patients. Efficacy depends on the patient's genotype. We are all unique genetically, as has been noted so often in my search for a cure. The difference in our genes explains why some people have a high affinity for Rituxan and others do not. Tests will be available soon to determine which of us would benefit from this and other Mabs. Subsequent modifications in the molecular structure of Rituxan may improve its affinity for greater numbers of patients.

Among the unknown possibilities for Rituxan are its interactions with other monoclonal antibodies and with other biological therapies. The success of Rituxan and other Mabs is only beginning. Clinical trials are already underway to test Rituxan's efficacy against other B-cell malignancies, such as chronic lymphocytic leukemia and multiple myeloma, as well as nonmalignant conditions such as rheumatoid arthritis and lympho-proliferative disorders associated with solid-organ transplant therapies.

• • •

After the first tiny infusion of Rituxan, my white-cell count dropped from 65,000 to 15,000. After the third infusion—which completed the first standard dose—the count leveled off at a normal 6,500. Rituxan was working—on mantle-cell lymphoma!

As an outpatient at the cancer clinic, I continued weekly with five more 700-mg doses and then followed with maintenance doses monthly. For the first two weeks I also took low-dose Cytoxan—one 50-mg pill daily. That happens to be the anti-angiogenesis dosage Giannoula Klement had told me about, although in such a short time, Cytoxan could not be expected to kill capillaries feeding tumors. (It would take ten times that dosage and delivered over a much longer period to make it a toxic chemo.) The reason for taking Cytoxan at all is because it works synergistically with Rituxan. Steve said, "Why endanger the immune system with longer or larger doses?"

Music to my ears. Ruzic music. I could take additional anti-angiogenics later to supplement the Celebrex, if needed. Meanwhile, I drank a gallon of water a day to flush my kidneys while the macrophages—those big eaters of the immune system—were cleaning up the litter of dead white cells.

As the weeks progressed, it became clear that Rituxan alone was keeping the white cell count down and also shrinking and stabilizing the lymph nodes, as revealed in several CAT scans. Such is the value of keeping your immune system intact by avoiding the toxins of chemotherapy. I signed up for a trial of Remitogen, just in case, but probably would need no other biotherapy to carry me over until the long-term vaccine was ready—in Spain.

• • •

Back in my office, I received more answers by computer and phone. One e-mail came from Maurizio Bendandi, and it could not have been more cordial.

"By definition, any friend of Dan Longo's is a friend of mine!" he wrote from the University of Navarra (or *Navarre,* as it is known in English) in Pamplona, Spain, near the southern border of France. Dr. Bendandi, an Italian M.D. and Ph.D., had come to the United States, where he worked with Larry Kwak making idiotype vaccines for lymphoma. Once again I was grateful for Ron Levy, who not only pioneered lymphoma vaccines at Stanford but then systematically fostered a protégé network. Kwak had been one of Levy's protégés and in turn became a mentor for others, including Bendandi. This process has begun the exportation to Europe of what in many cases may be considered an actual cure of lymphoma.

After a flurry of e-mails, Carl June agreed that it made no sense for me to wait for his clinical trial. He agreed that getting an idiotype vaccine in Spain was a good idea and would not preclude me from his protocol if I needed and wanted it later. Carl's laboratory called Federal Express to send 500 million of my frozen white cells to Maurizio Bendandi in Pamplona. At the same time I sent him three pounds of my medical records.

My records arrived in Spain first. The high tech of personalizing immunotherapies is one thing; the low tech of sending frozen cells is something else. Packed in dry ice, my diseased white cells, which (I hope) would never be available again, followed a circuitous route from Philadelphia to the FedEx sorting facility at Indianapolis, to another sorting facility in Newark, *back to Philly,* to Newark again, arriving during the night in *Paris,* where the package had to stay to await customs inspection in the morning. Tracking the shipment by computer, I called the sender at the U. Penn. laboratory, who at my request called Paris and asked a customs agent there to put the box in a freezer overnight. After inspection the next day, my cells traveled to Madrid for still-another customs inspection by the Spanish, and—finally—to Pamplona. Five days.

Once he received the frozen cells, Maurizio called and said he had begun the process of making the vaccine, which would take four or five months. Until then, Rituxan was keeping my white-cell count down and stabilizing the lymph nodes. Lymphoma patients probably can't continue to take Rituxan for the rest of their lives, because of the depletion of normal B cells that could occur. On the other hand, some members of the MCL Group have been on monthly maintenance of Rituxan for five years without harm. Dr. John D. Hainsworth and his group at Nashville's Sarah Cannon Cancer Center have studied sixty patients who took Rituxan as the first-line agent and then continued maintenance doses without harm for the three years of the study.

Instead of entering a clinical trial, which is the only way to get a lymphoma vaccine in the United States, I would become a private patient in Spain. I had always wanted to go there, to see the countryside and the pueblos and talk to the people as Shahid and I did on our trip throughout South America. (My Latin American friends tell me that in Spain they even speak a dialect of Spanish!) Yet the concept of being *required* to go to a less technologically advanced nation to get a vaccine developed in the United States —for no reason other than to avoid the prerequisite chemotherapy—smelled of the Inquisition in reverse. To get a vaccine in the United States, you first are questioned—and then your blood is tested—to make sure you have not had Rituxan or other Mab. If you pass, you are tortured with devastating chemotherapy.

Because idiotype vaccines are made from a patient's own cells, the Spanish equivalent of the FDA wisely does not regard them as drugs and thus sees nothing to regulate. The idea that in this respect the Inquisition had moved from fifteenth-century Spain to twenty-first century America made me mad as hell.

• • •

In most of the cancer clinics and hospitals I have visited during my four-year tour of laboratory research, chemotherapy patients recline on beds or stretch their legs on the footrests of easy chairs. Then they spend a few restless hours with heavy toxins dripping into their veins, miserable in the knowledge that when they get home, the vomiting will begin. When one patient leaves, another takes his or her place. The men are bald and the women wear wigs, looking like prey. Attempts at sunny humor trickle like chemo from smiling young nurses with avian laughs. Bad smells: tobacco breath, hairspray, perfume, hormones, sweat.

The cancer clinic in Michigan City where I went for my Rituxan infusions is a one-story brick building with ten rooms in which cancer patients recline on comfortable upholstered chairs with attached footrests. The similarity to the others I had seen ends there. This clinic is a clean, well-lighted place. The nurses and oncologists know about Rituxan, Herceptin, and other Mabs, although they rarely use them as first treatment.

A sign on the wall invites patients to ask their doctors about clinical trials that might be appropriate. There is no notice on the Rituxan IV bags spelling out "chemotherapy" or "toxic" or "biohazardous material," because Rituxan is none of those things. This clinic is not an assembly line. It is a CHOP shop in transition.

· · ·

If I had my way, I would scrap every big-brother FDA prohibition against scientific cancer therapies. Anyone suffering from cancer or any other incurable disease would be allowed to try to save his life by any means possible. If you can use "touch therapy" and other quack remedies in the United States with impunity, why can't you take modern scientific therapies? Whose lives are these, anyway? Who *are* these FDA bureaucrats to demand that we handicap our immune systems first with poisons before receiving an immune-*enhancing* vaccine?

I also would stop hobbling development of any new therapy—by insisting that their trials be fair trials instead of trials preceded by toxins. How can you adequately assess the efficacy of a drug if you give it only to sick people whose immune systems have been compromised? Instead of requiring the poisoning of a sick patient first, let's turn it around. The onus should be on proving efficacy *of the chemo toxins,* not of the biotherapies. If a vaccine, a Mab, an antisense agent, a kinase inhibitor, or an anti-angiogenic does not work, if all benign biotherapies have failed a patient, only then conduct clinical trials—but on the toxic therapies, not on the biotherapies! Make chemo advocates prove that their poisons do no serious ancillary harm and are more effective than biological agents over the long term, say five or ten years. At the same time, establish a rule of the "minimum effective dose" instead of the maximum tolerated dose.

I wonder how long it will take to bring about such fundamental changes in cancer treatment. Certainly the impetus is there: new genomic approaches to research; new bio-drugs; millions of cancer sufferers stirring, beginning to awaken and take responsibility for their own lives. Yet change is exceedingly slow, exceedingly frustrating, exceedingly deadly.

Remember the storyline of Joseph Heller's *Catch-22*? The only sane character in the book was the protagonist, who was trying to avoid almost-certain death while surrounded by pilots gung-ho to cross the sea and fly into intensive enemy flak. I feel like I have been shot down in that story, living now on the bottom of the ocean where far above I see the Chemo Culture riding the waves, oblivious to any dissent, hearing only my bubbles.

28

Cure!

IN DECEMBER 2002 CAROL AND I RETURNED TO PHILADELPHIA, BOTH
to attend the American Society of Hematology (ASH), conference and to have
my stem cells harvested at the University of Pennsylvania, a precaution suggested by Steve Schuster in the unlikely event that I might need a modern-
day transplant at some time during the rest of my life. (In such a case I would
use a radioactive monoclonal antibody instead of chemotherapy before stem-
cell reinfusion.)

The U. Penn. hospital was familiar to me by now, and as an outpatient I
entered the same apheresis ward as before, where the technicians performed
a procedure similar to the one before. That is, they drew blood from one arm,
passed it through a machine, and reinfused it into my other arm. But this
time, instead of taking out diseased white cells, the procedure harvested
normal white blood cells enriched in stem cells. These had been mobilized
from my bone marrow into circulating blood by a series of injections of G-
CSF (granulocyte-colony stimulating factor), or Neupogen, that I took in
Michigan City for a few days before coming to Philly. Collecting the required
two million stem cells normally takes three or four daily three-hour sessions.
In my case it took only three hours on a single day to harvest almost four
million stem cells.

"Why was my stem-cell harvest so fast?" I asked Steve, who was somewhat amazed.

"For two good reasons," he explained. "One is that you've had a splenectomy. Since stem cells hang out primarily in the bone marrow, spleen, and to a lesser extent, the blood, yours are concentrated in areas other than the spleen. More important, you have never had chemo, which definitely depletes the number—and impairs the quality—of stem cells. I don't think we've ever collected stem cells from a lymphoma patient who's never had chemotherapy. You are something of a first, Neil. Another reason—as if we need one—to hold off on chemo in favor of biotherapies."

Later Steve led Carol and me to a microscopy room in the pathology department where we were joined by two scientists to look at slides of my recent bone-marrow core that I'd had extracted and brought with me from Michigan City. It reminded me of the summer of 2000 in St. Louis when Jon Braun and the Celebrex pharmacologists noted the effects of anti-angiogenesis in slides of my blood. Now, as then, we peered into a series of microscopes linked to a series of light pipes so that we could view the slides at the same time. The five of us searched slide after slide but could find no cancer cells, just as in St. Louis two years before we had detected none in my lymph-node tissue. Would MCL return to plague me in the future? No one knows for certain. But it looked promising because the reason for the absence of cancer cells this time was vastly different. Back in 2000 my mutated genes had been pumping out lymphoma cells that were subsequently starved to death by anti-angiogenesis. It was remission then—not quite the same as absence of cancer—because my mutated 11 and 14 chromosomes had remained intact. (The 11-14 translocation, in which chromosome 11 actually switches places with chromsome 14, is a scientific definition of mantle-cell lymphoma.)

This time Rituxan antibodies had attacked the lymphoma cells directly. And it had wiped them out. In order to determine whether any cancer cells remained in my system, the scientists would have to do more-sophisticated blood tests. They would have to confirm the absence of the 11-14 translocation, as well as the absence of the partial translocations of several other chromosomes that had occurred when my white-blood-cell count was highly elevated.

Microscopic examination of bone marrow is the crudest method of look-ing for residual lymphoma, since it detects cancer cells present at a level of about one in fifty cells. Flow cytometry—the analysis of a cell suspension using a machine for counting cells stained to show tumor antigens—can detect about one cancer cell in ten thousand. Polymerase chain reaction can detect one cancer cell in a hundred thousand or sometimes one in a mil-lion. Unfortunately, the PCR primers used for detecting the 11-14 translo-cation are not the right primers for the breakpoints on my particular chro-mosomes (in fact, they are informative for fewer than half of MCL patients).

The scientists used flow cytometry and then "fished" for cancer cells in my collection of stem cells. FISH is "fluorescence in-situ hybridization," in which a DNA probe is labeled with fluorescent molecules so they can be seen in a microscope. The "fishing" is done "in situ," or "in place"—in other words, within the nucleus of the cells fixed to a slide. FISH tests, while not normally as sensitive (depending upon the number of cells examined) as flow cytometry in detecting cancer cells, possess a unique advantage. They can accurately detect whether any of the chromosomes have translocated. That's a vitally important determination in lymphoma because if some chro-mosomes still occupied the wrong places, their genes would renew the manu-facture of cancer cells.

Fortunately, the flow test detected not even one cancer cell in ten thou-sand of my blood cells. The FISH test—using my recently harvested stem cells—demonstrated that the 11-14 translocation defining mantle-cell lym-phoma and the other partial chromosomal translocations were *completely absent!*

"That's really great news," Steve Schuster said, "considering the vast numbers of these cells circulating in your blood before Rituxan."

Carol broke out into a broad smile. It truly would be a merry Christmas.

• • •

The next day the ASH conference was like old-home week, seeing hematolo-gists I had gotten to know: Phil Koeffler, Wolf Hofmann, who had come to the meeting from Germany; Sven de Vos; Mark Kaminski; Larry Kwak; and many others. We were invited to a Persian luncheon at the home of Abass Alavi and his wife, Jane. Abass, an M.D. at the University of Pennsylvania, was one of the inventors of advanced PET-scan instrumentation. These new PET scanners are so sensitive you can use one to determine the native language of a subject! The machine can do that by detecting differences in tongue-muscle activity when a person is speaking.

Steve, Carl June, Carol, and I tried to find Maurizio Bendandi, having arranged to meet him at a gathering of U. Penn. contributors where Steve and Carl would deliver lectures. We looked for a man in his late thirties who stood six foot three, weighed two hundred pounds, wore glasses, and doubtless showed signs of jet lag after his flight from Europe. He found us first and greeted Carol and me with hugs.

At dinner that night Maurizio said my hybridomas (cancer cells fused with a mouse cell line) were doing well after a first failed attempt, but he would like to have more of my cancerous white cells in case the hybridomas died during the lengthy process. Unlike Rituxan, which uses both murine and human cells for different functions, my idiotype vaccine, while hybridized with mouse cells, uses only the human portion of the hybridized cells. Since the vaccine consists entirely of my own human cells, there is no danger of a human antimouse antibody reaction (see chapter 27).

We thought of sending a container of my frozen diseased cells back with Maurizio when he returned to Spain a few days later. However, the Federal Aviation Administration is as regulation-bound as the FDA and has strict rules against carrying dry ice anywhere aboard a commercial airplane because it melts into carbon dioxide (let alone the problem of federal agents who might decide blood cells are a biohazard). Using liquid nitrogen, which is even colder than dry ice, would present containment problems. Once again we faced the predicament of shipping my blood. This time, however, Carl June found a company that specialized in transporting human organs for transplant.

• • •

In May 2003 Carol and I took a vacation in Pamplona, Spain.

After a commercial flight that stopped first in Madrid, the morning began as we descended into the sunny and vibrant capital of the province of Navarra, in the northeast corner of Spain. Pamplona, named for the Roman general Pompey in 75 B.C., lies at about the same latitude as Chicago, but the temperature was cool, not cold, more like northern Florida in the spring. A combination of old and new buildings, Pamplona blends the wet climate of the Atlantic a hundred miles to the north with the dryness of the Pyrenees Mountains, into which it is nestled on a low fifteen-hundred-foot mesa. Pamplona, a city of two hundred thousand, is tucked under France, a hundred miles south of the Bay of Biscay in the Atlantic and a little southeast of Basque country. It is where the "running of the bulls" festival takes place the second week of every July. In this festival, popularized by Hemingway, young men and bulls run freely together through narrow streets as marching bands play on every corner and parade up every street. It seemed a fine place for a vacation.

And a fine place to prevent the recurrence of cancer.

Carol and I greeted Maurizio Bendandi in his office at the university hospital. When we first met him at the ASH conference, he looked to me more American than European, and now I found he had played basketball in high school in his native Italy, like any tall youth might do in the United States. He had received both his doctor's degrees in Italy and worked there for eight years before coming to America to enter the world of research at the National Cancer Institute.

"I did not speak a word of English and had never seen a lab bench when I came to work with Larry Kwak and the NCI in 1995," he said. "Likewise, I had no Spanish when I returned to Europe to this wonderful University of Navarra," he added with an expansive gesture toward spacious green lawns and modern buildings that we could see through the window.

"We're thankful you did what you did," Carol said with a smile.

"We know why you came to Navarra," I said, "but what was your motivation to emigrate to the U.S. in the first place? Was it to work with Dr. Kwak?"

"No. I really left Italy to get away from the academic mafia that's almost as strong as the Cosa Nostra in Sicily. My boss did not help me advance as bosses in the States do routinely. So I came to the States, where you are blessed with the protégé system in medical research."

His marriage ended, Maurizio Bendandi is raising his ten-year-old daughter, Lavinia, himself. He is a devout Catholic who belongs to *Opus Dei* (God's Work), begun by Josemaria Escrivá during the Spanish Civil War and unique among Catholic organizations because it consists of 98 percent lay people and only 2 percent priests. Saint Josemaria was canonized in 2002, a process that normally takes hundreds of years.

"I work harder," Maurizio told us humbly, "because I believe my role in the world is a way to do God's Work wherever I am—no matter what my personal and inevitable shortcomings may be. My own particular job in life is to help everyone I meet achieve health. You, Neil and Carol, may be doing the same by running your research foundation or creating the businesses you have created, provided you do those things for others, not just for yourself—doing God's Work. Others can carry out his work by teaching in universities or serving in government or performing their jobs so as to help their fellow man."

He added in his forthright, unembarrassed manner, "It is the way we try to get into heaven."

I could not have imagined a better attitude for the man who had been customizing my immunotherapy these past five months and soon would inject the vaccine into me.

Maurizio showed us around the enormous campus, explaining as we went that the University of Navarra ranks first among the universities in Spain even though it is only fifty years old. Modern buildings surrounded an old chapel on the ultragreen campus. At the end of a glassed-in above-ground tunnel, we came to an enormous library where some of the twelve thousand students sat on the steps, sprawled on the grass, or hurried from one building to the next. Aside from the rolling *R* sounds of Spanish and the occasional tongue clicks of Basque, it was like being on any American campus, except that you saw no bluejeans or T-shirts bearing slogans. Young men wore sport coats or suits. Women wore skirts or elegant trousers.

The *Clínica Universitaria* is a tall, modern 450-bed hospital devoted primarily to cardiovascular treatment, transplant surgery, and oncology with state-of-the-art automated instrumentation and information systems. "For about forty-five years," Maurizio said, "the emphasis here was entirely on patient care. Only in the last five years has the policy changed, without renouncing what had been achieved earlier. By next year we'll have almost four hundred scientists—people like me from around the world to emphasize applied medical investigation. And of course, that means in my case personalized immunotherapy, or as you say, vaccine technology."

The idiotype vaccine that Maurizio had been preparing since October was ready for me, and I entered the hospital as an outpatient. The vaccine was made exactly the same way as are those by Larry Kwak at the NCI. It consisted of a clone made from those diseased white cells I'd had harvested at the University of Pennsylvania in September—a clone of my own tumor-specific immunoglobulin, which serves as the most specific antigen known. As in Kwak's method, the vaccine contained the immune-system carrier KLH—the hemocyanin protein extracted from the blood of limpet sea snails (see chapter 25). The body recognizes the limpet hemocyanin as foreign and therefore fights back with an immune response. The adjuvant, or aid, portion of the vaccine to stimulate neutrophils and other components of the immune system is GM-CSF (granulocyte macrophage-colony stimulating factor)—again, the same as used in Kwak's NCI vaccines.

Problems of transporting the frozen vaccine from Spain to the United States and the subsequent legal problems of reconstituting a foreign-made vaccine in the United States, while not insurmountable, are thorny. My answer was to turn the Spanish experience into five short vacations. On one of the trips, Steve Schuster and other friends joined us. We took the Al Andalus Express train through Andalusia, a unique region of southern Spain, the birthplace of flamenco dancers, rich with immense olive groves and villages consisting almost entirely of white buildings. On other trips we explored the Pamplona region north into southern France.

On our first visit to Pamplona, Maurizio vaccinated me with the idiotype vaccine in my upper left arm (where as a child I had received a smallpox vaccination). Once daily for the next three days, he injected at the same site the

GM-CSF adjuvant (tradenamed Leucomax). This genetically engineered immune stimulator commonly is used to restore white blood cells in patients who have had chemotherapy. Using it without first hamstringing your immune system—to enhance the personalized immunotherapy that is the vaccine—made a lot more sense to me.

A month later I returned to Spain for the same procedure and would continue to do so for a total of five times over a period of six months (skipping the fifth month). Choosing the same inoculation site on the arm allows direct contact with the idiotype vaccine, making it easier for the GM-CSF to stimulate antigen-presenting cells, which are abundant just under the skin. After six months of immunization Steve and Maurizio would collaborate in conducting a series of immune-function tests to determine whether I indeed had mounted an immune response.

Was it worth the trips to Spain?

Absolutely. It would have been worth it only for the vacations (when the population of Pamplona does *not* triple with the running bulls). It was worth it medically, too. My custom-made vaccine would function either as a specific immune enhancer or as a preventative, since as far as we knew, cancer cells no longer lingered in my blood or bone marrow. There were no good alternatives to traveling to Spain. Considering the problems we'd faced before in shipping the diseased white cells, it would have been next to impossible to transport the vaccine to the United States in good shape. Also, in view of FDA regulations, it would have been out of the question to arrange for an idiotype-vaccine expert here to monitor my reactions after the inoculations, in case I were to suffer some unforeseen reaction. That possibility is rare, yet anything can happen given the complexities of human cells.

After each inoculation Maurizio measured the quantity of antibodies in my bloodstream—and detected the desired anti-idiotype antibody response. The ultimate answer would involve counting the number of activated T cells, testing the specificity of my T cells against the tumor antigen, and using flow cytometry and BCL-1 staining to test for B-cell lymphoma proteins. Whether my cancer would remain cured would not be known for years—indeed, it might never known, since the generic vaccine that is Rituxan already had wiped out all detectable cancer cells in my body. I was reminded of the adage learned long before by Jonathan Said at UCLA: *Just because you don't find something doesn't mean it isn't there; it only means you haven't found it.*

Mantle-cell lymphoma is an extraordinarily relentless, fractious, truculent malignancy. If it were a human tyrant, it would rule the world. Most MCL patients who take Rituxan alone have relapsed. The only way I could prove the efficacy of my idiotype vaccine would be to continue cancer-free for the rest of my life. (Three or four years from now Steve, Maurizio, and I will write a scientific paper establishing proof of cure.)

The cost of the idiotype vaccine in Spain was markedly less than the average $50,000 in the United States, where cancer vaccines have not yet been FDA-approved and the expense reflects costs of clinical trials. At the University of Navarra my personalized idiotype vaccine cost me only $8,000, not much more than a single infusion of Rituxan in the United States (although Rituxan is FDA approved and its cost is therefore paid by Medicare). Even adding $12,000 or more for travel, it was still a bargain.

The beauty of this cancer vaccine is that in the unlikely event it ceases to bestow immunity and prevent a recurrence of my mantle-cell lymphoma, there is nothing to preclude my doing it all over again, since I have plenty of diseased white blood cells stored both at U. Penn. and UCLA. I even could try a different vaccine. For instance, I could enroll in the Carl June and Larry Kwak clinical trial when it starts (provided FDA regulations will allow me to skip the transplant-chemo portion of the trial). Or I could take the idiotype vaccine being tested by Large Scale Biology Corporation, the one made in tobacco plants instead of mice, now undergoing phase-three trials (see chapter 8).

Lymphoma victims like me, especially those who have not weakened their immune systems with chemo- or radiation therapies, can try vaccines and other biological therapies again and again. As with any vaccine, including those for diseases such as smallpox or polio, it is our cells' ability to remember that allows the vaccine to work. That memory can be prodded from time to time, if required by lymphoma patients (and victims of other cancers for which vaccines are being developed), simply by giving the patient booster shots of the initial vaccine or injections of a new preparation made from cancerous tissue or diseased white cells saved for this purpose.

In my case my sentence to hell was over. No chemo required.

. . .

What if in 1998, however, I had agreed to take chemo as first therapy, ignoring my screaming intuition that it was insane to poison the immune system? What if, instead, I had blindly followed the advice of Drs. A, B, C, and the rest of them by taking aggressive chemotherapy?

"The vast majority of relapses [of patients treated by chemotherapy for aggressive forms of lymphoma]," according a paper distributed by Genitope at the ASH conference in December 2002, "occur in the first two years following initial therapy, and for patients who experience such relapses, median survival is dismal, measured in just months." Had I taken the advice instantly meted out to me at the first four major cancer centers I visited, I would not be alive to write these words.

The cancer war is in collision with the future. Personalized vaccines and other biotherapies as first treatment—and probably the only treatment for cancer patients—soon will begin to enter mainstream practice. Some years from now the administration of these targeted agents may be regarded as one of the government's fundamental functions, such as defense of the nation. The fact that human and animal genomes have been mapped, the fact that animal cloning has been successful, that scientists finally can look at the interactions of thousands of genes at the same time, that almost half of some thirty-odd thousand human genes now have their functions understood . . . these facts have launched us into a new paradigm.

Knowledge (when you stop to think about it) has been the only *reliable* source of power among mankind throughout history. Not money, not armies, not bombs. The importance of knowledge in shifting power from one country or one person to another is becoming increasingly evident today. When I was a teenager on the streets of Chicago, I heard it said often, mindlessly repeated to this day, that it is not what you know that counts in life but who you know. If that maxim ever held merit, it doubtless vanished in the information age. Kings, presidents' widows, and celebrities, who might have spent their wealth on scientific teams to investigate and evaluate potential cures for themselves, die in their ignorance equally with the uninformed, without trying, without learning.

The war against cancer continues, but the smell of victory is in the air. For me, the prayer that once leapt out of the murky chaos of my nightmares has been fulfilled. I now am studying the fascinating fields of cancer research, watching the race to a cure up close, without having to do it for myself.

Now there will be time, that most precious of life's commodities, for enjoying the accomplishments of others. John McKenna lived through his transplant and has an excellent chance of being cured. David Cardin is doing well. Carl June and Lisa have gotten married. In the noncancer world, which I began to inhabit more and more, my son David was promoted to associate vice president of the University of Illinois. Brandon excelled in high-school sports while getting straight A's. Ryan scored in the Illinois ninety-ninth percentile in a nationwide scholastic aptitude test for college entrance and has begun at the University of Illinois; he will major in molecular biology. David, Ryan, and Brandon flew with me in Papa Whiskey to Cozumel, where we went diving, drifting with the current at eighty feet in a proliferation of undersea wildlife.

Jon Braun and I are making plans, postponed by my elevated cell-count detour, to go parachuting. We're scheduling it for May 2004, perhaps on the birthdate we share. Meanwhile, Shahid and I are planning to fly Papa Whiskey to Nova Scotia. On the way we'll stop in New York to meet the board members of some of the lymphoma organizations and then fly to Boston to see the Folkman researchers at Harvard.

Now there is time again for everything I have wanted to do. Energy enough and time. For family, for friends, for catalyzing research through the Ruzic Research Foundation with the goal of helping find cures for other cancer victims. God's Work, as Maurizio would put it. Graduating from the rigors of being a patient did more than renew my lease on time. Having been conscripted by force into the war on cancer, I was transformed into a student of the science behind that war, only to discover that learning about this new and vital field is intriguing. Once again, as in my youthful reporting in Costa Rica, I have been infused with life's passion. *Pura vida!* Pure life.

As Aristotle said, learning is not *part* of life. It *is* life!

Acknowledgments

THE SCIENTISTS WHOSE WORK IS REPORTED IN THIS BOOK ARE AC-
knowledged within. One of these scientists, however, Wolf-Karsten
Hofmann, M.D. and Ph.D., did more than test my blood and work on Project
Indolence. First at UCLA and later at the University Hospital in Frankfurt,
Germany, Wolf spent eighteen months on almost a daily basis as my science
editor, correcting shades of meaning and mistakes. If any mistakes remain,
they are mine alone.

Valuable advice also came from Ed Claflin, who began editing the manu-
script at Prentice-Hall, which had contracted to publish this book but then
terminated the division during the editing process. Ed was so intrigued by
the story that he continued offering constructive criticism even after leaving the company. He is now a freelance editor and writer in Nyack, New York.

Thanks are due to Terry Sinclair, chief editor, and Don Lewis, art director, both of my former magazines. Terry offered editorial suggestions, and
Don painted the cover for the book—both of them donating their time
without charge.

The book was indexed by Kathy Garcia, a professional indexer who also
offered her services free. Her much-appreciated work was her way of contributing to the fight against cancer; her husband suffers from chronic lymphocytic leukemia.

Considerable thanks are due to the staff members of the University of

Illinois Press, who gave unstintingly of their time to the editing and production of the book. I also want to thank my wife, Carol, who not only helped my search for a cure every step of the way but also read and offered improvements of every chapter as I wrote them. And my friend and sometimes co-pilot, Shahid Siddiqi, who helped immeasurably by questioning and updating the government's statistical data on cancer.

Notes

NON-HODGKIN'S LYMPHOMA, or NHL, as a designation of lymphoid malignancies is giving way to the single word *lymphoma,* since Hodgkin's is called *Hodgkin's disease,* leaving all the others grouped under non-Hodgkin's. At least thirty types of B-cell lymphomas include follicular, large-cell, small-cell, Burkitt's, mucosa-associated lymphoid tissue (MALT), splenic, marginal-zone, chronic lymphocytic, and mantle-cell. And there are T-cell lymphomas, such as cutaneous T-cell lymphoma. All lymphomas have many subsets. Some, such as chronic lymphocytic leukemia, are variously referred to as either lymphomas or leukemias, both being closely related "liquid" or blood cancers. Terminology is revised constantly owing to an evolving understanding of tumor physiology, immunotyping, and genetic analyses.

MISDIAGNOSES (discovered in autopsy and averaging 40% for all diseases, not only cancer) are of such enormity that, in a third of cases, physicians should have changed treatment, according to Atul Gawande, M.D., *Complications: A Surgeon's Notes on an Imperfect Science* (Metropolitan, 2002).

DRS. A, B, C, ETC.: It serves no good purpose to identify these chemotherapists, who are no different from thousands of others treating cancers with chemotherapy either indiscriminately or as first therapy while ignoring molecular-targeted and other nontoxic therapies.

QUOTED CONVERSATIONS with doctors, scientists, and others who appear in this book have been recorded or verified by the person involved or by an authorized colleague.

CANCER BOOKS especially useful in explaining the causes, treatments, and research involved in lymphoma and other cancers include Stephen S. Hall, *A Commotion in the Blood* (Henry Holt, 1997), which although somewhat dated is still worth reading for its detailed but easily understood information on a hundred years of research into all blood cancers; Mel Greaves, *Cancer: The Evolutionary Legacy* (Oxford, 2000); Robert Finn, *Cancer Clinical Trials* (O'Reilly, 1999); and James D. Watson, *A Passion for DNA* (Cold Spring Harbor Laboratory, 2000).

CANCER WEB SITES and newsgroups (in addition to those listed under specific subjects) include Cancer Lit Abstracts; to subscribe send an empty message to NHLlow-subsc@yahoogroups.com and then follow the reply instructions in an e-mail sent to you automatically. For in-depth information on anti-angiogenesis, access <www.groups.yahoo.com/group/angiogenesis>. For conferences and clinical trials, log onto <www.cancerconsultants.com>, and go to <www.phrma.org> for news of biotechnology therapies and Medicare prescription-drug coverage.

CHAPTER 2: WATCH AND LEARN

THE LARGEST CANCER CENTER in the United States outside of the NCI, defined by number of scientists and staff, is M. D. Anderson. However, Memorial Sloan-Kettering Cancer Center, founded in 1884 on Manhattan's upper East Side, has a larger (437-bed) hospital.

M.D. AND PH.D.: I refer to these degrees as a fast, vernacular way to portray the educational backgrounds of those who perform medical research. Those with M.D. degrees often choose to do science, although some of them also see a limited number of patients. Those with Ph.D. degrees, usually in immunology, molecular biology, physiology, or biochemistry, do not take patients but work with their M.D. colleagues at the forefront of medical research.

"HIS EXPERIMENTS": I value scientists of both sexes equally, even though I generally use male pronouns. The alternatives quickly grow tedious if not silly (as in "her or his") in our pronoun-deficient English language.

INDOLENT LYMPHOMA TREATMENT: Among countless other sources, P. H. Solal-Celigny's article "Increasing Treatment Options in Indolent Non-Hodgkin's Lymphoma," *Seminars in Oncology* vol. 29, no. 2, suppl. 6 (2002), says, "There is currently no first-line treatment for indolent non-Hodgkin's lymphoma because there is no curative treatment. . . . chemotherapy does not improve survival. . . . side effects of chemotherapy may outweigh the benefits." The paper suggests that Rituxan may become a first-line treatment following more randomized clinical trials. See also D. Voliotis and V. Diehl, "Challenges in Treating Hematologic Malignancies," *Seminars in Oncology* vol. 29, no. 3, suppl. 8 (2002).

CHAPTER 3: THE CHEMO CULTURE

CHEMOTHERAPY AND CHEMO are used interchangeably throughout this book to mean toxins employed to kill fast-dividing cells in an attempt to kill cancer cells as well. They do not refer to the same chemical toxins, such as cyclophosphamide or vincristine, given "metronomically"—that is, slowly and frequently to inhibit angiogenesis (the formation of tiny capillaries feeding the cancer cells). Nor does *chemotherapy* refer to biochemical therapies that are molecularly targeted or directed specifically to cell-surface markers or antigens. The latter are referred to as biological therapies or biotherapies.

HOW COMPLETE IS YOUR REMISSION if you are dead? The scientific paper referred to is Issa Khouri et al., "Hyper-CVAD and High-Dose Methotrexate/Cytarabine Followed by Stem-Cell Transplantation," *Journal of Clinical Oncology* vol. 16, no. 12 (Dec. 1998). Anderson continues to favor aggressive chemotherapy for MCL and other cancers, as witnessed by hundreds of papers written there since the one cited and tens of thousands of patients so treated, although molecular-targeted research conducted in hundreds of its own laboratories may be expected to change the Chemo Culture over time.

CANCER STATISTICS in the United States come mostly from SEER (the National Cancer Institute's "Surveillance, Epidemiology and End Results" program). The American Cancer Society's annual "Cancer Facts and Figures" defines *lifetime risk* as the "probability that an individual over the course of a lifetime will develop cancer or die from it." The ACS, a private cancer foundation based in Atlanta (<www.cancer.org>; 800-ACS-2345), uses SEER data to come up with the often-repeated statement that "in the U.S., men have a 1 in 2 lifetime risk of developing cancer, and for women the risk is 1 in 3." Since there are about half men and half women in the United States, the average is 41.6%, or 1 in 2.4. However, the ACS also states that only 1 of every 4 deaths in the United States is due to cancer, a severe discrepancy because it is unlikely that the tremendous number of claimed deaths are caused by accidents or by disease in which cancer plays no debilitating role. There are 285 million people in the United States, and 41.6% would amount to some *118 million with cancer*. The five-year survival rate for all cancers combined, after adjusting for normal life expectancy, is 62%, according to the ACS. Colleagues and I have come up with 12.7 million as a more-realistic number of cancer patients alive today in the United States (see the "12.7 million cancer victims" note to chapter 17).

CHEMO-CURE PERCENTAGES range widely, starting with Dr. John Cairns's famous article in *Scientific American* (Nov. 1985), which holds that chemo helps no more than 5% of cancer patients. In his book *Chemotherapie fortgeschrittener Karzinome* (Chemotherapy for advanced cancer) (Hippokrates, 1995), Dr. Ulrich Abel, a biostatistician at the University of Heidelberg, says, "The almost dogmatic belief in the efficacy of chemotherapy is generally based on false conclusions drawn from inaccurate data" (trans. by W.-K. Hofmann). In *The Politics of Cancer Revisited*, Samuel Epstein wrote that "five-year survival rates from 1974 to 1990 improved only minimally, from 49% to 54%"; this improvement reflects reduced smoking and all other causes. Ralph W. Moss, Ph.D., in his book *Questioning Chemotherapy* (Equinox, 2000), says that, amazingly, no one is keeping track of the number of people who receive chemotherapy each year. He extrapolated from 350,000 new cases of cancer treated in hospitals, identified by the National Cancer Data Base, to include private patients and estimates the figure to be around one million people (see the "Chemotherapy data" note to chapter 25).

CHEMO BRAIN information may be accessed via either <www.dogpile.com> or <www.brainland.com>. Loss of mental acuity discovered in a Dartmouth study is described further in a note to chapter 7.

TUMOR SHRINKAGE fails to correlate with survival of cancer victims, according to a statistical analysis pointed out by Samuel Epstein, M.D., in *The Politics of Cancer Revisited* (East Ridge, 1998). Technical reasons for preferring stability to shrinkage are explained in chapter 22.

BLOODLETTING persisted as late as the Civil War and, for some afflictions, well into the twentieth century. It was recommended in *Principles and Practice of Medicine* (1923), four years after the death of its author, Dr. William Osler, often considered the most influential physician in history.

CHAPTER 4: LIFE BEFORE CANCER

JOSÉ ("PEPE") FIGUERES not only rallied his side into the 1948 Costa Rican revolution almost single-handedly but later, during his second presidency in 1971, again proved his determination. Three gunmen who hijacked a Nicaragua-Miami flight and demanded it fly to Cuba landed at the capital city of San José for refueling after having killed one passenger. Figueres arrived at the airport to find two hundred of his country's civil guards standing by helplessly. He offered the hijackers safe conduct to Cuba if they would free the passengers and crew. The hijackers released fifty-four passengers, but they refused to let the crew go. Giving the murderers no time to reorganize, Figueres grabbed a submachine gun from a guardsman, opened fire, killed one of the hijackers, and led his men to subdue the others.

CLINICAL TRIALS for modern new cancer therapies are largely denigrated by uninformed physicians, such that only 3% of adult cancer patients enroll, according to HopeLink Clinical Trial Service, a database of cancer-trial listings (<www.hopelink.com>). In 2002 Hopelink said that 85% of cancer patients are unaware that they can participate. Physicians and families, however, enroll 60% of children with cancer (largely leukemia) in trials—contributing to an overall cure rate of pediatric cancer that, according to HopeLink, increased from 10% in 1970 to 70% in 2002.

THE R&D-100, as the IR-100 became known after the magazine's name was changed to *Research and Development* in 1984, remains the premier awards program for applied researchers, honoring the one hundred most significant developments each year.

MOON AND SPACE: I received U.S. patent number 3,355,050 for the lunar cryostat. My books *The Case for Going to the Moon* (Putnam's, 1965), *Where the Winds Sleep* (a "future history" of the scientific colonization of the moon, written as if in the year 2045) (Doubleday, 1970), and *Spinoff* (NASA, 1976) are available at libraries.

THE NATIONAL SPACE SOCIETY, headquartered at 600 Pennsylvania Ave., SE, Washington, D.C. 20003, may be accessed at <www.nss.org>.

SYMBIOSIS, as practiced in the Island for Science ocean polyculture system, where we grew seaweeds together with shrimp, each species contributing to the growth and health of the other, is common in nature. In fact, most life-forms evolve symbiotically, not individually, as did the bacteria in our intestines that help us digest our food. (The bacteria themselves are symbiotic colonies of originally separate strains of bacteria.) Other examples include legumes utilizing fungi to process the nitrogen they require from the air and pilot fish eating organisms that stick to sharks and whales, thereby cleaning these large bodies.

CHAPTER 5: OUR WAR WITHIN

THE PHYSICISTS Max Delbruck and Francis Crick created the field of molecular biology, according to "Bridging the Culture Gap," *Nature* vol. 419 (Sept. 19, 2002), which describes the U.S. Dept. of Energy's attempts to build a cross-disciplinary team at the Lawrence-Berkeley National Lab in California.

MONOCLONAL ANTIBODIES, first produced in mice, were based on N. R. Klinman's seminal discoveries in 1975, described in E. Haber and R. M. Krause, eds., *Antibodies in Human Diagnosis and Therapy* (Raven, 1977), beginning on p. 271.

BURSAS in chickens led to a huge set of data in mammals that support the existence of two-way communication between the immune and neuroendocrine (brain-blood) systems.

IMMUNITY and immune-inspired algorithms for computers to help unravel the immense complexities of cells are described in the easy-to-read article "Inspired by Immunity," *Nature* vol. 415 (Jan. 2002): 468, also accessible at <www.nature.com>.

THE TERRORISM ANALOGY is useful to focus "wars" against the blight of cancer, which kills 600,000 Americans each year. The analogy has been extended meaningfully by the patient advocate Karl Schwartz of Patients Against Lymphoma (<www.lymphomation.org>), who cites watchful waiting, mutation by unhealthy environments, and abandonment of rules that govern normal functions.

THE SWEDISH STUDY, "Risk for Lymphoma in Patients with Rheumatoid Arthritis," is by Anders Ekbom, of the Karolinska Institutet. Go to <www.ki.se> and enter the project number C8492.

COMBINATION DRUGS: Talking to the scientists will also help you find out whether experimentation is being done with the same drug in higher doses or in combination with others—for instance, the naked anti-CD20 Mab Rituxan in combination with the radioactive Mab Zevalin. Other naked Mabs for lymphoma include the anti-CD22 epratuzumab, which has entered clinical trials by Amgen; and an anti-HLA Mab called apolizumab now in trials by Protein Design Labs. Both include combination trials with Rituxan (see chapter 27).

DRUG INFORMATION today is accessed easily by computer once you know the name of the drug or the manufacturer. Using a search engine, such as Google, reveals such Web sites as Idecpharm.com, Genentech.com, and Corixa.com. Don't hesitate to call the pharmaceutical company and ask to talk to one of the scientists working on a drug and for references to their latest scientific papers. Not only are up-to-date papers invaluable for your own knowledge, but you can show them to your oncologist. New Mabs to attach to different cell-surface markers and many other targeted therapies are emerging so fast that it is hard to believe standard toxic chemotherapy will play any role in treating lymphoma in the next few years.

CHAPTER 6: A HALF-BILLION FOR PROOF

BOILING OIL to cauterize gunshot wounds left soldiers feverish, swollen, and in pain. In 1536 the French army surgeon Ambroise Paré applied a medicament normally used for digestion and found his patients experienced little pain and swelling and slept through the night. Paré's clinical trial changed gunshot treatment, at least in his area of France.

PHASE-THREE TRIALS are exceedingly expensive because they usually are conducted over tens of thousand of volunteers. They are often double-blind, randomized, controlled trials, the most rigorous type of investigation possible, in which a significant percentage of subjects get the drug while the remainder receive a placebo. Unlike phase-one and -two trials, phase-three trials are structured so that neither the subjects nor their doctors know who is taking the active medication—hence the "double-blind" designation.

HALF A BILLION dollars for proving a dramatic new drug's efficacy to the FDA is not unusual. "Unleashing Science," a *Wall Street Journal* editorial from Feb. 2, 2001, says, "Most of that $0.5 billion is spent proving efficacy, that a drug will perform as claimed, using massive, placebo-controlled clinical trials. This crude massiveness, with its indefensibly high cost, is increasingly inappropriate to the scientific and economic realities of modern drug discovery and needs to be rethought." A *Wall Street Journal* article from May 2, 2002, quotes Pfizer's chairman Henry McKinnel as saying that the often-cited statistic that only one in ten drugs in clinical trials goes into production understates the rate of failure. Pfizer claims that only "*one of many thousands*" of chemical compounds that its scientists discover make it to market."

ZEVALIN was approved in Oct. 2001. It and other radio-Mabs in various combinations continue to be the subject of hundreds of trials comparing better safety and higher efficacy measured against the standard of chemotherapy. Clinical trials are accessed easily via <www.nci.nih.gov/clinicaltrials>. Bexxar was not approved by the FDA until 2003, despite benefiting about a thousand people worldwide since its inception twenty years ago. The extended caution was attributed to the radioisotope used in Bexxar, iodine-131, which emits gamma rays in addition to beta rays. Gamma rays are like X rays but with longer range and significantly higher energy.

RADIATION FEAR is so pervasive in the United States that in Oct. 2002 the FDA began allowing food companies to petition it to avoid printing the word *irradiation* on their labels, using instead terms such as *cold pasteurization.*

HIGH-DOSE RITUXAN (rituximab) patients, who are treated with six times the usual dose on the second, third, and fourth weeks after an initial infusion of 375 mg per m^2, suffered no unusual toxic reaction and showed greatly improved remissions, according to Michael Keating and Susan O'Brien, "High-Dose Rituximab Therapy in Chronic Lymphocytic Leukemia," *Seminars in Oncology* vol. 27, no. 6, suppl. 12 (Dec. 2000): 86. (The designation "mg per m^2" means milligrams per square meter of skin area.)

ANTI-ANGIOGENESIS has became a hot topic in cancer research since Harvey Black's article "Angiogenesis—Promoting and Blocking—Comes into Focus," *The Scientist,* Apr. 27, 1998. Two periodicals, *Angiogenesis* and *Angiogenesis Research,* are both issued by the Dutch firm Kluwer Academic Publishers, Dodrecht. See <www.jimmunol.org/v160n3/1402>, as well as notes to chapter 22.

CYCLINS were discovered in 1982 by the Nobel-laureate physiologist Tim Hunt, Clare Hall Laboratories, South Mimms, U.K., who named them after noting that certain proteins in sea-urchin eggs were highly expressed only to decline precipitously before the eggs divided. Researchers have found about ten different cyclins in humans, which regulate various CDs. The quantity of cyclin D1 expressed can be used to approximate residual cancer cells.

FOREIGN SCIENTISTS: The number of Americans entering the sciences and engineering decreases every year even as society depends increasingly on technology. Only half of high-school seniors have a basic grasp of science, according to a recent U.S. Dept. of Education compilation of test scores. The more-difficult questions were answered correctly by 18% in 2001, down from 21% in 1996. It is a serious problem, made all the more so because it is generally ignored. (See chapter 12 for a science quiz given to university journalism students.) More than 40% of graduate students at MIT come from abroad, and eight of the eleven U.S. residents who shared Nobel prizes in physics and chemistry between 1998 and 2000 were born elsewhere, according to a front-page article in the *Wall Street Journal,* Mar. 1, 2001.

CHAPTER 7: THE LANGUAGE OF MEDICINE

LEADING DRUG COMPANIES, worldwide, after the four listed, are Roche Holdings, Merck, Bayer, and Lilly; all these firms rank among the world's thirty-six largest companies of any kind as reported annually in the *International Science Yearbook* (Schonfeld and Associates).

MEDICAL DICTIONARIES are a necessity for cancer patients reading scientific papers. *Taber's Cyclopedic Medical Dictionary* (ed. F. A. Davis, M.D.) defines most words except those in the field of genomics, which may be found in *A Dictionary of Gene Technology Terms,* ed. Yong-he Zhlang, M.D. (Parthenon). Try to get the latest editions.

THE GRANET MCL GROUP may be accessed by contacting mantelcell@ucsd.edu. and asking to be placed on the list.

CHEMO BRAIN has been verified in at least two studies. In 2000 Tim Ahles, a psychologist at Dartmouth Medical School in Hanover, N.H., tested seventy-one patients who were cancer-free ten years after chemotherapy for lymphoma or breast cancer and compared them with fifty-eight who had been treated with radiation or surgery alone, finding the chemotherapy patients scored significantly worse (see the "Chemo brain" note to chapter 3 for Web sites). An earlier study in the Netherlands compared cognitive impairment in breast-cancer patients treated with chemo to that in patients who had only surgery and radiation (F. S. van Dam et al., "Impairment of Cognitive Function in Women Receiving Adjuvant Treatment for High-Risk Breast Cancer," *Journal of the National Cancer Institute* vol. 90 [Feb. 4, 1998]: 210–18). High-dose chemo patients had 3.5 times more cognitive problems than women receiving standard-dose chemo and 8 times more than those who received no chemotherapy. Also see C. B. Brezden et al., "Cognitive Function in Breast Cancer Patients Receiving Adjuvant Chemotherapy," *Journal of Clinical Oncology* vol. 18, no. 4 (July 18, 2000): 2695–2701.

CHAPTER 8: CANCER VACCINES

RONALD LEVY'S Karnofsky Lecture is an excellent step-by-step account of the development of monoclonal antibodies and cancer vaccines; see Levy, "Immunotherapy of Lymphoma," *Journal of Clinical Oncology* vol. 17, no. 11, Nov. suppl. (1999): 7.

ADJUVANTS today include cytokines—proteins produced by immune-system cells, such as interleukins, interferons, and blood-cell growth factors—as well as other stimulators, including DETOX, made from the cell walls of bacteria, and keyhole limpet hemocyanin (KLH), extracted from sea snail. KLH is one of the adjuvants used in the NCI vaccine trials described further in chapters 10 and 25.

AGE OF ONSET of non-Hodgkin's lymphoma was extrapolated from the NCI's Surveillance, Epidemiology, and End Results (SEER) data of 1998 and the 2001 Hoffmann-LaRoche publication on NHL. These data, given separately for men and women per age group, were averaged according to percentages among male-female victims (53% male) and then six months was subtracted to estimate age of onset (55) instead of age of diagnosis (55.5). A "roll call" of the Granet MCL Group conducted in 2002 averaged the same age of onset as other lymphomas, but consisted of 71% males—consistent with data from other sources indicating that mantle-cell lymphoma afflicts far more men than women. The youngest woman in the group was diagnosed at age 21. Incidence of NHL has almost doubled during the last two decades, and new diagnoses currently are increasing between 5% and 10% annually in the United States and Europe, according to both SEER and Hoffmann-LaRoche.

LYMPHOMA EPIDEMIC: Non-Hodgkin's lymphoma has increased in frequency by 4% a year since 1950. In 2003 new cases will number about 60,000 in the United States and about 300,000 worldwide, according to ACS and NCI data.

TOBACCO VACCINES: A close Australian relative of American tobacco is being used to grow fragments of tumor because that plant is a cheap and relatively fast vehicle. Dozens of biotech companies, including Large Scale Biology Corp. (<www.lsbc.com>), and the NCI are working on lowering the cost of personalized cancer vaccines.

Seventy vaccines under development by biotech companies for various cancers include twenty-nine in late-stage trials, according to *Business Week,* Nov. 26, 2002.

CHAPTER 9: PREMATURE RESULTS

TIME ARTICLES at the end of 1998 and a more-detailed earlier story, "I Wasn't Going to Curl Up and Die" (Oct. 12, 1998), described Duke University's dendritic vaccine as though it were an accomplished fact. An article by S. K. Nair et al. (including Eli Gilboa), "Induction of Cytotoxic T Cell Responses and Tumor Immunity against Unrelated Tumors Using Telomerase Reverse Transcriptase RNA Transfected Dendritic Cells," *Nature Medicine* vol. 6, no. 9 (Sept. 2000), reports progress at Duke on RNA-transfected dendritic cells.

RNA types include messenger (nRNA), transfer (tRNA), and ribosomal (rRNA), which, respectively, carry the genetic code from the DNA for making proteins, transfer the amino acids to the cell, and assist in protein synthesis.

AMGEN/IMMUNEX, Seattle (<www.amgen.com>), produced the Flt-3 "ligand" (small molecules bound to another), which stimulates production of large numbers of dendritic cells and has caused regression of tumors in mice.

CHAPTER 10: CO-STIMULATING T CELLS

THE NCI's "intramural" facility (for the research it conducts in-house) comprises several campuses combined in Jan. 2001 and called the "Center for Cancer Research," the largest basic and clinical cancer research facility in the world. It is located in Gaithersburg, Bethesda, Frederick, and Rockville, Maryland.

THE NIH was started in 1887 when Congress authorized an annual budget of $300 for Joseph Kinyoun, a young bacteriologist trained in German methods. Kinyoun was charged with setting up a one-room laboratory in the Marine Hospital on Staten Island, N.Y., to look into cholera, which had been infecting arriving ship passengers. The laboratory (and its one employee, Dr. Kinyoun) moved to Washington, D.C., in 1891.

CYTOKINES, the chemical messengers secreted in the co-stimulation of T cells, consist of more than a hundred distinct proteins produced primarily by white blood cells. They function during both inflammation and specific immune response.

CELLPRO'S shares, formerly valued at $100 million, dropped to zero, and its cell-purification system was lost to humanity. The full story is told in *Patient Number One* (Crown, 2000), by Rick Murdock and David Fisher. In later years other cell separators and blood irradiators were devised by various companies, among them one by MDS Nordion in Canada.

ARTIFICIAL APCs (antigen-presenting cells) are explained in two articles: Marcela Maus et al., "Ex Vivo Expansion of Polyclonal and Antigen-Specific Cytotoxic T Lymphocytes by Artificial APCs Expressing Ligands for the T-Cell Receptor, CD28 and 4-IBB," *Nature Biotechnology* vol. 20 (Feb. 2002): 143–48; and Mark Dudley, "A

Stimulating Presentation," *Nature Biotechnology* vol. 20 (Feb. 2002): 125–26. For his T-cell co-stimulation research, Carl June was honored at the Leukemia and Lymphoma Society's annual banquet in March 2002.

CHAPTER 11: DO THEY HAVE TO DIE?

THE MCL WEB SITE is now run by Ron Edwards's son Vince in England. Named for the aid of MCL (and other lymphoma) victims, the site can be accessed at <www.MCLaid.users.btopenworld.com>.

HIGH-DOSE RITUXAN: See relevant notes to chapters 6 and 21.

BARBERS AND DOCTORS: The title *doctor* was applied originally to teachers and scholars and then, in the fourteenth century, to those with the highest degree awarded by a university. Around the time of Columbus's voyages, the title came into widespread usage for physicians but not surgeons, the latter still considered barbaric in their evolution from barbers. (The red and white stripes on today's barber poles are symbolic of white bandages wound around red limbs.) As late as the nineteenth century in most countries, physicians were addressed as "doctor" while surgeons were still called "mister." (*Sources:* dictionary.com and *Encyclopedia Britannica*)

THE EVOLUTIONARY EXPLANATION of cancer is presented by Prof. Mel Greaves, a cell biologist at the Institute of Cancer Research in London, in his excellent book *Cancer: The Evolutionary Legacy* (Oxford, 2000). Greaves describes how cancer preceded mankind and then accelerated as the human lifestyle changed. He explains the "wholesale failure of chemotherapy" and discusses how modern therapies are beginning to emerge out of molecular biology.

POLLUTANTS, such as polychlorinated biphenyls (PCBs), entering the water years ago from paper mills along Michigan's Kalamazoo River made fish there unsafe to eat, according to Chuck Ide, Ph.D., director of environmental research at Western Michigan University (<www.deq.state.mi.us/documentsdeq-erd-pm-020701>). Coal-fired utilities spew sulfur dioxide and other pollutants in the Great Lakes and rivers, according to an annual list of the nation's most endangered rivers (<www.amrivers.org>).

INHERITED GENES contribute in only a minor way to most cancers, according to a study of twins in Scandinavian countries: P. Lichtenstin et al., "Environmental and Heritable Factors in Causation of Cancer," *New England Journal of Medicine* vol. 343 (2000): 78.

Lymphoma increase: Ken Garber, "Lymphoma Rate Rise Continues to Baffle Researchers," *Journal of the National Cancer Institute* vol. 93 (Apr. 4, 2001): 194–96, gives statistics for the United States. The British medical journal *The Lancet* (Mar. 9, 2002) reports worldwide figures.

Causation of lymphoma: An article by Adi Gazdar, "UT Southwestern Researchers Link Human Lymphomas to Polio Vaccine Tainted with Monkey Virus" (*The Lancet*, Mar. 9, 2002), implicated a monkey virus. University of Texas Southwestern Medical Center scientists who examined 400 tumors found the viral footprint for simian virus-40 in 43% of non-Hodgkin's lymphoma patients but to be almost totally absent in healthy patients. The study confirms earlier research on hamsters that linked SV-40 with NHL, mesothelioma (cancer in the lining of the lungs), and brain and bone tumors. Dr. Janet Butel, Baylor College of Medicine, Houston, independently obtained almost identical data (lori@bcm.tmc.edu). The researchers estimated that between 1955 and 1963, some thirty million people were vaccinated with batches of polio vaccine contaminated with SV-40. Some persons born after 1963 also carry the virus; its transmission route to them is uncertain.

Suspected carcinogens are identified frequently. A study in Sweden recently suggested a known carcinogen, acrylamide, can result from frying potatoes or baking bread at high temperatures; such foods are staples of the human diet throughout the world (see <www.ens.lycos.com/ens/may2002>). The World Health Organization has undertaken a study of acrylamide. Exposure to organic solvents was found to be a cause of lymphoma in a Brazilian study; see M. A. Vasconcelos Rego, "Non-Hodgkin's Lymphomas and Organic Solvents," *Journal of Occupational and Environmental Medicine* vol. 44, no. 9 (Sept. 2002): 874–81. Smoking was implicated in lymphoma causation via its role in mutating the $p53$ tumor-suppressor gene, according to a news release issued by the Comprehensive Cancer Center of Northwestern University, Nov. 1, 2002.

Samuel Epstein's book is *The Politics of Cancer Revisited* (East Ridge, 1998).

H. pylori and its role in MALT lymphoma and stomach cancer may be explored via the Helicobacter Foundation, <www.helico.com>.

A. N. Whitehead (1861–1947) was an English mathematician and philosopher who collaborated with Bertrand Russell on *Principia Mathematica* and later taught at Harvard.

Sleep research For discoveries on the importance of sleep, see especially publications by Joseph Takahashi, Northwestern University Center for Sleep and Circadian Biology; James Krueger, Washington State University at Pullman; Eve van Cauter, University of Chicago; Michael P. Stryker, University of California at San Francisco; and David Dinges, University of Pennsylvania's Division of Sleep and

Chronobiology. An apparently contrary view, that people live longer when averaging seven hours of sleep instead of the commonly recommended eight hours, came from a University of California at San Diego study of data on one million Americans collected by the ACS; see D. Kripke et al., "Mortality Associated with Sleep Duration and Insomnia," *Archives of General Psychiatry* vol. 59 (2002): 131. The two bodies of research need not conflict, since it is difficult for cancer patients to obtain even seven hours of quality sleep.

CHAPTER 12: ALTERNATIVE MAGIC

LACK OF TIME SPENT BY ONCOLOGISTS: Cancer physicians averaged 1.3 minutes informing their patients, although the patients believed it to be ten minutes, according to a study quoted in I. Lerner et al., "The Prevalence of Questionable Methods of Cancer Treatment in the U.S.," *CA: A Cancer Journal for Clinicians* vol. 42 (1992): 181. This study also measured patients' passivity; they spent only eight seconds asking their oncologists questions. The greater variety of treatments available now may have increased the time spent in discussing options.

CSICOP—the Committee for the Scientific Investigation of Claims of the Paranormal—publishes one of the best sources for distinguishing sound from fallacious medical practices in its quarterly, *Scientific Review of Alternative Medicine*, distributed through Prometheus Books (800-421-0351; mfrench@prometheusmail.com). In 2001 data available at <www.nccam.nih.gov/research/grants> revealed that between 1993 and 2000 the NIH spent about $110 million on its National Center for Complementary and Alternative Medicine, with no reports confirming or refuting herbal and other alternative medicines. *The Skeptical Inquirer,* a patient and thorough debunker of pseudoscience, is published bimonthly by CSICOP (<www.csicop.org>).

ASTROLOGY—or its underlying belief that there is a connection between the motion of stars and human lives—has been invalidated by scientists since the seventeen century. Not only is the theory ridiculous, but it suffers from internal discrepancies. For instance, astrologers track the calendar, not the precise movement of stars in constellations, and they consider dates of birth more momentous than dates of conception. Yet horoscopes and meaningless astrological "signs" are embedded in society, even in the technologically advanced United States, largely due to the scientific ignorance of the most significant purveyors of adult education: the popular media.

THE FAILURE OF CHEMO to cure lymphoma has led many people to reject established medicine totally. This nihilistic attitude should change with the advent of biological agents, according to P. McLaughlin, "Progress and Promise in the Treatment of Indolent Lymphomas," *Oncologist* vol. 7, no. 3 (2002): 217.

ALTERNATIVE THERAPIES are used by 70% of adults with cancer, according to a Hutchinson Cancer Center survey reported in "Research on Paradigm, Practice, and Policy," *Journal of Alternative and Complimentary Medicine* (Sept. 10, 2002), but 65% of these were vitamin or herbal supplements. Only 17% indulged in naturopathics, massage, hypnotism, crystals, chelation, or magnets.

ANTISCIENCE attitudes among talk-show hosts are just a small part of the absurdities to which Americans are exposed, as explained in Kurt Butler's *Consumer's Guide to "Alternative Medicine"* (Prometheus, 1992).

THE SCIENCE POLL OF AMERICANS is conducted biannually by the National Science Foundation. The May 2002 survey of 1,574 adults chosen at random revealed that 48% thought the earliest humans lived at the same time as dinosaurs (which died off millions of years before humans appeared); 54% knew that the earth orbits the sun in one year (only 50% had known this two years before); and 51% thought that antibiotics kill viruses as well as bacteria. Alarmingly, the NSF report found that U.S. reliance on foreign-born scientists and engineers is growing at all degree levels, with the highest ratio, 45%, in engineering.

SCIENCE QUIZ FOR JOURNALISTS: In 2002 seventy-two journalism students at Northwestern University took our simple test, the questions chosen to span a variety of sciences. The average score was 33.9%; that is, 5.08 correct out of 15—closer to "scientific imbecility" on the idiot-to-genius scale of 2 to 14 (approximating a "science I.Q." of 20 to 140). The quiz given to journalism students at the University of Illinois produced similar scores. Engineering and science students at Illinois, however, scored "high genius," averaging 14.2 correct answers.

Answers:

1. Most of the Northwestern students (86%) knew that the molecule consisting of two atoms of hydrogen and one of oxygen is water.

2. Only 39% knew that the most common element in the universe is hydrogen. (Wrong answers were mostly carbon, nitrogen, or oxygen.)

3. Only 28% knew that the number pi is the ratio of the circumference of a circle to its diameter (or mentioned circles at all).

4. Only 7% knew that the setting sun is reddish because we view it horizontally at such times. There is thus more atmosphere and more matter (molecules, dust, or other particles) between us and the sun at sunset than there is at noon, and this matter scatters away light at the blue end of the spectrum, leaving the red. (Most wrong guesses said there is greater pollution at sunset than at noon.)

5. A tiny minority (6%) had any idea (within 100,000 miles) that the mean distance from the earth to the moon is 239,000 miles. (Many put the distance in the millions of miles.)

6. Only 15% knew that legumes get their nitrogen from the air.

7. Only 15% knew that the solar system is 4.5 billion years old (within 3 billion years). (Many, perhaps "creationists," said that it is debatable.)

8. Most, 60%, knew that bacteria are larger than viruses. (The fact that viruses are immensely smaller explains why they can get inside a cell, where they can't be killed as easily as bacteria, which reside on the surfaces of cells.)

9. Only 21% knew that air is almost entirely a mixture of 21% oxygen and 79% nitrogen. (Most thought that the two major gases in the air were oxygen and carbon dioxide.)

10. Only 19% knew that the shape of a wing's airfoil causes the air on top to travel farther and faster than the air under it, resulting in less pressure on top and thus forcing the wing upward.

11. A majority (51%) knew three of the four states of matter—solid, liquid, and gas—but only 39% knew all four, including plasma.

12. Only 36% knew that sand is geologically older than rock, because sand has been ground up from rock over time. (One student said, "it must be rock because of 'rock of ages' being old.")

13. None described mammals as having a four-chambered heart, but 24% knew they have hair, that they give birth to live young (with few exceptions, such as platypuses), and that the females nourish their young with milk or possess mammary glands. (Most wrong guesses mentioned legs and lungs.)

14. Only 7% knew that the air pressure at sea level is 14.7 psi—in other words, that the air presses against each square inch of us at 14.7 pounds.

15. Only 42% realized that the star closest to the moon is the sun. Four named the second-closest star, Alpha Centauri. The most popular of the other wrong guesses were the North Star (or Polaris), Betelgeuse, Arcturus, Mars, Venus, and the earth—the last three, of course, being planets.

The nonscientific bent of novice journalists explains why, as their careers develop, so many of them favor pseudoscience or treat stories of the paranormal equally with those of real science, thereby abetting superstition among the public.

CHAPTER 13: ALLIES IN THE QUEST

PEREGRINE PHARMACEUTICALS (<www.peregrineinc.com>), like most biotech companies, has numerous alliances with university researchers. See the Web pages for Philip Thorpe (<www.swmed/edu/cancer/Labs/Thorpe>) and Alan Epstein (<www.peregrineinc.com/Epstein>). The remarkable new radioactive antibody Cotara is now in clinical trials for a variety of solid tumors, including lung, brain, and other cancers.

THE LYMPHOMA RESEARCH FOUNDATION, resulting from the 2002 merger of the LRFA in Los Angeles and the Cure for Lymphoma Foundation in New York, is accessible at 212-213-9595 or LRF@lymphoma.org. The foundation's Web site is <www.lymphoma.org>.

UCLA SCHOOL OF MEDICINE: <www.medsch.ucla.edu>.

THE BURNHAM INSTITUTE, which is headed by John Reed, may be accessed at <www.burnham.org>.

THE HUTCHINSON CENTER, the University of Washington, Children's Hospital, and the Regional Medical Center together form the "Seattle Cancer Alliance." They are pioneers in bone-marrow transplants.

STEM-CELL RESEARCH: Adult stem cells could rival embryonic stem cells as a source for therapy, according to Yuehua Jiang et al., "Pluripotency of Mesenchymal Stem Cells Derived from Adult Marrow," *Nature* vol. 418 (July 4, 2002): 41–49. For problems involved also see J. B. Cibelli et al., "Somatic Cell-Nuclear Transfer in Humans, *Journal of Regenerative Medicine* vol. 2 (2001): 25; and R. Kline, "Whose Blood Is It Anyway," *Scientific American,* Apr. 2001. Also check out the American Society for Bone and Mineral Research in Washington, D.C. (<www.asbmr.org>).

CHAPTER 14: FALSE ALARM

A DESMOID TUMOR, also called aggressive fibromatosis, is a soft-tissue tumor that does not metastasize but usually is aggressive locally. When you are diagnosed with a desmoid, you should rule out "familial adenomatous polyposis" (FAP), or "Gardner's syndrome," which usually is inherited (hence "familial"). The disease often shows up as multiple polyps in the intestines that could become malignant, according to the Desmoid Group (desmoid-request@listserv.acor.org), an e-mail information and support club of patients analogous to the Granet MCL Group.

PILL CAMERAS go a long way to eliminate the need for exploratory surgery. The first, called the "Gut Cam," was developed by an Israeli company, Given Imaging, Ltd. The FDA approved it for clinical use in the United States in Aug. 2001. See <www.givenimaging.com/usa>.

CHAPTER 15: DOES PRAYER WORK?

THE POLL OF SCIENTISTS belonging to the National Academy of Sciences was published in *Nature,* July 25, 1998; a similar 1916 study showed about the same percentages of belief in God among American physicists, biologists, and mathematicians.

"POWER OF PRAYER in the Practice of Medicine," an internet article by Larry Dossey, M.D. (available at <www.win-winresourcecenter.com/the-power-of-prayer>), cites evidence that prayer is therapeutic "whether you believe the power comes from within, or from the external power of the God of your faith." In "Can Science Prove That Prayer Works?" *Free Inquiry* vol. 17, no. 3, Hector Avalos ascribes prayer to "supernatural ignorance" and warns of "a dark side to prayer" when critically ill patients wait too long for God to answer (<www.secularhumanism.org/avalos>). Other relevant sources include Debra Williams, D.D., "Scientific Research of Prayer" *The PLIM Report* vol. 8, no. 4 (<www.plim.org/PrayerDeb.htm>); Herbert Benson, M.D., *Time Healing* (Scribner's, 1996); and Robert Wright, *Three Scientists and Their Gods* (Times Books, 1988).

BRAIN-IMMUNE COMMUNICATION: Shared receptors are used as a common chemical medium for communication within and between the immune and neuroendocrine systems, suggesting an immuno-regulatory role for the brain and a sensory function for the immune system, according to J. Blalock, "Associations between the Neuroendocrine and Immune Systems," *Immunology Today* vol. 15 (1994): 504. You may contact Astrid Linthorst, of the Max Planck Institute of Psychiatry, Germany, who has studied the subject (linthors@mpipskykl.mpg.de). See also "The Mind-Body Link" (Society for Neuroscience, 2002), available by sending e-mail to webmaster@sfn.org.

LAUGHTER as a stimulant to the immune system has been studied for many years. The Mayo Foundation for Medical Education and Research's "Laughter and Medicine: How Humor Can Help You Heal" (available at <www.mayoclinic.com/ invoke.cfm>) reveals a host of studies since the 1930s, including a year-long inquiry by the Oakhurst Health Research Institute into the status of 240 heart-attack victims; those who watched comedy videos had fewer recurrences than did a control group.

EXPRESSIVE WRITING also has been cited as beneficial to helping the immune system fight cancer, according to an editorial by David Spiegel, a psychiatrist at Stanford University's School of Medicine; see Spiegel, "Emotional Expression and Disease Outcome," *Journal of the American Medical Association* vol. 281, no. 14 (Apr. 1999): 1328–29.

JUDEO-CHRISTIAN prayer intercession and its effects on patients with various ailments has been studied from time to time by the Complementary Medicine Research Group at the California Pacific Medical Center in San Francisco and at San Francisco General Hospital (<www.godandscience.org/apologetics/smj1>). Duke University prayer research was reported in the *Christian Science Monitor,* Mar. 25, 1998.

CHAPTER 16: PROJECT INDOLENCE

NATURE'S BLUNDERS: The mutation of even a single copy of a pair of genes (such as Myc, Dmpl, or p27 genes) at the beginning of the biochemical pathway that leads to lymphoma and leukemia may be enough for some forms of these cancers to start, according to the tumor-cell biologist Charles Sherr at St. Jude's Research Hospital in Memphis and others quoted in article 536 of *Lymphoma Newsline* (Nov. 29, 2001), published online by the Lymphoma Research Foundation. Scientists have been look-ing at tumor-suppressor genes such as p21 for years; in mid-2002 a drug called "CYC202," developed by Cyclacel, Ltd., in Dundee, Scotland, entered phase-two trials in the United Kingdom and France.

GENE-EXPRESSION PROFILING in mantle-cell lymphoma resulted in a flurry of UCLA papers, notably Wolf-K. Hofmann et al. (including Sven de Vos, Jonathan Said, and Phil Koeffler), "Altered Apoptosis Pathways in Mantle-Cell Lymphoma Detected by Oligonucleotide Microarray," *Blood* vol. 98, no. 3 (Aug. 2001): 787–94.

FORCING APOPTOSIS is the approach of Myriad Genetics, Inc., Salt Lake City (<www.myriadgenetics.com>), which is subjecting chemo-refractory cell lines to a drug the company calls "MPI-176716."

GENECHIPS (also called biochips, DNA chips, and oligonucleotide- or hybridiza-tion-array assays) are manufactured by several companies employing a unique mar-riage of semiconductor technology and the life sciences. The chips used by the Project Indolence team were designed by Affymetrix, Inc., Santa Clara, Calif. (<www.affymetrix.com>).

LYMPHOMA STATISTICS quoted are from "Cancer Facts and Figures 2002," pub-lished annually on-line by the American Cancer Society's Surveillance Research branch (<www.cancer.org>). The year 2002 saw 60,900, new cases of lymphoma in the United States (53,900 non-Hodgkin's lymphoma and 7,000 Hodgkin's), with 25,800 new deaths from lymphoma. New leukemia cases in 2002 numbered 30,800, with 21,700 new deaths.

POLYMERASE CHAIN REACTION, or PCR, is explained fully in articles published online by the NIH National Center for Human Genome Research, such as "New Tools for Tomorrow's Health Research" (1992). Also see <www.highveld.com/pcr.htm>.

CHAPTER 17: CURE CANCER IN TEN YEARS

CONGRESSIONAL TESTIMONY before the House Committee on Appropriations: Subcommittee on Labor, Health and Human Services, Education, and Related Agen-cies was given on March 14, 2000, and is available from the U.S. Government Print-ing Office.

THE SCARIEST AIRPORT is Reagan International in Washington, D.C., according to Kevin Garrison's book *Congested Airspace* (Belvoir, 1993).

NON-HODGKIN'S LYMPHOMA is considered an epidemic. Among others, the epidemiologist Susan Fisher, University of Rochester, said there were 56,200 new cases in 2001 and 24,000 deaths. When you add Hodgkin's and other lymphomas on the borderline with leukemia, there are about 87,000 new cases annually, according to the Lymphoma Research Foundation and other sources.

12.7 MILLION LIVING CANCER VICTIMS: The number of people living with cancer in the United States has been updated to 2003 using NCI's SEER data for 1997, which totaled 8.3 million cases. A linear interpolation of the 17 million newly diagnosed cases reported by SEER in the thirteen years since 1990 suggests that since 1997 there would have been 3,636,364 new cases added. Subtracting deaths, the number of people in the United States living with cancer comes to 12.7 million, according to Shahid Siddiqi and the statisticians he consulted at SEER and elsewhere. This is a low estimate; in 2003 the American Cancer Society reported 1, 284, 900 new cases of cancer in the United States during 2002. (See "Cancer statistics" note to chapter 3.)

SIX HUNDRED THOUSAND DEATHS: The number of deaths due to cancer in the United States has been extrapolated to the year 2003 by continuing the trend, and rounding, from the 2001 figure of 553,400. In countries where reliable data are estimated, cancer is proportionate to population. Cancer deaths for the somewhat larger European Union in 2002 was estimated at 750,000. According to Sally Goodman's "E.U. Ponders Joint Action on Cancer," *Nature* vol. 419 (Sept. 12, 2002): 101, the "EU has no coordinated research approach and most of its national programs are small and fragmented."

HUMAN-GENOME mapping by the Dept. of Energy and NIH Human Genome Project was vastly accelerated by J. Craig Venter's nonprofit Institute for Genomic Research (TIGR) and Celera Genomics Corp., in Rockville, Md. The project met its goal—to discover all human genes and render them accessible for biological study by the end of 2003—years ahead of first projections, primarily because of Venter's efforts. Venter, who utilized his own DNA to ease fears that such sequencing would lead to genetic discrimination, also sequenced, for comparison, the genomes of the mouse, the fruit fly, and other organisms. Venter gave the number of human genes as a little more than 30,000, consisting of some three billion base pairs. But William Haseltine, CEO of Human Genome Sciences, writing in *Discover* (Apr. 2003, p. 74), came up with a number "around 90,000" using a method completely different from Venter's.

SIMULATING the way cancer cells express antigens to make a template for previously undifferentiated natural killer cells has met with success at the University of Illinois, Urbana, where Steven Zimmerman and Kenneth Suslick have developed a way of creating artificial antibodies. The first example of a process in which "a single molecular template is imprinted into a single macromolecule" results in a synthetic molecular shell that binds specific molecules and rejects all others, just as a natural antibody does. See Zimmerman et al., "Synthetic Hosts by Monomolecular Imprinting inside Dendrimers, *Nature* vol. 418 (July 25, 2002): 399–403. Other laboratories are working to produce virtual libraries of three-dimensional antigen shapes in order to be able to treat patients with antibodies that will attack only their own highly unique malignant cells.

ECONOMIC VALUE OF CURING CANCER: The astounding estimate of $46.5 trillion in the United States alone was calculated by Robert Topel, professor of economics at the University of Chicago Graduate School of Business, and Kevin Murphy, professor of finance at the Marshall School of Business, University of Southern California.

"WAGE PEACE," an article originally published in the March 1971 issue of *Industrial Research,* advocated what might be described today as nation building, but with an important difference: the United States would declare peace on a nation by invitation only and *before* unrest and ignorance turned a country into an enemy. Reprints are available from the author (neilruzic@attbi.com). The follow-up article mentioned is "A Force for Peace," written by the research historian Dean Babst and published in the April 1972 issue. Babst defines "freely elected governments" throughout history and concludes that *freely elected governments do not go to war against each other.*

CHAPTER 18: THINK TANKS

LACK OF COORDINATION among clinical trials was found in a study conducted between Nov. 2001 and Jan. 2002; the study looked at 108 universities working under contract with drug companies. Only 1% of the contracts required that researchers, who typically work at a single medical site, have access to clinical data at other sites in the same trials, according to J. M. Drazen, "Institutions, Contracts, and Academic Freedom" (editorial), *New England Journal of Medicine* vol. 347, no. 17 (Oct. 24, 2002): 1362–63.

THE ANTI-CD20 monoclonal antibody Rituxan's efficacy is detailed in an especially clear paper on the results of a phase-two trial of retreatment with the same Mab. See T. A. Davis et al. (including Ronald Levy), "Rituximab Anti-CD20 Monoclonal Antibody Therapy in Non-Hodgkin's Lymphoma," *Journal of Clinical Oncology* vol. 18, no. 17 (Sept. 2000): 3135–43. Among a host of papers attesting to the value of anti-CD20 antibodies for many lymphomas, including CLL, is J. Golay et al., "CD20 Levels Determine in Vitro Susceptibility to Rituximab," *Blood* vol. 98, no. 12 (Dec. 1, 2001). A good source for upcoming papers is the Medscape Resource Center (<www.medscape.com>).

ANTISENSE DRUGS are small modified strands of DNA called "oligo-nucleotides" that have been engineered in a sequence exactly opposite (hence "anti") to the coding sequence ("sense") of messenger RNA. The drug Genasense is designed by Genta, Inc., Berkeley Heights, N.J. (908-286-9800; <www.genta.com>).

KINESIN INHIBITING is like "freezing a car motor by throwing a monkey wrench into it," according to Cytokinetics' founders, who left Stanford University to start the company in 1988 (<www.science.gsk.com/press/press.htm>).

FABER'S BOOK OF SCIENCE, edited by John Carey and published by Faber and Faber (1995), is one of those priceless books that highlight science history in many disciplines by excerpting short key writings by the famous scientists themselves.

LABORATORY ANIMAL deaths pale in comparison with the billions of farm animals slaughtered annually for food, even though vegetable protein, which is far less fatty, would better serve a nation endangered by obesity; see *Discover,* Mar. 2002, 76. U.S. hunters and trappers kill 7.4 million deer each year, and drivers kill another 1.8 million; the deaths of other wild animals, such as squirrels and raccoons, are at least as numerous, according to the *Wall Street Journal,* Aug. 1, 2002, p. 1.

BREAST-CANCER patients had been routinely advised to take chemotherapy following mastectomies, until oncologists began to consider the risk for contracting leukemia to be greater than that of the recurrence of breast tumors. The Mab Herceptin was partly responsible for the change; see "Doctors Start to Rethink Wisdom of Chemo for Breast-Cancer Patients," *Wall Street Journal,* Oct. 8, 2002. Eighty-five percent of cancer patients are unaware of clinical trials for their specific disease. (See "Clinical trials" note to chapter 4.)

ANNUAL ASH MEETING: The American Society of Hematology is typically attended by 25,000 medical participants, family members, company representatives, and others. According to the ASH public relations department, 10,000 of these are scientists: hematologists (28%), hematologist-oncologists (44%), and scientists working in various other biological disciplines (28%).

CHAPTER 19: TRANSPLANTS

TRANSPLANT SUCCESS: Fewer than half the 4,500 transplants performed in the United States each year are successful, according to a Dec. 12, 2002, release from Tufts School of Medicine, Boston. The Tufts study indicated that the transplant success rate could be doubled using ultraviolet-light treatment combined with pentostatin. Among ninety elderly patients with advanced lymphoma, leukemia, and multiple myeloma who underwent transplants incorporating the ultraviolet treatment, only 20% contracted graft-versus-host disease, while the rate for current regimens stands "between 40% and 50%."

THE TRANSPLANT STUDY at M. D.Anderson and the Medical College of Wisconsin (MCW) determined a 40% long-term survival of chronic lymphocytic leukemia patients undergoing bone-marrow transplants; the rate for chemotherapy alone was 26%. The data come from a Dec. 20, 2001, MCW news release, which did not define "long term."

GLEEVEC'S FAST APPROVAL was not quite as speedy as the beleaguered FDA made it out to be at the time of its approval (May 10, 2001), for the drug had entered trials in 1998. Gleevec is an entirely new class of drugs, a growth-factor inhibitor called imatinib, and at first the FDA didn't know how to handle it. Only after smaller trials were repeated in a larger combined phase-one and -two trial— and showed once again that Gleevec resulted in normal blood counts in 95% of participants—did the FDA rush approval. Starting at the point when the new clinical trial began, it took only two and a half months for approval, but it had been three years since the first trial.

GLEEVEC'S EFFICACY for CML was said to increase with prolonged use, reported widely in the scientific press during 2001. Brian Druker explained that the drug works by blocking the enzymes known as tyrosine kinases, which are triggered by the DNA mutation caused when the two chromosomes translocate their fragments of genetic information. Three months after Gleevec was approved for treating gastrointestinal stromal tumors (Feb. 1, 2002), Gleevec's manufacturer, Novartis, moved its worldwide research center from Switzerland to Cambridge, Mass., in one of the most significant defections of a European pharmaceutical company to the United States. The move was made primarily because of greater opportunities in researching and marketing Gleevec (*Wall Street Journal,* May 7, 2002, p. A3).

CHRONIC LYMPHOCYTIC LEUKEMIA (CLL) is the target of hundreds of research studies. One that Ellen Cohen and I discussed at length investigated a kind of apoptosis that Marika Sarfati, M.D. and Ph.D., had induced at the University of Montreal (see V. Mateo et al., "CD47 Ligation Induces Caspase-Independent Cell Death in Chronic Lymphocytic Leukemia," *Nature Medicine* vol. 5, no. 11 [Nov. 1999]: 1277–84). Sarfati and her group used purified B cells from forty-two lymphocytic leukemic patients and then added the CD47 antibody—in culture dishes—which caused many characteristics of apoptosis, such as cell shrinkage. But it was not "classic" apoptosis; that is, it did not depend on the usual enzymes that cleave key cell proteins. Electron micrographs showed the cancer cells were programmed to die, but via an entirely different, undiscovered pathway. The Sarfati team is now working to determine efficacy, first in lab animals and then in humans.

PENTOSTATIN is given during transplants (often with Rituxan) to reach a balance between rejection and the desired graft-versus-tumor effect. Pentostatin, a common treatment for hairy-cell leukemia and cutaneous T-cell lymphoma, belongs to the class of purine nucleoside analogs. The drug, developed by SuperGen and trade-named "Nipent," inhibits the work of a critical enzyme called ADA, which clears T cells of certain waste products and leads to apoptosis.

"MINI" (MINIMAL) TRANSPLANTS, also called "nonmyeloablative," are explained by Barbara Lackritz in her book *Adult Leukemia* (O'Reilly, 2001).

STEM-CELL TRANSPLANTATION: See Oliver W. Press, "Treatment of Mantle Cell Lymphoma," in *Educational Book 2002*, ed. M. Perry (American Society of Clinical Oncology, 2002), for a comprehensive overview of transplant technology.

THE VALUE OF TRANSPLANTS: For a dramatic article about the bad and good of bone-marrow transplants by one who performs them, see Jerome Groopman, "A Healing Hell," *The New Yorker*, Oct. 18, 1998 (jgrooma@caregroup.harvard.edu).

FAMOUS PEOPLE who have died of lymphoma, many of them following transplants (as did King Hussein of Jordan), are listed at the Web sites <www.datafork.com> and <www.lymphomation.org>.

JOHN ULTMANN'S many contributions to lymphoma research are told in the lead editorial, "In Memoriam," of the *Journal of Clinical Oncology* vol. 19 (Jan. 1, 2001), a publication he had founded.

CHAPTER 20: PATHWAYS TO SUCCESS

CELL SIZES vary, but an average cell diameter of 7 microns (7-millionths of a meter) yields a volume of 1.8×10^{-10} cc—that is, 18-billionths of a cubic centimeter. Assume a 150-lb. (68.2 kg) person and further assume the weight of a human is equal to that of water. The volume of a human being is then 68,200 cc, which yields a cell-to-human ratio of 379 trillion to 1. The volume of water in all the Great Lakes (the largest source of fresh water in the world) is about is 23,000 cubic kilometers, or 337 trillion times that of a human being. Therefore the ratios of a cell to a human and of a human to the Great Lakes are roughly equivalent.

EXTREME COMPLEXITY of tiny cells is explained clearly by W. W. Gibbs in "Cybernetic Cells," *Scientific American*, Aug. 2001.

EPITHELIAL GENES: See J. Braun, "Unsettling Facts of Life: Bacterial Commensalism, Epithelial Adherence and Inflammatory Bowel Disease," *Gastroenterology* vol. 122 (2002): 228.

THE TCL1 GENE is explained further by S. French et al. (including Mike Teitell) in "A Modeled Hydrophobic Domain on the TCL1 Oncoprotein Mediates Association with AKT at the Cytoplasmic Membrane," *Biochemistry* vol. 41, no. 20 (2002): 6376–82. Teitell has developed the first animal models for three common lymphomas: Burkitt's, diffuse large B-cell, and follicular.

ONCOGENES, as mutated forms of proto-oncogenes that regulate cell cycles, are explained on-line by the Genetics of Cancer Resource Center (<www.intouchlive.com/cancergenetics>).

APOPTOSIS—programmed cell death, as opposed to necrosis, or nonprogrammed cell death—is explained well in Alison C. Lloyd, "Cell Senescence and Cancer," in the Reviews/Cancer section of *Nature* vol. 1 (2001). In preclinical studies of chemotherapy-resistant cancer cells, including those from prostate tumors and lymphomas, Myriad Genetics's small-molecule drug MPI-176716 killed cancer cells selectively by inducing apoptosis. See <www.myriad.com>.

TUMOR-SUPPRESSOR GENE P53: Easy-to-understand reports of current p53 (and p73) research include three one-page reviews: Cath Brooksbank, "Drifting Downstream," *Nature Reviews Cancer* vol. 2, no. 2 (Feb. 2002): 79; Kristine Novak, "Age Activator," *Nature Reviews Cancer* vol. 2, no. 2 (Feb. 2002): 81; and Alison Mitchell, "From Damage to Death," *Nature Reviews Molecular Cell Biology* vol. 3, no. 3 (Mar. 2002): 148. (Also see "Swedish drug" note to chapter 21.) A report on experiments at the University of Illinois at Chicago using bacteria to stabilize p53 appears in T. Yamada et al., "Baterial Redox Protein Azurin, Tumor Suppressor Protein p53, and Regression of Cancer," *Proceedings of the National Academy of Science* vol. 99, no. 22 (Oct. 29, 2002): 14098–103.

BIOTECH COMPANIES, which need not emphasize blockbuster, billion-dollar drugs as do the giant pharmaceutical companies, are leading the way in a variety of new approaches. Among those seeking to treat end-stage refractory lymphoma is BioTransplant, Inc. Its drug Allomune is an antibody that binds specifically to the CD2 antigen receptor found on T cells and natural killer cells, thus permitting the engraftment of donor bone marrow. In 1998 the FDA awarded Allomune orphan-drug status (a designation for drugs having few customers). Another approach is to design bio-informatic software for more-precise drug development. For instance, a joint effort between LeadScope, Inc., and the NCI relates gene expressions to 27,000 compounds previously tested for their effect on tumor growth. This technology may be extended to protein profiles, according to O. P. Blower et al., "Pharmacogenic Analysis: Correlating Molecular Substructure Classes with Microarray Gene-Expression Data," *Pharmacogenomics Journal* vol. 2 (2000): 259. Other software techniques speeding screening are described in "In-Silico Screening Needed for Drug Discovery," *Research and Development*, Aug. 2002, p. 31.

CHAPTER 21: FROM INDIA WITH RESULTS

HIGH-DOSE RITUXAN still has not become standard therapy for lymphoma despite studies showing its safety and efficacy. (See "High-dose Rituxan" note to chapter 6.) Rituxan for rheumatoid arthritis has entered phase-three trials sponsored by the manufacturers IDEC Pharmaceuticals and Genentech, as well as the drug's comarketer, Hoffmann–La Roche.

CELEBREX AS ANTI-ANGIOGENIC had appeared in the literature at least a dozen times by 1999; see the "Cox-2" note to chapter 22.

HYPERTHERMIA AND HYPOXIA: See R. Issels et al., "Hyperthermia and Hypoxia for Cancer-Cell Destruction," *The Lancet* (the world's longest running medical journal, London) vol. 2 (Sept. 2001): 521. Issels obtained remarkable 5-year survival improvement in cancer patients with soft-tissue sarcomas.

EPRATUZUMAB, tradenamed "LymphoCide" by Immunomedics and Amgen, is a yttrium-90-labeled monoclonal antibody, or radioactive Mab, shown to be effective in phase-two clinical trials against various non-Hodgkin's lymphomas, especially in combination with Rituxan.

A SWEDISH DRUG to repair DNA damage due to defective p53 genes in mice grafted with human cancer of the skeleton was announced in 2001 by K. Wiman of the Karolinska Hospital, in Stockholm; see V. J. N. Bykov et al., "Restoration of the Tumor Suppressor Function to Mutant p53 by a Low-Molecular-Weight Compound," *Nature Medicine* vol. 8, no. 3 (Mar. 2002): 282–88.

AN IMCLONE SYSTEMS drug shrank tumors 50% in 30 of 120 patients with chemoresistant, end-stage colon cancer at Memorial Sloan-Kettering, according to a report that B. Saltz gave to the American Society of Clinical Oncology meeting, May 2001.

MOLECULAR NANOGENERATORS at Memorial Sloan-Kettering consist of actinium-225 delivered inside a "molecular cage" and attached to an antibody to home in on cancer cells. Results with work on mice were reported by D. Scheinberg; see M. R. McDevitt, "Tumor Therapy with Targeted Atomic Nanogenerators," *Science* vol. 294, no. 5546 (Nov. 16, 2001): 1537–46.

METHYLGLYOXAL: See Manju Ray et al., "Implication of the Bioelectronic Principle in Cancer Therapy: Treatment of Cancer Patients by Methylglyoxal-Based Formulation," *Indian Journal of Physics* vol. 75b, no. 2 (2001): 73. This paper is the latest in a series dating back to 1991.

CUTANEOUS T-CELL LYMPHOMA (CTCL) is the fastest-growing cancer in the United States, according to Madeleine Duvic, "Current Treatment of Cutaneous T-Cell Lymphoma," *Dermatology Online Journal* vol. 7, no. 1 (<www.dermatology.cdlib.org/ DOJvol7num1>). The terms *cutaneous T-cell lymphoma* and *mycosis fungoides* often are used interchangeably, but the latter (which Thayer Sheets had) is really a subset of the former. Photopheresis is being used against both. See M. Duvic et al., "Photopheresis Therapy for CTCL," *Journal of Dermatology* vol. 35 (1996): 573. (These are but two of Prof. Duvic's 200 scientific papers.)

CHAPTER 22: ANTI-ANGIOGENESIS

THE VALUE OF ANGIOGENESIS: R. Jain and P. Carmeliet's article "Vessels of Death or Life," *Scientific American*, Dec. 2001, presents the two faces of angiogenesis—the harmful and beneficial effects of blood-vessel formation.

COX-2 IN ANIMALS was inhibited to slow angiogenesis throughout the 1990s, stopping cancers in the epithelium, gastrointestinal tract, breast, and elsewhere. See especially J. Masferrer et al., "Antiangiogenic and Antitumor Activities of Cyclooxygenase-2 Inhibitors," *Cancer Research* vol. 60 (Mar. 1, 2000): 1306; and H. Sawaoka et al., "Cyclooxygenase Inhibitors Suppress Angiogenesis and Reduce Tumor Growth in Vivo," *Laboratory Investigation* vol. 79, no. 12: 1469.

COX-2 IN HUMANS has been found overexpressed in virtually all cancers, including prostate, bladder, breast, neck, lung, pancreatic, gastric, cutaneous, and cervical cancer, a phenomenon demonstrated in dozens of studies described by A. Koki and J. Masferrer in "Celecoxib: A Specific Cox-2 Inhibitor with Anticancer Properties," *Cancer Control* vol. 9, no. 2, suppl. (Mar.–Apr. 2002). Jaime Masferrer and three of his colleagues won the Pharmacia Research Manufacturing Association's 2002 Discovery Award for their research on celecoxib.

COX-2 INHIBITORS—now classified as a separate class of NSAIDs called "coxibs"—include the "truly specific" celecoxib (Celebrex) and rofecoxib (Vioxx), as well several "preferential" Cox-2 inhibitors, such as nabumetone, nimesulide, and meloxicam. The specific inhibitors are about 100 times more selective for Cox-2 than the preferential group. For bleeding and other side effects of NSAIDs versus coxibs, see "Selective Cox-2 Inhibitors" at <www.home.eznet.net/-webtent/coxi>.

COX-2 CONFIRMATION: That Cox-2 inhibitors reduce prostaglandin production and the risk of many cancers is presented in E. Hawk et al., "Cox-2 in Cancer: A Player That's Defining the Rules," *Journal of the NCI* vol. 94, no. 8 (Apr. 17, 2002). The authors note that Celebrex and other Cox-2 inhibitors are "being tested in advanced clinical trials against a variety of epithelial malignancies (e.g., colon, esophagus, skin, and bladder cancers)." A paper in the same issue by X. Song, "Cyclooxygenase-2, Player or Spectator" (585), questions whether the mechanism at work is apoptosis or something else.

The FAP study—revealing the effect of Celebrex on familial adenomatous polyposis—was conducted between Dec. 1996 and Dec. 1998 at M. D. Anderson and at St. Mark's Hospital in London. For the results of this double-blind, placebo-controlled clinical trial, see G. Steinbach et al., "The Effect of Celecoxib, a Cyclooxygenase-2 Inhibitor, in Familial Adenomatous Polyposis," *New England Journal of Medicine* vol. 342, no. 26 (June 29, 2000): 1946–52. The authors note that FAP diagnoses almost always are followed by colorectal cancer. The study concluded that in patients with FAP, six months of twice-daily treatment with 400 mg of Celebrex (800 mg daily) "leads to a significant reduction in the number of colorectal polyps." The study led to FDA approval of Celebrex for FAP in 1999.

Chemo used incorrectly: Dr. Tim Browder, a pediatrician working in Judah Folkman's pioneering laboratory at Children's Hospital of Boston, is quoted in Robert Cooke, *Dr. Folkman's War* (Random House, 2001), 344. Browder suggested that some of the standard chemo drugs were in fact anti-angiogenic when used in small and frequent doses (anti-angiogenically) to kill the vasculature feeding the tumors instead of trying to poison the tumors directly (and in the process also killing normal fast-dividing cells).

University of Toronto papers include J. L. Yu et al. (including R. Kerbel), "Effect of p53 Status on Tumor Response to Antiangiogenic Therapy," *Science* vol. 295, no. 5559 (Feb. 22, 2002): 1526–28; J. L. Yu, J. W. Rak, G. Klement, and R. S. Kerbel, "Vascular Endothelial Growth Factor Isoform Expression as a Determinant of Blood Vessel Patterning in Human Melanoma Xenografts," *Cancer Research* vol. 62, no. 6 (2002): 1838–46. Also see the chapter by R. Kerbel and G. Klement, "Low-Dose Metronomic Anti-Angiogenic Chemotherapy," in *Breast Cancer Management*, 2d ed., ed. J.-M. Nabholtz et al. (Lippincott, Williams, and Wilkins, 2003).

Metronomic dosing was the phrase coined by Prof. Doug Hanahan "to convey the regularity of the dosing strategies, with no pauses, like a metronome, an unrelenting regular assault with no time for rest, repair, and recovery" (private communication). Anti-angiogenesis is a growing field; every week about forty scientific papers on it are published; there were only about three per year in the 1970s, when Judah Folkman started the field.

Angiogenic inhibitors in clinical trials: kinase inhibitor "SU011248," the signal-transduction kinase inhibitor that produces anti-angiogenesis, may have direct antitumor activity, according to Jerry McMahon, the president of Sugen, Inc. (<www.sugen.com>). Access <www.cancer.gov/clinical_trials> and then search for the word *angiogenesis*. The Web site lists Celebrex in phase-one trials for prostate cancer; phase-one and -two trials for cervical cancer; and phase-two trials for basal-cell metastatic breast cancer. Also listed are clinical phase-one and -two trials of thalidomide for dozens of cancers.

THALIDOMIDE'S devastations in childbirth and subsequent revival as an anti-angiogenic for cancer and 130 other diseases are described in Trent Stephens and Rock Brynner, *Dark Remedy* (Perseus, 2001). Brynner used the drug against his own lupus, an ulcerating progressive skin disease. Also see "Treatment with Rituximab Plus Thalidomide Shows Marked Anti-Tumor Activity," *Hematology Journal* vol. 3 (2002): abstract 1199.

CHAPTER 23: THE MYSTERY OF SPLENECTOMY

FRENCH STUDY: See T. Molina (of the Hôtel-Dieu de Paris) et al., "MCL in Leukemic Phase with Prominent Splenomegaly," published on-line at <www.virchowsarch> and in *Medline/Health Star Abstracts* vol. 437, no. 6 (2000): 591.

THOMAS WITZIG'S research was reported first in a one-page abstract on *ASCO On-Line Shortcuts* (2000), which stated that five patients untreated by chemo "maintained diseased stabilization up to more than 89.4 months" (7.4 years). The full paper said, "Their disease process remains stable . . . at last contact for up to 164 months (13.7 years)" (Y. Yoong et al., "Efficacy of Splenectomy for Mantle Cell Non-Hodgkin's Lymphoma," *Leukemia and Lymphoma* vol. 42:1235).

TWO-DECADE-OLD RESEARCH: For a description of the splenectomy mouse experiments, see Brian L. Kotzin and Samuel Strober, "Role of Spleen in Growth of a Murine B-Cell Leukemia," *Science*, n.s., 208, no. 4439 (Apr. 1980): 59–61. Dr. Strober is now the director of immunology at Stanford.

INTERLEUKIN-12 used with Rituxan for lymphoma patients is described in an article by S. Ansell, T. Witzig, et al., "Phase-1 Study of IL-12 in Combination with Rituximab in Patients with NHL," *Blood* vol. 99, no. 1 (Jan. 2002): 67.

CCI-779, the Wyeth-Ayerst Lab drug originally tried on renal-cell-carcinoma patients, blocks the replication of certain cell types by targeting mTOR, a protein kinase central to cell growth. The drug is in development for use against a variety of tumor types (see <www.wyeth.com>).

RADIO FREQUENCY energy combined with MRI scanning is explained in "Radio Frequency Energy Sizzles Tumors without Surgery," a news release from the Warren Grant Magnuson Clinical Center, NIH, Nov. 26, 2001. Jonathan Lewin, director of magnetic-resonance imaging at the University Hospitals of Cleveland, reported success in treating a man whose kidney cancer had metastasized.

CHAPTER 24: THE STREP CONNECTION

CATARACTS, MACULAR DEGENERATION: Esoteric connections between these conditions and Cox-2 are elucidated in C. Hutnik et al., "Cataracts in Systemic Diseases and Syndromes," *Opinion in Ophthalmology* vol. 9, no. 1 (Feb. 1998); and P. Penfold et al., "Immunological and Aetiological Aspects of Macular Degeneration," *Progress in Retinal and Eye Research* vol. 20, no. 3 (May 2001): 385.

THE INFECTION CONNECTION: Exposure to common infections may produce severe proliferative stress in bone marrow years later, according to Greaves's *Cancer: The Evolutionary Legacy* (Oxford, 2000), and may underlie lymphomas and other cancers. Infections from the common stomach bacterium *H. pylori* and from HIV are linked more directly to cancer, according to Greaves and to studies reported in popular publications such as *On Health* (e.g., Aug. 2002).

IL-12 is a potent stimulator of the immune system and an anti-angiogenic but has limited therapeutic uses and severe side effects; see C. Halin et al., "Enhancement of the Antitumor Activity of Interleukin-12 by Targeted Delivery to Neovasculature," *Nature Biotechnology* vol. 20, no. 3 (Mar. 2002): 264.

IL-10 is a focus of research on non-small-cell lung cancer by Prof. Steven Dubinett, director of lung-cancer research at UCLA's Jonsson Cancer Center. Prof. Harvey Hershman, who discovered the Cox-2 molecule, is the director of basic research at Jonsson.

DNAX, a biochemical company located in Palo Alto, Calif., may be accessed at <www.dnaxresearch.com>.

STAT-3 IN MCL: See R. Lai, J. Medeiros, et al., "Expression of STAT-3 and Its Phosphorylated Forms in Mantle Cell Lymphoma Cell Lines and Tumors," *Journal of Pathology (European)* (in press). See also M. Onciu et al. (including Medeiros and Lai), "Cytogenetic Findings in MCL," *American Journal of Clinical Pathology* vol. 116 (2001): 886.

RED WINE and grape skins contain resveratrol, which metabolizes into the antileukemic agent piceatannol. According to G. A. Potter et al., "Wine Consumption Associated with Lower Risk of NHL in Men," *British Journal of Medicine* vol. 86 (2002): 774, this naturally occurring antibiotic can be converted to a compound that is antioxidant, antiplatelet, and antiatherogenic. The conversion is effected by an enzyme found in human tumors, called "CYP1B1." With more evidence than similar previous suggestions have had, the authors suggested that "if one is going to imbibe alcohol, red wine would be the best choice" for cancer prevention.

RUZIC RESEARCH FOUNDATION is a 501(c)3 tax-deductible scientific and charitable nonprofit foundation. See <www.ruzicresearchfoundation.org>.

CHAPTER 25: PATIENT RAGE

HODGKIN'S DISEASE, considered curable by standard toxic chemotherapy and radiation, was the focus of a huge study in which long-term survivors developed cancers of the breast, esophagus, stomach, and most other organs. Out of 32,591 patients studied between 1935 and 1994, 2,153 developed second malignancies. See G. Dores, "Risk of Second Cancer Remains High 25 Years after Hodgkin's Disease," *Journal of Clinical Oncology* vol. 20 (Aug. 15, 2002): 3484.

BRAIN IMPAIRMENT of chemotherapy patients had been observed even before the Dartmouth study (see the "Chemo brain" note to chapter 7). Earlier studies revealed lingering intellectual problems in people receiving high-dose chemotherapy, such as those who undergoing transplants. See <www.brainland.com>. William Wood, a surgical oncologist and the chairman of surgery at Emory University, in Atlanta, noted that patients with early-stage cancer are often given aggressive chemotherapy, even though statistically it offers only a percentage point or two improvement in survival. See also "Chemotherapy's Effect on the Brain," *American Cancer Society News Today,* Mar. 2000.

CHEMOTHERAPY DATA: Dr. Ulrich Abel, the University of Heidelberg biostatistician whose book is referenced in the "Chemo-cure percentages" note to chapter 3, says chemotherapy-remission data often are misleading if not false. The cancers said to be "mostly curative" by chemotherapy—childhood leukemia, Hodgkin's disease, large B-cell lymphoma, Burkitt's lymphoma, choriocarcinoma, embryonal testicular cancer, Ewing's sarcoma, lymphosarcoma, retinoblastoma, rhabdomyosarcoma, and Wilms's tumor—account for fewer than 5% of all cancers, according to Abel. The ten most lethal cancers (according to SEER data)—lung, colon, breast, prostate, pancreas, ovary, stomach, and brain cancers, as well as non-Hodgkin's lymphoma and leukemia—are not considered curative by chemotherapy. There are 1.3 million new cases of cancer per year in the United States.

INDISCRIMINATE USE OF CHEMO for many cancers is only part of widespread medical mistakes. An editorial, "Medical Malpractice: Blame the System" (*Wall Street Journal,* Mar. 15, 2002), estimated that 44,000 Americans die each year as a result of other medical mistakes. (The figure was extrapolated by the editorial writer from two 1991 papers in the *New England Journal of Medicine* that documented a 4% rate of treatment complications in the United States.)

PATIENT-ADVOCACY GROUPS: The Patients Against Lymphoma (PAL) Web site is <www.lymphomation.org>. The Center Watch Web site, which lists clinical trials for all medical conditions, is <www.centerwatch.com>. The MCL Web site is <www.MCLaid.users.btopenworld.com>. Center Action Now, another nonprofit group, helps patients determine whether they can gain access to experimental drugs (<centeractionnow.org>).

THE VACCINE PETITION may be accessed at <www.cancerdrugsnow.org>. The *Nightline* program referred to aired Sept. 12, 2002.

THE ADJUVANT used in personal, or idiotype, vaccine trials is usually GM-CSF, or "granulocyte macrophage-colony stimulating factor" (also called filgrastim, or Neupogen), although a variety of others have been tried. See M. Bendandi et al., "Complete Molecular Remissions," *Nature Medicine* vol. 5, no. 10: 1171.

CONTROL GROUPS in lymphoma vaccine trials are placed at greater risk than those who get the idiotype vaccine in two ways:

1. If idiotype vaccines are proved effective and later receive FDA approval on the basis of these trials—which, after all, is the point of conducting them—a control patient would want a vaccine. But because the immune system has a memory, control-group patients will have developed a strong established response to the KLH carrier, such that their B and T cells may not recognize the idiotype portion as something new to which they should respond. Such an occurrence, long recognized, is called "carrier suppression." The opposite also could happen: the immune system may overrespond to the idiotype ("carrier potentiation"). No one knows.

2. The adjuvant used to boost the immune system, GM-CSF (see the "adjuvant" note to this chapter), is a naturally occurring signaling protein that stimulates neutrophils and other components of white blood cells. By itself GM-CSF has been reported to mobilize lymphoma cells in patients being prepped for stem-cell transplants. In this way, people with stable disease could be at risk of further proliferation of their lymphoma without any benefit.

Patient advocates are concerned for the patient *and* for scientific data to confirm vaccines for future cancer victims. Karl Schwartz, of PAL, argues that the two need not be entirely incompatible if patients are fully informed. For instance, the Genitope and NCI trials aim for 75% of participants to be eligible for the vaccine in a two-to-one randomization. However, because the Genitope protocol requires immediate "partial remission" after the chemotherapy phase, and because the NCI trial requires "complete remission," the odds of a participant's actually getting the vaccine are not two to one but 50% in the first trial, and 42% in the other.

STALLED BIOTHERAPY DRUGS: Twenty-five Mabs and other molecularly targeted drugs were stalled at the applications stage by the FDA, which approved only eighteen of the more than one hundred in human trials (as noted in the Peregrine Pharmaceuticals annual report, Sept 2002).

COGNITIVE DISSONANCE THEORY is explained in R. Wickland and J. Brehm, *Perspectives on Cognitive Dissonance* (Halsted, 1976).

SAMUEL EPSTEIN, *The Politics of Cancer Revisited* (East Ridge, 1998).

COLLUSION between oncologists and the drug companies is claimed by Ralph W. Moss in *Questioning Chemotherapy* (Equinox, 2000).

CLINICAL TRIALS in the United States, according to Center Watch, a patient information group that monitors clinical research, numbered 80,000 in the year 2001 and enrolled some 20 million people, three times the number a decade ago ("Medicine," *Time*, Apr. 22, 2002).

JAMES WATSON, *A Passion for DNA* (Cold Spring, 2000), 113.

CHAPTER 26: THE BIOTHERAPY REVOLUTION

CUTANEOUS T-cell lymphoma patients now may use an FDA-approved agent called "denileukin diftitox" (tradenamed "Ontak"). One of the new molecular agents, it is produced by genetically fusing protein from diphtheria toxin to interleukin-2, a natural protein in the immune system. The manufacturer is Seragen, Inc., Hopkinton, Mass. (<www.seragen.com>).

AIDS vs. cancer incidence: AIDS cases reported to the United Nations agency UNAIDS in the United States and Canada totaled 980,000 in 2002 (including 141,048 females and 9,074 children under age 13). Total AIDS deaths were 15,000 in the United States and fewer than 500 in Canada. Total annual new cancer cases in the United States, extrapolated from SEER data for 2003, were about 1.3 million, for a total of about 12.7 million living cancer victims and an annual death rate of cancer patients of about 600,000.

CHAPTER 27: DETOUR

DRUG SPECIFICITY diminishing over time has been elaborated by Natalie Ahn, University of Colorado, in discussing protein enzymes, or "kinases," as quoted by J. M. Perkel in "Researchers Are Getting Specific about Protein Kinase Inhibitors," *The Scientist*, Sept. 2, 2002. Even "target-specific" drugs such as protein-kinase inhibitors, once thought unlikely to develop resistance, turned out to become resistant in patients as time passes. It is a major reason for combination therapy using several drugs at the same time.

REMITOGEN, or apolizumab, has been shown effective for solid tumors, including breast, colon, kidney, ovary, and stomach cancers, as well as chronic lymphocytic leukemia—for those patients expressing the particular antigens that this naked Mab targets—according to its developer, Protein Design Labs (<www.pdl.com>).

GENASENSE, developed by Genta, Inc. (<www.genta.com>), is an 18-base antisense drug that inhibits Bcl-2 expression by being exactly complementary to RNA. Binding of the antisense strand to messenger RNA results in cleavage of the message, thereby preventing translation of the protein.

TELOMERASE-INHIBITOR research has been led by Geron (<www.geron.com>), a biotech company in Menlo Park, Calif. Preclinical studies (not in humans) have indicated antitumor activity in more than a dozen different cancers, with low toxicity.

RITUXAN kills cancer cells by at least three mechanisms: by direct antibody action, by inducing apoptosis, and by "complement-dependent" cell killing. Glucocorticoids such as dexamethasone significantly increase cell sensitivity to complement-dependent cytoxicity (A. Rose, B. Smith, and D. Maloney, "Glucocorticoids and Rituximab in Vitro," Blood vol. 100, no. 5 [Sept. 1, 2002]: 1765–78). The radioactive monoclonal antibody Zevalin, which is "hot Rituxan," does nothing to preclude taking chemotherapy as a last resort. Its most common side effect, low blood-cell counts, did not affect the tolerability of subsequent chemotherapy, including autologous stem-cell transplants, according to a study conducted at the Mayo Clinic; see S. Ansell et al., "Subsequent Therapy Well Tolerated in Patients Treated with Zevalin," Journal of Clinical Oncology vol. 20 (2002): 3885.

HAMA REACTIONS: Human antimouse—or antimurine—antibodies now can be produced in transgenic mice or other murine animals engineered to synthesize human antibodies instead of murine antibodies. Such "fully human" antibodies also can be produced in vitro using bacteria. However, there has been no convincing demonstration that they are superior to humanized antibodies such as Rituxan. (See <www.abmaxis.com>.) Although discussions of HAMA usually refer to mice, the animal actually used is a Chinese hamster (the same as is used in Rituxan). Experimental murine animals commonly include mice, rats, hamsters, guinea pigs, and rabbits.

A MAB FOR ARTHRITIS, in addition to a post-Rituxan anti-CD20 Mab for lymphoma, was announced by Applied Molecular Evolution, Inc., San Diego, in a Jan. 6, 2003, news release. The arthritis antibody, called AME-157, binds to and neutralizes tumor necrosis factor–alpha to treat rheumatoid arthritis. In 2003 neither Mab was yet available in clinical human trials.

RITUXAN MAINTENANCE DOSES are evaluated in J. D. Hainsworth et al., "Rituximab as First-Line and Maintenance Therapy for Patients with Indolent Non-Hodgkin's Lymphoma," Journal of Clinical Oncology vol. 20, no. 20 (Oct. 15, 2002): 4261–67.

CHAPTER 28: CURE!

GM-CSF AND G-CSF: GM-CSF, or granulocyte macrophage-colony stimulating factor, is trademarked Leucomax (also called Molgramostim) by its developer,

Genentech. G-CSF, or granulocyte-colony stimulating factor, is trademarked Neupogen (also called Filgrastim) by its developer, Amgen. Both are human immune stimulators produced by recombinant DNA technology. They are used not only as adjuvants with cancer vaccines but also separately to boost white cells.

SENSITIVITY OF FISH (fluorescence in-situ hybridization) is described by the National Human Genome Institute at <www.accessexcellence.org/AB/GG/fish.html>. Use of PCR in detecting the characteristic chromosomal translocations mantle-cell lymphoma is explained in R. Luthra et al. (including Jeff Medeiros), "Real-Time 5' → 3' Exonuclease-based PCR Assay for Detection of the t(11;14) (q13;q32)," *American Journal of Clinical Pathology* vol. 112, no. 4 (Oct. 1999): 524–30.

PET'S EXTREME ACCURACY is explored in A. Alavi and S. J. Schuster "Utility of FEG-PET Scanning in Lymphoma by WHO Classification," *Blood* (in press).

VACCINES IN SPAIN for lymphoma are available on both a private-patient and clinical-trial basis. Send inquiries via e-mail directly to Dr. Maurizio Bendandi, mbendandi@unav.es. See also M. Bendandi, "Complete Molecular Remissions," *Nature Medicine* vol. 5 (1999): 1171.

CHANGING FDA RULES governing placebo-controlled trials for desperately ill patients who might otherwise have been saved by cancer vaccines and other biotherapies have been the subject of countless editorials in the scientific and lay press, such as "Now for the Real Cancer Vaccines," *Wall Street Journal*, Nov. 26, 2002.

DISMAL SURVIVAL or the vast majority of patients relapsing from chemotherapy is taken from an unpublished December 2002 Genitope, Inc., paper entitled "Idiotype Immunotherapy Backgrounder," distributed at the ASH conference that month.

Glossary

Angiogenesis: The sprouting of new microvessels from pre-existing blood vessels or their formation from embryonic stem cells to provide nutrients to growing tissue after an injury. Tumor cells produce molecules that stimulate local angiogenesis, so that the resultant vessels feed the expanding tumor mass. Anti-angiogenesis is the process of stopping new blood vessel formation in order to starve cancer cells to death.

Antibodies: Proteins made by B cells to bind with and destroy antigens. Each antibody is produced in response to a specific antigen, fitting it like a glove to a hand.

Antigens: Molecular structures, typically originating from foreign, infectious, and cancerous agents, that are capable of provoking an immune response.

Apoptosis: Programmed cell death—unlike necrosis, which is the death of cells surrounded by healthy tissue. If apoptosis is suppressed, the cell becomes immortal, resulting in cancer.

ATP (adenosine triphosphate): A compound bearing chemical energy in the form of phosphate bonds. It is present in all cells but particularly in muscle cells. When ATP is split by enzyme action, energy is released, providing the power source used by the cell for its activities.

B cells: Lymphocytes that mature into antibody-producing cells.

CDs: "Clusters of designation" that identify the surface markers of T cells.

CHOP: A standard, widely used chemotherapy combination consisting of the chemical toxins cyclophosphamide, hydroxydoxorubicin, and Oncovin and the steroid prednisone. (See also *Toxins.*)

Co-stimulation of T cells: A method of helping T cells recognize cancer by stimulating them with both anti-CD3 and anti-CD28 antibodies.

Cox-1 and -2 (Cyclooxygenase-1 and -2): Enzymes that speed the production of chemical messengers called prostaglandins. The prostaglandins made by Cox-1 protect the stomach lining and clot the blood; when Cox-1 is inhibited, inflammation is reduced but the protective mucus lining of the stomach is also inhibited. The prostaglandins made by Cox-2 cause the pain and swelling of arthritis. Nonsteroidal anti-inflammatory drugs such as aspirin block both Cox-1 and -2 but primarily Cox-1 and can lead to ulcers and intestinal bleeding. Specific Cox-2 inhibitors such as Celebrex (celecoxib) and Vioxx (refocoxib) provide the anti-inflammatory benefits without the drawbacks of relatively high doses of NSAIDs. Celebrex and Vioxx are different compounds both of which reduce inflammation, but of the two only Celebrex has been shown to be a powerful anti-angiogenic.

Cyclin D1: One of a group of enzymes important in regulating cell division. Also called Bcl-1 (for B-cell lymphoma), it is produced in high quantities in mantle-cell lymphoma and some other cancers.

Cytokine: One of more than a hundred distinct proteins produced primarily by white blood cells. Cytokines provide signals to regulate cell function and cell growth during both inflammation and specific immune responses.

Endothelium: A form of epithelium consisting of flat cells that line the blood and lymphatic vessels, the heart, and various body cavities.

Enzyme: An organic catalyst or protein that changes the rate of chemical reactions without requiring an external energy source or itself being changed. Enzymes are produced by living cells but can act outside the body, for instance, in a laboratory dish.

Epithelium: The layer of cells forming the epidermis of the skin and the surface layer of mucous membranes.

Genomic: Pertaining to the genome, or the complete set of chromosomes, and thus the entire genetic information present in a cell.

GM-CSF: Granulocyte macrophage-colony stimulating factor, a naturally occurring cytokine (an immunological signaling protein) that stimulates neutrophils and other components of white blood cells. A manufactured version is called Leucomax. G-CSF is granulocyte-colony stimulating factor, the manufactured version of which is Neupogen.

Granulocyte: Any of three types of white blood cells containing granules that help destroy invading pathogens. The three types are basophils, eosinophils, and neutrophils.

HLA (human leukocyte antigens): A set of six surface proteins that appear on white blood cells. Like blood-group antigens on red cells ("blood type"), the HLA proteins are slightly different in each person. Two monoclonal antibodies target these HLA proteins (see *Remitogen* and *Oncolym* under *Monoclonal antibody*).

Hyper-CVAD: A highly toxic chemotherapy combination consisting of hyper-fractionated cyclophosphamide, vincristine, dexamethasone, and doxorubicin. *Hyper-fractionated* means the total dose is spread over an extended period.

Interferons: Natural substances produced by the body to stimulate the immune system against viral infections and used therapeutically to stimulate the immune system to fight cancer.

Interleukins: Natural hormonelike proteins in the body, numbered from IL-1 to IL-14 (at last count), that control the growth and activity of various kinds of lymphocytes and other cell types.

Kinases: Enzymes central to pathways that regulate genes.

Leukocytes: White blood cells.

Lymph: The usually colorless liquid containing white blood cells and carried in the vessels of the lymphatic system.

Lymph nodes: Glandlike masses of tissue located throughout the body that contain immune cells and serve as filters for antigens in the blood and lymph. The number of lymph nodes in the body ranges from about 600 to 1,000. Their normal size is about one centimeter or less.

Lymphatic system: The veinlike system that includes the lymph vessels, which collect tissue fluid and return it to the blood; the bone marrow; and the organs made of lymphatic tissue—primarily the spleen, the lymph nodes and nodules, the thymus, and tonsils.

Lymphocytes: Cells present in the blood and lymphatic systems, including B cells, T cells, and natural killer cells. Lymphocytes constitute about a third of total white cells.

Mab: Monoclonal antibody. (Also abbreviated MAb, mAB, or MoAb.)

Macrophage: Literally "big eater," a large, mature phagocyte that can ingest and destroy invading microbes, foreign particles, cancerous or otherwise diseased cells, and cellular debris. Macrophages can alert lymphocytes to the presence of antigens and produce cytokines, or messengers that facilitate the immune response.

Methylglyoxal: A common organic chemical used uncommonly as a nontoxic cancer therapy. It has been known since the 1930s that methylglyoxal inhibits the electron flow of mitochondria—the tiny threads of cells containing enzymes necessary for cell respiration and production of ATP—thereby blocking the electrical energy of living cells.

Monoclonal antibody: A bioengineered antibody cloned from a single B cell that works in several ways: by activating enzymes to punch holes in the cancer cells, by serving as a bridge between killer cells of the immune system and cancer cells, and by causing apoptosis. Some of the more than seventy Mabs in various stages of development, in clinical trials, or FDA approved include the following (with their tradenames given first):

Avastin (bevacizumab): a Mab that promotes anti-angiogenesis by inhibiting VEGF, developed by Genentech and currently in clinical trials for metastatic breast cancer, non-small-cell lung cancer, and colorectal cancer.

Bexxar (tositumomab): a radio-Mab conjugated with iodine-131 to bind to and attack malignant cells marked by CD20 antigens, which usually are overexpressed in lymphoma, and also to deliver the iodine radioisotope to kill surrounding cells. Developed by Corixa, it was FDA approved in 2003.

Campath (alemtuzumab): a Mab that targets the CD52 antigen prevalent in chronic lymphocytic leukemia. Developed by Berlex Laboratories, it was FDA approved in 2001.

Epratuzumab: a not-yet-tradenamed Mab that targets the CD22 antigen overexpressed in some lymphomas, currently in clinical trials by its developers Amgen and Immunomedics.

Herceptin (trastuzumab): a Mab that targets the Her-2 receptor on cells overexpressed in almost a third of women with metastatic breast cancer. Developed by Genentech, it was FDA approved in 1998.

Oncolym (lym-1): a radio-Mab combined with iodine-131 to bind to and attack the HLA-DR10 and other closely related antigens expressed in many lymphomas and leukemias. The Mab, said to attach to antigens almost exclusively in cancerous cells, is still in preclinical development at Peregrine Pharmaceuticals.

Remitogen (apolizumab): a naked (nonradioactive) Mab that binds to the 1D10 antigen, which is an HLA-DR determinant found on many B-cell lymphomas, developed by Protein Design Labs and now in clinical trials.

Rituxan (rituxumab): called Mabthera outside the United States, this Mab targets the CD20 antigen expressed on most lymphoma cells. Developed by Genentech and IDEC, Rituxan was FDA approved in 1998.

Zevalin (ibritumomab): a radio-Mab conjugated with yttrium-90 to bind to and attack malignant cells marked by CD20 antigens, which usually are overexpressed in lymphoma, and also to deliver the yttrium radioisotope to kill surrounding cells. Developed by IDEC Pharmaceuticals, it was FDA approved in 2002.

Neutrophil: The most numerous and important of the granulocytic white cells that migrate to the site of infection to destroy bacteria and other invaders. One of the more significant lymphocytes involved in immune responses, neutrophils normally make up between 42% and 78% of the white blood cells. A normal neutrophil count is between 3,000 and 7,000 in a microliter of blood.

Phagocyte: Any cell that ingests and destroys foreign particles such as bacteria and cell debris, such as a macrophage.

Platelet: A platelike cell fragment in the blood that helps the blood clot and also activates certain immune responses. The normal count is between 130,000 and 400,000 per cubic millimeter. High platelet counts occur after violent exercise, tissue injury, and operations, especially splenectomies.

Polymerase chain reaction (PCR): A process that allows laboratories to make unlimited numbers of copies of genes beginning with a single molecule of DNA. A hundred billion clones can be made in a few hours.

Proteins: Complex compounds constituting a large portion of the mass of every life form. They are synthesized by plants and animals to provide the amino acids essential for growth and repair of tissue.

Radio-Mab: A radioimmunotherapy consisting of a monoclonal antibody conjugated or labeled (combined) with a radioisotope. The Mab delivers the radioisotope to the antigens of cancerous cells, where it kills not only the cells attacked but also additional cells in the vicinity.

Red blood cells: Cells (also called erythrocytes) that contain hemoglobin and carry oxygen to the tissues and return carbon dioxide to the respiratory organs. Types of red blood cells are designated by A, B, O, or their combinations. Normal red-cell counts average 5 million in a microliter of blood in men and 4.5 million in women.

Stem cells: Immature cells originating in bone marrow that upon division replace their own numbers and from which specialized mature blood cells, such as the immune system's B or T cells, "stem," or are generated.

T cells: A type of lymphocyte, the strongest fighters during an immune response. Mature T cells are "antigen specific"—that is, each T cell responds to only one antigen identified by cell-surface markers, called CDs. Cancer cells evolve rapidly to evade recognition of T cells.

Toxins: Organic poisons.

Tumor-necrosis factor: A cytokine released by macrophages and T cells that helps regulate the immune response. The functions of TNFs are similar to those of interleukin-1.

Vaccines: Usually preventative preparations containing a weakened form of a disease-causing agent used to stimulate production of antibodies and provoke immunity. Idiotype vaccines—administered *after* cancer has been diagnosed—are immunotherapies custom-made for each person. They consist of cloned antibodies specific to a patient's own cancer antigens.

VEGF (vascular endothelial growth factor): A protein that plays a critical role in tumor angiogenesis and maintenance of established tumor blood vessels. Since VEGF stimulates angiogenesis, anti-VEGF genetically engineered proteins, such as those of the naturally occurring angiostatin and endostatin, are anti-angiogenic.

White blood cells: Also called leukocytes, they are colorless immune cells that include lymphocytes, granulocytes, and phagocytes. Types of white blood cells are designated by HLA markers. Normal white-cell counts are between 4,000 and 11,000 in a microliter of blood.

Index

136; remission, splenectomy and, 269; stage-four, 4; statistics, 384*n;* SV40 virus and, 135–36; symptoms of, 5, 21, 37; terminology, 83; victims of, 241–42; waxing and waning of, 227. *See also* Non-Hodgkin's lymphoma; *specific types of lymphoma*

Lymphoma Research Foundation: "Celebration of Life Ball," 161–64; merger, 307–8, 382*n;* Neil Ruzic as boardmember, 167, 207, 209, 226, 243; research funding, 170, 201–2, 233, 243; startup, 158–59; think tank, 219–24. *See also* Cohen, Ellen Glesby

Lymphoma vaccine. *See* Vaccines

Lymph system, indolent, 169

Mabs. *See* Monoclonal antibodies

Mabthera. *See* Rituxan

Macrophages, 83

Macular degeneration, 295, 296, 394–95*n*

Magnetic resonance imaging (MRI), 290

Malpractice lawsuits, 227

MALT lymphomas, 137, 378*n*

Mantle-cell lymphoma (MCL): aggressiveness, 254–55, 360; causation, 133–34; chromosome translocations, 335; confirming diagnosis of, 335; cyclin D1 overexpression in, 162; development, 250–51; diffuse stage-four, 5; experimental therapies for, 256–57; gene-expression profiling and, 384; male-female ratio, 134; morphology of, 271–72; progression, 303; remission rates, 14; Rituxan for, 341; scientific definition of, 353; survival rates, 8, 27, 269; terminology, 6

Mantle zone of lymph node, 6

Maris, Roger, 242

Markers, 54, 57. *See also specific markers*

Marx, Nancy, 308

Masferrer, Jamie, 269, 270–71

Mason, David, 221–23, 328, 329

Maximum tolerated dose (MTD), 276

Mayo Clinic, 68, 269, 285, 288, 289

McGuire, Phil, 177

McKenna, John, 132–34, 266–69, 274–75, 291–92, 296, 311, 343, 362

McKenna, Michele, 132–34, 291, 293

MCL. *See* Mantle-cell lymphoma

MCL Group, 374*n;* anger of members, 308; Celebrex usage and, 274–75; cell-purging devices and, 117–18; deaths of members, 125–26, 240, 242; decision making and, 238, 239; founding of, 127; growth of, 126–27; lack of resources, 133; Levy's vaccine research and, 81; messages from, 127–29; research funding and, 229, 304–5; Ruzic, Neil, and, 310; splenectomy and, 288. *See also specific group members*

MCL laboratory, 302–4

MCL Web site, 128, 377*n*

M.D. Anderson Cancer Center, 12, 14, 18, 31, 291, 302–5, 317

M.D. degrees, 368*n.*

Medeiros, Dr. Jeffrey, 20–21, 73–75, 162–63, 170, 264, 302–6, 334–35

Media, pseudoscience and, 151–52

Medical dictionaries, 82, 374*n*

Medical laboratories, 4

Medical terminology, 82–83

Megavitamins, 16

Meinert, Curtis, 65

Melanoma, 83, 136

Mesothelioma, 16

Methotrexate, 6

Methylglyoxal (pyruvic aldehyde; pyruvaldehyde), 258–63, 326, 343, 391*n*

Metronomic dosing, 277, 393*n*

Midway Plaisance, 130

Migraines, 139

Minimum effective dose, 350–51

Mini-transplants, 237–38, 389*n*

Misdiagnosis, 3, 8, 367*n*

MoAs. *See* Monoclonal antibodies

Mohrbacher, Ann, 158, 326

NEIL RUZIC is the founder and publisher of several worldwide scientific magazines, including *Industrial Research* and *Oceanology International.* He is also the author of more than two hundred articles and eleven books, which serve as a bridge between various science disciplines and lay readers, including *The Case for Going to the Moon* and *Where the Winds Sleep.* He holds the first U.S. patent for a device to be used on the moon, a lunar cryostat, and originated the R&D Annual Awards Program for applied physical research scientists. Later he spent fifteen years developing the island of Little Stirrup Cay in the Bahamas, first as the Island for Science and later as a cruise-ship port of call, and wrote an adventure novel set on the island, *The Shallow Sea.*

The University of Illinois Press
is a founding member of the
Association of American University Presses.

Composed in 11/16 Minion
with Helvetica Neue display
by Jim Proefrock
at the University of Illinois Press
Manufactured by Thomson-Shore, Inc.

University of Illinois Press
1325 South Oak Street
Champaign, IL 61820-6903
www.press.uillinois.edu